Flow of a Long River

Tributes to SAVIO L-Y WOO
ON HIS 70TH BIRTHDAY

Dear Mimi,

Thank you for taking such great care of us during our many visits — you are the best! Hope you'll enjoy browsing through this book — especially Chapters 7 and 8 —

With my compliments,

Savio Woo
Sept. 2013

Flow of a Long River

Tributes to SAVIO L-Y WOO ON HIS 70TH BIRTHDAY

Edited by

Zong-Ming Li
Cleveland Clinic, USA

Jennifer S Wayne
Virginia Commonwealth University, USA

Chih-Hwa Chen
Chang Gung University, Taiwan

Kirstin Woo
Palo Alto Medical Foundation, USA

World Scientific

NEW JERSEY · LONDON · SINGAPORE · BEIJING · SHANGHAI · HONG KONG · TAIPEI · CHENNAI

Published by

World Scientific Publishing Co. Pte. Ltd.
5 Toh Tuck Link, Singapore 596224
USA office: 27 Warren Street, Suite 401-402, Hackensack, NJ 07601
UK office: 57 Shelton Street, Covent Garden, London WC2H 9HE

British Library Cataloguing-in-Publication Data
A catalogue record for this book is available from the British Library.

TRIBUTES TO SAVIO L-Y WOO ON HIS 70TH BIRTHDAY
Copyright © 2012 by World Scientific Publishing Co. Pte. Ltd.

All rights reserved. This book, or parts thereof, may not be reproduced in any form or by any means, electronic or mechanical, including photocopying, recording or any information storage and retrieval system now known or to be invented, without written permission from the Publisher.

For photocopying of material in this volume, please pay a copying fee through the Copyright Clearance Center, Inc., 222 Rosewood Drive, Danvers, MA 01923, USA. In this case permission to photocopy is not required from the publisher.

ISBN 978-981-4405-88-1

Printed in Singapore by Mainland Press Pte Ltd.

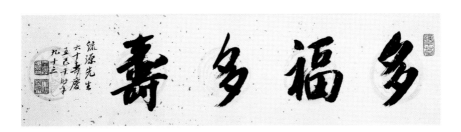

Calligrapher: Chi-Chien Wang 王智简
A 60th birthday gift from cousin Mr. Alan Woo

Foreword

Chancellor Mark A. Nordenberg

Chancellor of the University and Distinguished Service Professor of Law
University of Pittsburgh
Pittsburgh, Pennsylvania, 15213, U.S.A.

Savio Woo's always-cheerful, ever-youthful appearance would leave almost anyone doubting that his 70th birthday is approaching. However, his extraordinary record of high achievement and meaningful impact creates just the opposite impression. With all that he has accomplished, it is hard to believe that his time on this earth does not span a much longer period. Clearly, he has made the most of that time.

To share just some of the basic numbers, Savio has published 315 refereed journal articles, 141 book chapters and 834 abstracts and extended abstracts. He has edited 12 books and 19 Congress proceedings and has served on more than two dozen editorial boards. He also has given over 900 lectures and supervised over 460 graduate and undergraduate students and post-doctoral research fellows.

Savio has been elected to membership in both the Institute of Medicine of the National Academy of Sciences and the National Academy of Engineering. Either, standing alone, would be the honor of a lifetime even for very accomplished researchers. However, in Savio's case, there is even more. He also was elected to membership in Academia Sinica and is a founding member of the IOC Olympic Academy of Sports Medicine.

His leading role in that latter group came one year after the International Olympic Committee honored him as an Olympic Gold Medalist and presented him with the IOC Prize for Sports Science. Among the many other honors that he has received are the Muybridge Medal from the International Society of Biomechanics, the H.R. Lissner Medal from the American Society for Mechanical Engineers, the Kappa Delta Award for Outstanding Orthopaedic Research from the Orthopaedic Research Society of the American Academy of Orthopaedic

Surgeons, the O'Donoghue Sports Injury Research Award from the American Orthopaedic Society for Sports Medicine, and the Biovanni Borelli Award from the American Society of Biomechanics.

Savio has provided leadership to a wide-ranging group of important scientific societies. Those roles have included President of the Orthopaedic Research Society, the American Society of Biomechanics and the International Society for Fracture Repair. He also served as Chairman of the Bioengineering Division of the American Society of Mechanical Engineers and was a Founding Chair of the College of Fellows of the American Institute for Medical & Biological Engineering.

Savio earned his undergraduate degree in mechanical engineering from the California State University at Chico and then earned graduate degrees in mechanical engineering and bioengineering from the University of Washington. He spent the next two decades as a professor of surgery and bioengineering at the University of California at San Diego. Then, to our good fortune, he was recruited to the University of Pittsburgh.

At Pitt, Savio has served as Director of our Musculoskeletal Research Center for more than twenty years. He has held principal academic appointments in two different departments, Bioengineering and Orthopaedic Surgery, and secondary appointments in three others, Civil and Environmental Engineering, Mechanical Engineering, and Rehabilitation Science and Technology. He currently holds the rank of Distinguished University Professor and earlier in his career held two different named professorships. I am proud to report that he also has received our Chancellor's Distinguished Research Award.

However, Savio's colleagues, at Pitt and in other locations, honor him not only as a distinguished professional, but as a very special person. His successes almost certainly are a product not only of his love for his work, but also of his love for the people with whom he works. He is a kind, considerate and engaging colleague, as well as an amazingly attentive mentor. Even without the benefit of an exact count, I can confidently state that no other faculty member has introduced me to nearly as many junior colleagues, post-docs or students over the course of the years that we have known each other. Because he is a devoted Panther fan, those introductions often have taken place at a Pitt basketball or football game.

Savio's successes, of course, also are a credit to the support that he always has received from his regular game-day companion and wonderful wife, Pattie, who has been a constant source of encouragement, whether Savio was pursuing exciting possibilities or dealing with daunting challenges. Together, they are the proud parents of Kirstin and Jonathan, a daughter and son who possess the same strong values and warm human qualities as their mother and father.

Savio's special touch in the lab has helped him build a remarkable career. His special touch with people sits at the heart of his equally remarkable life. As the testimonials in this tribute book so clearly demonstrate, Savio is a person who not only is respected, but is beloved. He has added richness to the lives of countless others, and in countless ways.

As Savio counts the candles on his 70th birthday cake, then, we all want to deliver a message of birthday greetings that includes both heartfelt thanks and our best wishes for continued happiness and success in all of the years that lie ahead.

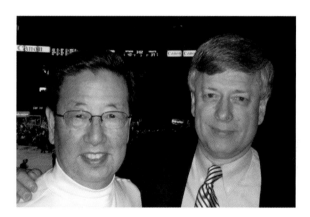

Preface

This Book of Tributes represents the collective feelings of many colleagues, students, family, and friends who have come together to honor Professor Savio Lau-Yuen Woo on his 70th birthday. As detailed in the various tributes, Professor Woo's international stature in the orthopaedic research community is second to none. He is considered not only to be an outstanding scholar with unwavering high standards, but is also a sincere and earnest gentleman who takes personal pride in seeing others become accomplished themselves. He teaches many valuable lessons in the laboratory about research and in personal conversations about life.

The co-editors of this book represent four different manners of individuals who have been profoundly influenced by Professor Woo. Dr. Kirstin Woo has had the longest and most personal relationship with the honoree, as his daughter. Dr. Jennifer Wayne was mentored for her doctoral work with the honoree at the University of California at San Diego (UCSD). Dr. Chih-Hwa Chen was practising orthopaedic surgery in Taiwan before he became a research fellow with the honoree in the Musculoskeletal Research Center (MSRC) at the University of Pittsburgh. Dr. Zong-Ming Li was faculty with the honoree in the MSRC at the University of Pittsburgh. Of course, the connections did not end with the initial relationships, but have continued to flourish in subsequent years. The sentiments expressed in the tributes collectively represent those of the co-editors. We feel privileged to have been a part of this journey.

This book has been organized in chapters to present the different groups that have been touched by Professor Woo. It begins with those closest and dearest to Professor Woo — his family. It is followed by tributes from the students, residents and staff members who were influenced by Professor Woo during his 20 years at UCSD as Director of the Orthopaedic Bioengineering Laboratory. In 1990, Professor Woo moved to the University of Pittsburgh to establish the MSRC and the next chapter contains tributes from those who made the cross-country move with him. Chapter 4 presents tributes from the many who have passed through the doors of the MSRC and how Professor Woo has been an influence in everything from sparking new careers in bioengineering to indirectly arranging marriages. The next chapter contains tributes from Professor Woo's colleagues and friends. These friendships span the decades as we hear from those who knew Professor Woo back in graduate school and at the beginning of his career as well as those he has met more recently. Finally, there is an autobiography written by Professor Woo and personal photos from Mrs. Pattie Woo.

Our sincere appreciation goes to Mrs. Diann DeCenzo and Mrs. Serena Chan Saw of the MSRC at the University of Pittsburgh for their editorial assistance in the production of this tribute book. Diann and Serena have worked tirelessly and put tremendous time, energy, enthusiasm and love into this book volume. We are grateful to Ms. Joy Quek and Ms. Sandhya Devi at the World Scientific Publishing Co. for their guidance in the preparation of this book. And of course, we are thankful to the authors for offering their tributes and making this book memorable for years to come.

Co-Editors
Zong-Ming Li
Jennifer S. Wayne
Chih-Hwa Chen
Kirstin Woo

Contents

FOREWORD.. vii
    Chancellor Mark A. Nordenberg

PREFACE... xi

CHAPTER 1
    Tributes from Family and Relatives 1

Some Important Truths... 3
    Kirstin Woo

Baseball Through the Evolution of a Father/Son Relationship 7
    Jonathan Woo

A Dedicated Educator, Devoted Family Man and Doting
Grandfather... 11
    Pattie Woo

In Memory of Gung Gung 15
    Antonio Cheong

Happy 70th Birthday, Brother & Uncle............................... 19
    Liu-Yun Woo and Family

Happy 70th Birthday, Ah Xi Dö.. 21
    Sister Bernadette Woo

Happy 70th Birthday.. 23
    Sister Agnes Au

Happy 70th Birthday, Savio 24
    Paulo and Anna Cheong

Happy 70th Birthday, Savio 26
    Vang and Eileen Cheong

More Than a Special Friend, He's Family 27
    Linda and Mark Saxon

Remembrances and Tribute to Savio Woo on His 70th Birthday 28
    Bruce Simon

Happy 70th Birthday, Uncle Savio 30
    Nancy, Irene, Helen and Kevin Chan

The Importance of Family 31
    James Lai

An Unforgettable Experience 32
    Joshua Lai

Our Tribute - A Limerick 33
    Bob and Holly Frymoyer

CHAPTER 2
Tributes from Students, Residents and Fellows (University of California, San Diego) 35

Showing Me the Way 37
    Cy Frank

A Tribute to Dr. Woo: A Bioengineering Pioneer 39
    Mark A. Gomez

Demand for Excellence 41
    J. Marcus Hollis

From Student to Professional: Moulding Young Careers 42
    Jennifer S. Wayne

Happy Birthday, Dr. Woo... 44
   Thay Q. Lee

Fond Memories.. 46
   Lynnette Fleck

A Great Mentor.. 48
   Shuji Horibe

My Sincere Congratulations and Best Wishes on the Occasion
of His 70th Birthday 50
   Shinro Takai

Long Time Mentor and Collaborator.. 52
   Jack Winters

One of a Kind 54
   Erin McGurk and Ron Dieck

Tribute to Dr. Woo 55
   Robert A. Hart

Birthday Wishes for Dr. Woo... 56
   Caroline Wang

Hau`oli Lā Hānau to Dr. Woo! Wishing You All the Best for
Many More Wonderful Years to Come 57
   Linda Kitabayashi

Thanks Dr. Woo from a Mentee at UCSD in the Mid-1980s 59
   David Hawkins

A Sincere Thank You from One of Your Students........................ 60
   Jeff Weiss

Congratulations and Thank You! 61
   Edmond (Ned) Young

Thank You!.. 62
   Roger Lyon

CHAPTER 3
Tributes from Students, Residents and Fellows (University of California, San Diego and University of Pittsburgh) 63

"Life Is a Journey, Not a Destination" - Ralph Waldo Emerson 65
Karen Ohland

Warm Words of Encouragement 67
Hiromichi Fujie

The Past Isn't Dead. In Fact, It's Not Even the Past. - William Faulkner 69
Glen Livesay

My Friend, My Teacher, Thank You for the "Opportunity" 71
John Xerogeanes

Warmth 73
Meena Joshi

CHAPTER 4
Tributes from Students, Residents and Fellows (University of Pittsburgh) 75

My Career in Orthopedic Research and Dr. Savio Woo 77
Patrick J. McMahon

Dr. Woo, My Teacher and Mentor 79
Chih-Hwa Chen

Woo-Dapest, Woo-Ashington DC 81
Christos D. Papageorgiou

20+ Years and Counting 83
Diann DeCenzo

To Dr. Woo, an Exemplary Engineer, Thinker and Teacher 85
Jorge E. Gil

An Opportunity for a Young Student, an Appreciation from a
Less-Young Student 87
   Duane Morrow

Thank You Dr. Woo 89
   Duy Tan Nguyen

A Great Educator in the Field of Bioengineering 91
   Ryan Prantil

Dr. Woo, A Great Man I Always Look Up To 93
   Wei-Hsiu Hsu

A Great Scientist and Global Educator 94
   Rui Liang

Leading Me into the Wonderful Research World 96
   Yin-Chih Fu

Mentoring to Perfection: A Tribute to Dr. Savio L-Y. Woo on the
Occasion of His 70th Birthday 98
   Matthew Fisher

My Fond Memories of Dr. Woo - His Mentorship, Uncanny
Insights, and My Good Fortune 100
   Todd Doehring

Teacher, Mentor and Guide 102
   Serena Chan Saw

An Inspiration to Generations of Engineers, Scientists, and
Physicians 104
   Kristen L. Moffat

A Provident Decision 106
   Kwang Kim

Happy Birthday Dr. Woo 108
   Maria Apreleva-Scheffler and Sven Scheffler

Making Something out of Nothing 110
  Steven Abramowitch

The Importance of an Advisor 112
  Akihiro and Jennifer Kanamori

Bringing Us Together 114
  Alejandro Almarza and Sabrina Noorani

Marriages and Lifelong Friendships 116
  Carrie (Voycheck) Rainis

Coming Full Circle: Dr. Woo as a Mentor and a Colleague 118
  Mininder S. Kocher

贺胡流源教授 70 岁生日 120
  Guoan Li

The Confucius of Biomechanics 121
  Daniel K. Moon

Strive for Excellence 122
  Thomas W. Gilbert

We Are Getting Mature 124
  Yoshitsugu Takeda

祝古稀 126
  Masataka Sakane

Nice to Meet You 128
  Yukihisa Fukuda

Congratulations for Dr. Woo's 70 Years Young Birthday from a Japanese Fellow 130
  Kazutomo Miura

A Great Mentor 132
  Sinan Karaoglu

....You Are My Teacher You Are My Family 134
  Fabio Vercillo

Quickly Learn to Use Chopsticks 136
  Louis E. DeFrate

An Incredible Inspiration 137
  Mara Schenker

Chinese Food and Dr. Woo 139
  Noah Papas

You Don't Have to Be an Einstein… 141
  Xia Guo

My Eternal Professor! 143
  Greg Carlin

Happy Birthday, Dr. Woo 144
  Guoguang Yang

An Education and Experience of a Lifetime 145
  Richard Debski

Milestone and Testament 147
  Kevin Hildebrand

A Real Leader 149
  Dimosthenis Alaseirlis

Reflections on My Time at the MSRC with Dr. Woo 150
  Ken Fischer

Tribute to Savio L-Y. Woo on His 70th Birthday 152
  Christopher Schmidt

Dr. Savio Woo – the Researcher, Teacher and Olympic Medalist .. 153
  C. Benjamin Ma

Discipline & Inspiration - A Brief Story of Good Mentorship 155
   Christopher A. Carruthers

Lunchtime in the Library: The Talented Storyteller 157
   Katie Farraro

Dr. Woo's 70th Birthday Tribute - Ties in Pittsburgh and Tokyo 159
   Takatoshi Shimomura

Commitment, Dedication and Pride 161
   Andrew Feola

Thank You from Northeastern Japan 163
   Yasuyuki Ishibashi

A Fantastic Leader 164
   Stefano Zaffagnini

Almost Like a Father 166
   Masayoshi Yagi

Celebrating with Family and Friends 167
   Becky (Levine) Leibowitz

Dr. Woo: My Mentor Forever 168
   Yuhua Song

To My Lifetime Mentor on His Seventieth Birthday 170
   Fengyan Jia

The Days of Our Years - A Tribute To Dr. Woo on His 70th
Birthday 171
   Changfu Wu

The Best Teacher 173
   Sarita Maheedhara

Compassionate Instructions 174
   Yuji Yamamoto

A Wise Mentor 175
  Ben Rothrauff

The Last "Real" Teacher 177
  Matteo Maria Tei

A Priviledge to Meet Dr. Woo as a Person and as a Professional ... 178
  Gustavo Miguel Azcona Arteaga

Happy 70th Birthday Dr. Woo! 180
  Eiichi Tsuda

Heartiest Congratulations 181
  Rajesh Jari

Tribute to Dr. Woo from the Stehle's 182
  Jens Stehle

"Uncle Savio" 183
  Chee-Hahn Hung

Happy Birthday Dr. Woo! 184
  David Provenzano

My Tribute to Dr. Woo 185
  Eric Wong

CHAPTER 5
Tributes from Colleagues and Friends 187

A Toast to Savio 189
  Y. C. and Luna Fung

Happy 70th Birthday, Dear Savio! 191
  Shu Chien

Congratulations Savio on Your 70th Birthday!! 193
  Albert and Betty Kobayashi

In the Presence of Greatness 195
  Chancellor Michael Lovell

O! What a Beautiful Day 197
  President H.K. Chang

A Tribute to Professor Savio L-Y. Woo on the Occasion of
His 70th Birthday 199
  Provost Emeritus James V. Maher

A Most Accomplished Scholar, Family Man and Friend 201
  Dean Gerald Holder

Esteemed Friend and Colleague 203
  Dean Cliff Brubaker

For Celebration of the Seventieth Anniversary of
Dr. Savio L-Y. Woo 205
  Theodore Wu

To My Birthday Twin and Grandmaster of the ACL
Reconstruction 207
  Sheldon Weinbaum

A Friend Indeed! 209
  Ed Chao

The Bioengineering Family 210
  Robert M. Nerem

Have a Wonderful 70th Birthday and Many Happy Returns 212
  Albert King

Savio Woo: We Applaud a Pioneer in Bioengineering 214
  Geert W. Schmid-Schönbein

A Tribute to Savio L-Y. Woo 216
  Thomas Budinger

Leadership, Research Excellence, and Great Chinese Food............ 217
　Steven Goldstein

An Extraordinary Investigator and Educator.................................. 218
　John Watson

Happy 70th Birthday, Savio 219
　Kerong Dai

Congratulations Savio! 220
　Tingye Li

Chico - It Is Next to Paradise... 221
　Tim Thomassen

Memories from College Life 223
　Jeremy and Barbara Jones

Tribute to Savio Woo 224
　Wayne Akeson

Our Special Partnership and Friendship 226
　David Amiel

It Started with a Bump.. 228
　Peter Chen

Three Cheers for Dr. Woo's Birthday 230
　Michael Yen

Professor Savio Woo - Pioneer and Promotor of Soft Tissues 233
　Albert J. and Elizabeth Banes

An Exemplary Role Model... 236
　Eva and Wen-Hwa Lee

Good Health, Good Luck and Happiness Always.......................... 238
　Winston and Priscilla Tsang

Happy 70th Birthday to a Dear Friend.. 239
Brad and Loretta Sowers

To the Celebration of Savio's 70th Birthday!................................. 241
Ikuko Seguchi

A Tribute to Dr. Savio L-Y. Woo for His Distinguished Career
and Happiness.. 242
Tin-Kan Hung and Shunan Cho Hung

Congratulations x 70! 243
Kai-Nan An

Congratulations Savio: The Field is a Better Place Because
of You... 244
Thomas Andriacchi

A Tribute to Savio Woo on His 70th Birthday 246
Jody and Kitty Buckwalter

Happy 70th Birthday to My Friend and Mentor 247
Steven P. Arnoczky

A Tribute to My Good Friend, Savio Woo....................................... 248
David Butler

A Tribute to Dr. Savio Woo 249
Malcolm Pope

Vision, Knowledge and Wisdom... 250
Richard Steadman

Un Grande Maestro 252
Giuliano Cerulli

Savio L-Y. Woo – A Distinguished Professor, Teacher, Scientist,
Tennis Player and Friend.. 253
Per Renström

In Friendship for Savio Woo 256
    Werner Mueller

Very Happy Birthday Savio from All Your Friends in Australia.... 258
    John Bartlett

Tribute to a Dear Friend 260
    Mahmut Nedim Doral

Thanks for What You Have Done & Are Still Doing 262
    Jose Huylebroek

Professor Savio Woo on His 70th Birthday...................................... 264
    Arnold Caplan

A Long History Together 266
    James C.Y. Chow

Thank You, Savio.. 268
    Peter Katona

Congratulations and Happy 70th Birthday 270
    Ron Zernicke

Tribute to a Colleague, Collaborator & Friend:
Dr. Savio L-Y. Woo 273
    Mario Lamontagne

The Highlight of Dr Woo's Contribution to Hong Kong 275
    K.M. Chan

An Ageless Sage.. 277
    Bruce Reider

The Best Is Yet to Come... 279
    John Feagin

Happy 70th Birthday Savio 280
    Rene Verdonk

Smart, Approachable, Kind 281
    David B. Root

The Scientific Olympian 282
    Benno Nigg

Sharing Good Times 283
    Ben and Betty Kibler

Happy 70th Birthday to My Good Friend, Savio 284
    Robert J. Johnson

A National Treasure 286
    Scott F. Dye

Sabio 287
    Ramon Cugat

To My "Old" Friend Savio Woo 288
    Giancarlo Puddu

Tribute to Savio Woo 289
    Peter and Linda Jokl

A Youthful Dr. Woo 290
    Zong-Ming Li

Mazel Tov and L'Chaim 292
    Harvey Borovetz

Professional Debt of Gratitude 294
    Sanjeev Shroff

A Tribute to Dr. Woo: From Recruitment to Pittsburgh to a
Valued Mentor and Friend 296
    David Vorp

A Partner in Triumph – Bioengineering at the University of
Pittsburgh 298
    Jerome S. Schultz

A Significant Success Story 300
   James Herndon

A Tribute to Dr. Woo 301
   Mark S. Redfern

Long May You Run 302
   Patrick Loughlin

"Engineering Nobility" 303
   Alan Russell

You Are the Best 304
   Jag Sankar

A Teacher and Mentor 305
   William T. Green, Jr.

A Remarkable Scientist and Person 306
   Marc J. Philippon

Happy 70th Birthday Savio! 307
   Larry J. Shuman

A Mentor, a Colleague and a Friend
   Harry E. Rubash 308
   Jon JP Warner 308
   James Kang 309

回憶科學耕耘二十年 310
   Cheng-Wen (Ken) Wu

A Great Teacher 312
   Monto Ho

A Tribute to Savio Woo 314
   Chien Ho

A Lifetime Mentor 316
   Daisy Tsai

Thank You for Your Inspiration 318
   Zhi-Pei Liang

A Privilege to Know You 320
   Kam W. Leong

The Savio I Know – Mentor, Connoisseur, Scholar 322
   Abraham "Abe" Lee

A Leader with Foresight and Conviction 324
   K. Kirk Shung

A Role Model and Friend 326
   Richard Cheng-Kung Cheng

Your Legacy Continues 327
   Jeremy Mao

Savio - A Giant in His Own Right 328
   Wei-Shou Hu

Dr. Savio Woo's Singapore Connection 329
   James Goh

Professor Savio L-Y. Woo – Our Honorary Doctorate 331
   Arthur Mak

My Mentor and Friend 333
   Shiyi Chen

A Great Leader in Bioengineering 335
   Fong-Chin Su

An Extraordinary Career and Legacy 337
   Lori Setton and Farshid Guilak

Knowledge, Humility, Leadership & Friendliness 339
   Javier Maquirriain

Celebrating Dr. Woo, Research Pioneer and Inspirational Mentor . 341
  Helen H. Lu

Tribute to a Pioneer and Mentor: Dr. Savio L-Y. Woo 343
  Catherine K. Kuo

Happy Birthday Savio! 346
  Mitsuo Ochi

A Tribute to Savio Woo 348
  Robert Hsu

A Mentor for Us All 350
  Braden C. Fleming

Hard Work, Dedication and Commitment 352
  Lou Soslowsky

福如东海长流水，寿比南山不老松· 354
  Nigel Zheng

Mentorship and Inspiration Buon Compleanno! 356
  Michael Torry

An Extraordinary Teacher, a Kind Man 358
  João Espregueira-Mendes

A Special Friend 360
  Gian Luigi Canata

My Special Mentor 362
  Norimasa Nakamura

The Highest Levels of Science 364
  Nicola Maffulli

A True Innovator in Our Field 366
  Scott Rodeo

Savio Woo at 70 367
   Michael Turner (UK) and Babette Pluim (NED)

Healthy, Energetic and Cordially Friendly 369
   Milan Handl

A Tribute to Dr. Woo - Savio the Savior 371
   King H. Yang

To a Pioneering Bioengineer and Leader - Happy Birthday,
Dr. Woo 373
   X. Edward Guo

A Leader and Giant 375
   James Tibone

A Great Heart in Savio Woo 376
   Rogerio Teixeira da Silva

Happy 70th Birthday and Warm Wishes 377
   Noshir A. Langrana

You Are a Leader 378
   Moises Cohen

A Great Leader in Orthoapedic Biomechanics 379
   Toru Fukubayashi

Tribute to My Friend, Savio Woo 380
   Ken Kuo

"The Age of Rarity" 381
   Michael Lai

Thank You Professor Savio Woo 382
   Ching-Jen Wang
   PC Leung

A Gentleman and a Scholar 383
    Steve Burkhart
    Gideon Mann

A Special Mentor and Friend 384
    Evan Flatow

CHAPTER 6
The Story of One Blessed Academic 385
    Savio Lau-Yuen Woo

CHAPTER 7
Journey down Memory Lane 435
    Contributed by Pattie Woo

APPENDIX
Members of Dr. Woo's Team 473

AUTHOR INDEX 489

Chapter 1

Tributes

from

Family and Relatives

SOME IMPORTANT TRUTHS

Kirstin Woo

San Carlos, California, 94070, U.S.A.

Dearest Dad,
Happy, Happy 70th Birthday! This year has been all about celebrating your achievements and your ability to touch lives - both in simple personal interactions and in large lecture halls. It is challenging to condense my feelings into a few succinct and print-worthy paragraphs, but I will try my best to do so.

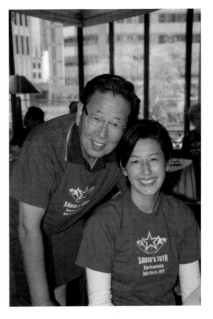

Many people have written sincere and precious words in your honor for this book. While previewing these tributes, I felt more and more proud to learn about how your hard work and morals have influenced others in such a profound way. Then, having the opportunity to read your own personal account gave me a bit more insight into our family history and the context of your life that I never had before. It is not just from reading all this sentimental material that I am feeling greater motivation to understand and connect with you. There is a recent transition that has come about in me - perhaps with motherhood, perhaps with age (eek!) - and it is my heartfelt wish to make you feel happy.

As you wrote in your piece and have wished aloud many times, in the ideal world your daughter would be "nicer to her Daddy". You often lament how attending Brown corrupted me - as I became much more messy, less obedient, and more opinionated after going there. It is true that I wanted to declare independence as most teenagers do at age 18.

And although I genuinely admired you for many things, I did not want to feel like my character was predetermined. As an adult, I have continued to struggle to find my own answers and pathways while being ever-conscious of your and 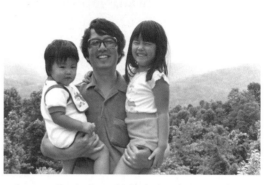 Mom's approval. However, whereas I tried to deny it in the past, I now freely admit that your respect and acceptance are extremely important to me. I have spent many years trying to fight against the similarities between us in order to establish an identity of my own, but now I am proud of the characteristics we share. I am proud that indeed, we are very much alike (although now I always drink fully-caffeinated coffee). Spending less energy on keeping an arm's length between us means I have greater energy to see positive aspects of our relationship. I continue to learn new things from you and I find that the more I open myself to those lessons, the more value they have.

In addition to taking genuine interest in the stories and experiences you have to share, I more deeply appreciate your emphasis on certain values than ever before. Some family values do change from generation to generation (especially when weathering drastic cultural change such as immigrating from the "Far East" to the U.S.), but your philosophy of gradual growth, courtesy, and integrity are personal characteristics that I hope to pass on to our children.

The adventures of parenting have made me feel more vulnerable - and at times needy - than I have ever felt or wished to admit. Work-life balance is something that I strive to achieve every day. Knowing how difficult it is to be away from my children, I see what an emotional sacrifice it was for you to work outside the home in order to financially support my education and ambitions. As Adam and I devote ourselves to the same goal (albeit within a different family construct), my appreciation for what you have done grows deeper and more sincere.

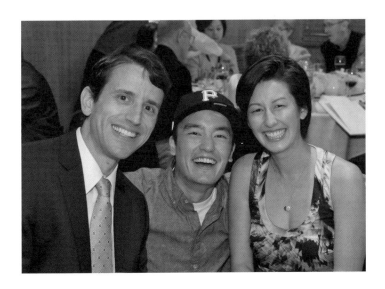

You have gone on to make other sacrifices to support my family (including taking initiative to help out with the girls and living solo in Pittsburgh while Mom helps us), which is truly touching. But above all, seeing you interact with Zadie and Arden - your sentimentality, your generosity, and deep love - just fills my heart with warmth. I will never ever take for granted your and Mom's active participation in their lives. Nonetheless, you *will* continue to hear my resistance to unnecessary spoiling - although I know it is never heeded!

Dad, I hope you can feel the sincerity of my words. There has always been love in my heart, and I hope with each year you will come to know it more and more.

Kirstin

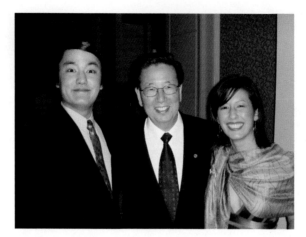
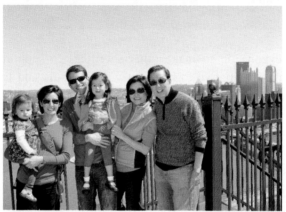
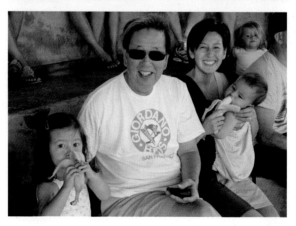

BASEBALL THROUGH THE EVOLUTION OF A FATHER/SON RELATIONSHIP

Jonathan Woo

*San Francisco, California, 94118, U.S.A.
Email: wooeleven@yahoo.com*

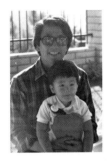

It is fitting that my contribution to this book is revolves around sports, since I have worked in a Pittsburgh sports bar for the past four years. I have grown and matured in that time, as has my relationship with my father. In terms of work ethic and loyalty, I have learned much from my father. This is the most important thing that I could have taken from him as a role model and an example of how to live my life. He has taught me from childhood to work hard and to apply all of myself to whatever job I had. Now that I have found a job that I am passionate about, I realize how my father dedicated himself to what he was doing. When I was younger (yes, I can say that now), I was confused as to why my father traveled so much and worked at his desk before he went to work and after dinner. But now I realize that my father loved and truly believed in what he was doing. He applied the majority of his energy in this way not just to provide for our family, but also to educate his students and others.

So now that I have sung my father's praises for his work ethic and guidance, I will move on to the real reason why I am writing this. My father and I have not had the smoothest of relationships through the years. This is probably to be expected, considering we are both extremely stubborn people. I have particularly vivid childhood memories of going to baseball games. These memories date back to our time in San Diego, when we would go to Jack Murphy Stadium to see the Padres play - watching guys like Steve Garvey, Tony Gwynn, Gary Templeton, and Dave Dravecky. Then when we moved to Pittsburgh, where the Buccos were actually in contention with guys like Barry Bonds (pre-steroids), Bobby Bonilla, Mike LaValliere, Stan Belinda (I got his autograph - actually, I think my father got it), and Doug Drabeks. Did I really almost forget Andy Van Slyke? So what do the Pirates and Padres have to do with my relationship with my father? Some of my earliest memories include my entire family at Jack Murphy all the way up in the nosebleed section watching the Beach Boys perform on the field and my mother and sister sleeping through the game. Then in Pittsburgh, watching a playoff game from 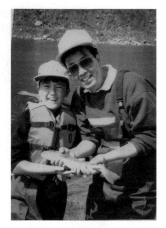 the Department of Orthopedics seats; sitting across from the Braves wives and children as they chanted and "tomahawk chopped" in Three Rivers Stadium. In middle school, while walking to the that stadium, we got into an argument in front of two of my friends about the legality of selling peanuts in the parking lots of the stadium. Go figure. Things have changed and so has my relationship with my father. I now look forward to my annual trip home in the middle of summer. Since I cannot leave my responsibilities at my job during the fall and winter and into spring (assuming the Pens do well in the playoffs), I return home now, almost full circle to enjoy a night or day at the park with my father to watch the Buccos. I have found that going home now and walking to the park with my father brings back all the old memories of what having a very special connection through sports that a father and a son are supposed to share - no matter what age. Among other things, hoping that one day the Buccos will have an over .500 season and getting hot dogs (my father likes his with mustard and relish) and soda (he only drinks Diet Coke). These are the things I appreciate every year when I go home. Now that I am older and have grown into the sports fan that I am, I realize the importance of the times that fathers and sons spend together at the ballpark.

Since the birth of my nieces, I have taken a backseat to them. I know and actually encourage this. However, when I come home and we get to the ballpark, the distractions of the outside world - work, nieces/grandchildren, and other issues - all seem to disappear. We are once again taken back to Jack Murphy Stadium and we are just a

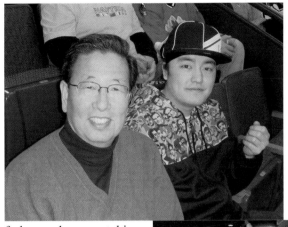

Home for a Penguin's and a Pirate's game

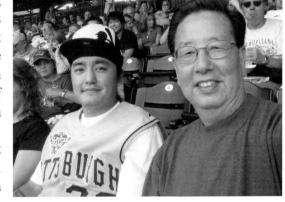

father and son watching baseball. We may miss a year here or there but I hope we will continue to meet in Pittsburgh regularly - regardless of where we are - for a long, long time.

My father has taught and guided many lives. Earlier, I reviewed a copy of what I wrote to honor him and his teachings when he received an honorary degree from the Hong Kong Polytechnic University. I spoke about him teaching me about how to solve problems on my own. I know that he has passed this lesson on to many of the students, fellows, and residents who have come through his lab. To honor my father now, I wanted to give everyone a glimpse into the bond with him that he and I share. Our bond is different from any other person that we are now connected to.

He is my father.
I am his son.

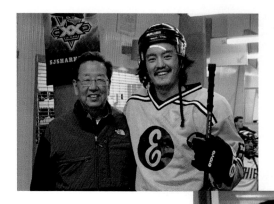

After playing hockey

Surprising dad for his 60th birthday

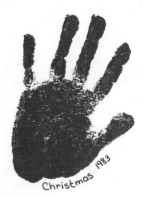

Sometimes you get discouraged
Because I am so small
And always leave my fingerprints
On furniture and walls.

But every day I'm growing...
I'll be grown up someday.
And all those tiny handprints
Will surely fade away.

So here's a final handprint
Just so you can recall
Exactly how my fingers looked
When I was very small.

Handprints from when I was 4

A DEDICATED EDUCATOR, DEVOTED FAMILY MAN AND DOTING GRANDFATHER

Pattie Woo

Fox Chapel, Pennsylvania, 15238, U.S.A.
E-mail: pattiewoo@yahoo.com

Seventy years sounds like such a long time, but when I think back, the big celebration for Savio's sixtieth birthday seems like it happened just a week ago. The love and respect expressed by friends everywhere for both events have been overwhelming.

We all wish to pay tribute to Savio on this very happy occasion because we want to let him know how much we appreciate him. I myself would like to first salute his parents for giving me such a gift. They successfully raised a family of nine children with very limited means amid great social turmoil - during the Japanese invasion and Chinese civil revolution. Savio's siblings are all very loving, caring, and hardworking. I can see how the high moral standards, compassion and work ethic that their parents instilled in each and every one of them has made such positive impact on their lives.

I still vividly remember the evening I went downstairs in my rooming house at the University of Washington and met our "ride" to the Ice Capades show. I saw a very clean-cut and intelligent looking young man with a pair of black-rimmed glasses and white turtleneck sweater. What impressed me most was his broad smile, nice straight teeth and soft-spoken nature. I remember thinking that it would be a pleasant evening. You may think of me being ridiculously naive for not realizing that this was supposed to be a blind date! But, if you knew what a sheltered life I had led before coming to the U.S. for college, you would understand.

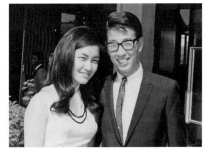

Savio and I in Seattle (1967)

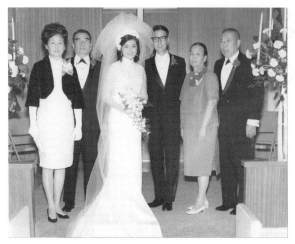

Our wedding day with our parents (1969)

We all crammed into Savio's little Volkswagen Beetle with me sitting in the roomy front seat. (I still did not get it!) When we arrived at the ice rink, I think I paid for my own ticket. Inside, I chose to sit at the end of our row and my friend Susan sat down next to me. Her boyfriend, Jim sat next to Savio on the other end. I enjoyed the show thoroughly since it was the first live ice-skating show I had ever seen. We might need to check with Savio some other time for his opinion.

On our first "real" date, Savio took me ice-skating. Then, at the International Pancake House, he talked nonstop for over an hour. He told me at length about his family and his personal philosophy.

It was evident from the beginning that he loves to talk and I like to listen. I have never needed to second-guess his words because he is so honest and direct. This is very energy efficient for any kind of relationship. We have kept this going for more that forty-four years now.

Efficiency is one thing Savio believes in wholeheartedly. I remember that many years ago I came across a sign and felt compelled to get it for him. It reads: "Your efficiency scares the hell out of me." He truly is gifted in being able to totally focus and complete each task. He can think clearly because he can compartmentalize and organize efficiently, and the neatness of his desk is a reflection of the way his mind works.

Sharing is another virtue that comes from growing up in a large family. Savio loves to share his time, his thoughts and his happiness without reservation. What is most touching to me is how generously he shared his love and respect for my parents, treating them as his own. From a professional standpoint, he created "open-lab" to encourage communication. He encourages the group to take lunch together. He

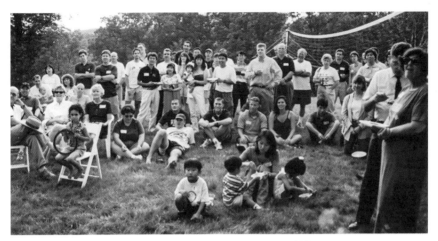

MSRC summer party at our home (1998)

further fosters social connections within the lab by organizing parties to welcome new comers, say good-bye to those departing, as well as to celebrate good news and professional accomplishments. I have enjoyed meeting everybody through these gatherings: ice cream taste tests, dumpling-making parties, Thanksgivings, Heritage Dinners, and the annual summer picnic at our house. Savio gets very excited for each and every event. He is passionate about sharing time with his students and colleagues.

Our two beautiful offspring are most important to Savio. He cares deeply and would do anything for them at any time. We made a conscious decision for me to stay at home to raise our children. We divided our responsibilities so that each of us could focus and work more efficiently. Our primary goal was to provide them with a stable home environment. So, that was what Savio did - focusing on what he did best to provide for the family.

We have traveled mountains and valleys together - literally and figuratively. His work has brought us to all corners of the world. We treasure the friends we have made, the sights we have seen

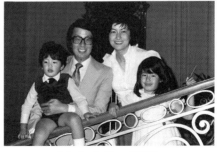

Mother's Day (1982)

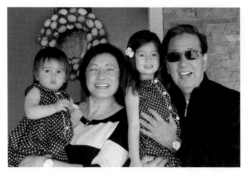

With our two grandchildren (2012)

and the many valuable experiences we have had. We are truly blessed with a great wealth of friendship everywhere. I believe this may have been the result of Savio's genuine honesty, gentle nature and willingness to share.

Now that we have two beautiful, sweet and just perfect little granddaughters, Savio has set his next goal to be the most doting and best grandfather he can be. They have him completely wrapped around their tiny little fingers.

Personally, I love getting up to a gentle "morning call" for coffee each day – not being offered a cup, but rather being requested to make a fresh pot from our favorite Peet's coffee beans. Then we sit down to enjoy our coffee time and plan the day together. I love being greeted by his broad smile and his cheerful face every morning. This is ALWAYS the best time of our day.

Savio, I look forward to many, many more years of making you a good cup of Peet's coffee in the morning.

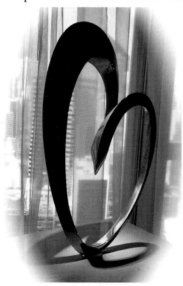

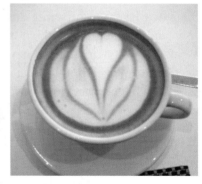

IN MEMORY OF GUNG GUNG

Antonio Cheong
Posthumous

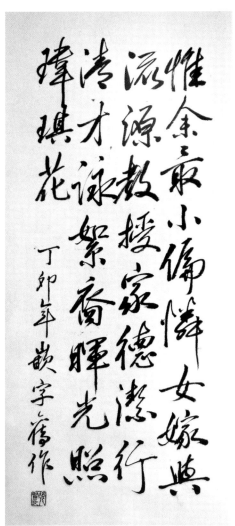

Poem written by Gung Gung that incorporates the Chinese names of Dr. and Mrs. Woo, Kirstin and Jonathan.

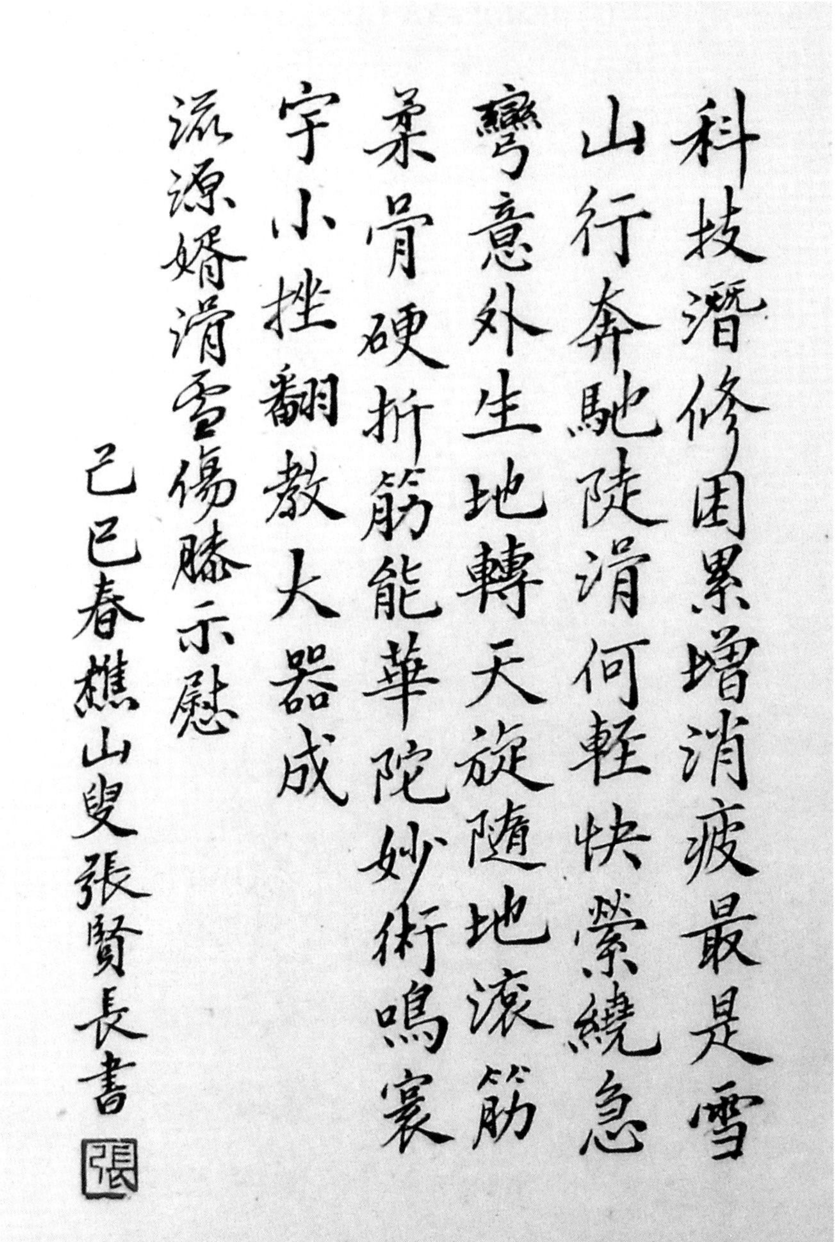

科技潛修困累增消疲最是雪
山行奔馳陡滑何輕快縈繞急
彎意外生地轉天旋隨地滾筋
柔骨硬折筋能華陀妙術鳴寰
宇小挫翻教大器成
流源婿滑雪傷膝示慰
己巳春樵山叟張賢長書

Poem that Gung Gung wrote after Dr. Woo injured his ACL. The poem was written for comfort and encouragement for him and for a positive outcome after adversity.

Tributes from Family and Relatives 17

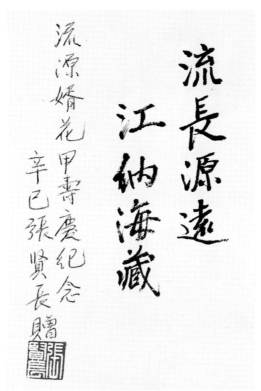

Poem written by Gung Gung (when he was 88 years old) in honor of Dr. Woo's 60th birthday celebration.

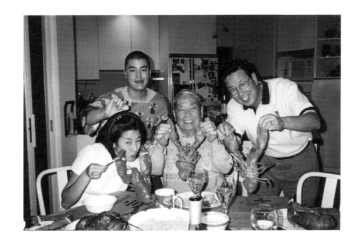

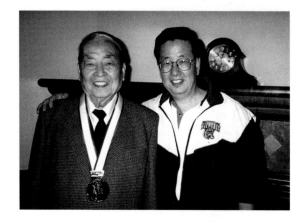

Sharing the Olympic Gold medal in 1998

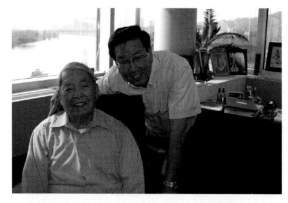

In Dr. Woo's office overlooking the Monongahela River

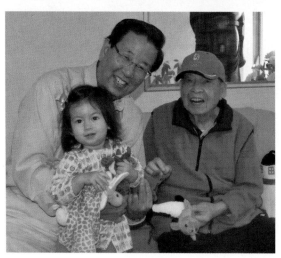

The last photo of Gung Gung

HAPPY 70TH BIRTHDAY, BROTHER & UNCLE

Liu-Yun Woo and Family
Marubeni Hong Kong & South China Limited
Hong Kong
E-mail: ek-woo@marubeni.com

同慶流源七十大壽
炫耀歷程

流源始幼孝爹娘
勤奮好學乃自強
圖謀鵬程漂過海
願作細佬領頭羊
智慧努力結合緊
美國學府奇葩新
學士碩士博士後
四料院士胡宅尋
為家為國俱增光
雙親恩情素未忘
賢內子女好支撐
溫馨家庭幸福嘗

三哥盡興拙作
二零一一年於上海

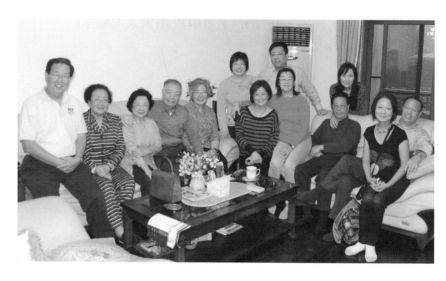

恭祝四叔叔七十大寿
Happy Birthday
您是我们胡家的光荣、是我们的自豪。
四叔叔(四叔公），您好嘢！！！

Angela, EK, Cindy and Eugene Woo

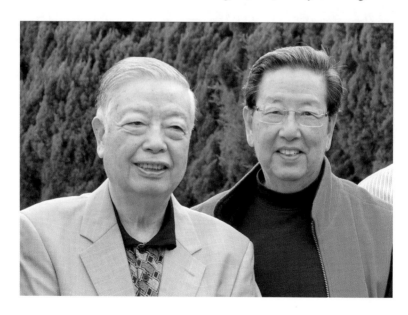

HAPPY 70ᵀᴴ BIRTHDAY, AH XI DÖ

Sister Bernadette Woo

Precious Blood Convent
Kowloon, Hong Kong
E-mail: bernadette.woo@gmail.com

生日之所以值得慶祝，因為生命寶貴，生活美好！
生命寶貴，因為每個日子都是全新的，永不重複！
生日是生命的起點，每個生日都周而復始地為生命創造羅旋式嶄新起點！
看來近似，絕不重叠！生命人人一樣，生活各自精彩！

10年前曾隆重地慶祝你圓滿地完成第一個豐盛的甲子！
今年慶祝你甲子重開後第一個10年！
歡迎你加入「從心所欲」的行列！

願偕所有親朋同心合意地祝親愛的流源70大壽滿心稱意！
祝願你在第一個甲子的穩固基礎上不斷開展生命的新里程！

二姊祝禱
2011.7.5. 香港

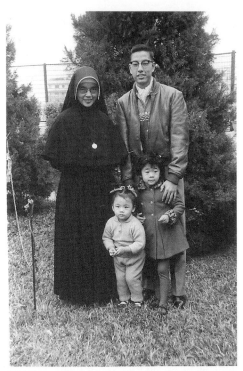

Bid Farewell to sister before leaving for the U.S.
(with nieces, Nancy & Winnie)

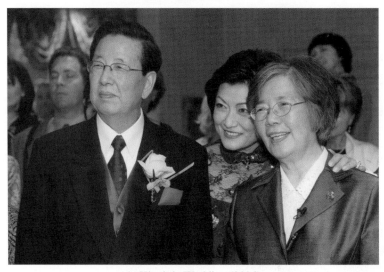

At Kirstin's Wedding (2006)

HAPPY 70TH BIRTHDAY

Sister Agnes Au

Precious Blood Secondary School
Chai Wan, Hong Kong
E-mail: sisterau@hotmail.com

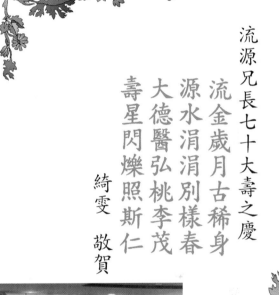

流源兄長七十大壽之慶

流金歲月古稀身
源水涓涓別樣春
大德醫弘桃李茂
壽星閃爍照斯仁

綺雯　敬賀

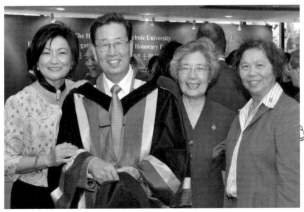

HAPPY 70ᵀᴴ BIRTHDAY, SAVIO

Paulo and Anna Cheong
Concord, California, 94520, U.S.A.
E-mail: paulocheong88@gmail.com

流源妹倩七十大寿致慶

從古稱稀尊上壽

自今叹始樂餘年

辛卯夏於舊金山張錫鈞

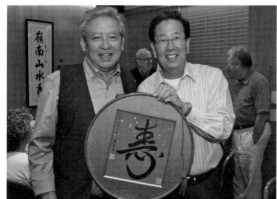

The Chinese character "longevity"

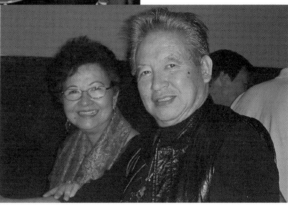

HAPPY 70TH BIRTHDAY, SAVIO

Vang and Eileen Cheong
Hsingju, Taiwan
E-mail: vangc@hotmail.com

賀流源妹倩七十之慶
杏林譽滿　桃李遍天下
四海名揚　嘉惠濟蒼生

弘發翊菱同賀
二〇二一年七月

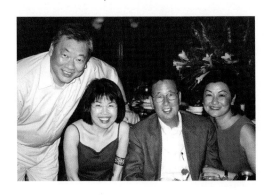

MORE THAN A SPECIAL FRIEND, HE'S FAMILY

Linda and Mark Saxon
Rancho Sante Fe, California, 92067, U.S.A.
E-mail: saxonlm@yahoo.com

Dear Savio,

We want to wish you all that life has to offer on your 70th birthday! You have been such an important force in our lives - not as the world renowned Dr. Savio Woo, but as Kirstin and Jonathan's dad - along with Pattie, our dear and treasured friend!

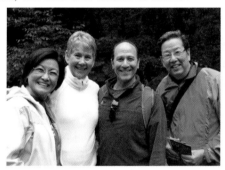 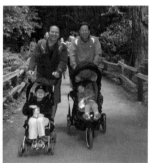

We have been blessed to consider you as a member of our family for over 30 years. It has been wonderful to watch our children grow up as though they were siblings and we know Shana and Brandon will always have a close and loving bond with you and Pattie. We have always been honored to be the Godparents for Kirstin and Jonathan, who we love dearly. And, it is so exciting to watch the next generation of Woos and Saxons growing strong.

We will always have very fond memories of so many experiences with your family, including skiing in Park City, Thanksgiving in Pittsburgh, our children's weddings, and important celebrations in San Francisco.

We are so happy to be a part of your birthday celebration!

With our love, Linda and Mark

REMEMBRANCES AND TRIBUTE TO SAVIO WOO ON HIS 70TH BIRTHDAY

Bruce Simon

The University of Arizona
Tucson, Arizona, 85721, U.S.A.
E-mail: simonb@email.arizona.edu

Savio Woo and I have been good friends since 1965 when we were graduate students in Mechanical Engineering at the University of Washington. We both worked with Dr. Albert Kobayashi during the pioneering years of bioengineering and biomechanics. Savio studied the eye and I studied large arteries. It is my recollection that Savio developed one of the first finite element models of a biological structure: a simulation of the wall of an arteriole. We were also 'suite mates' in a dormitory at UW. During that time, we both married and had two children of similar ages. Since then, the Woo and Simon families have continued to be close (almost relatives). Even though time and distance often have separated us, when we do meet, it is as if we had never been apart!

There are too many stories about Savio to tell in this short space. Here I offer a few personal and professional remembrances. Savio was in my wedding party and I sang at Savio and Pattie's wedding. Some years later, I sang for his daughter - Kirstin's - wedding. Savio and I have made several trips to northern Idaho, where I grew up. It was there that he was initiated in the ways of "big Idaho men". During the early years of our careers, we collaborated on grants to study optimal designs for internal fixation plates. This also provided opportunities for many memorable visits with the Woos in San Diego. Savio moved from UCSD to the University of Pittsburgh and I remained at the University of Arizona for 34 years until becoming emeritus in 2006. I am wondering when Savio will do the same.

Savio and I have attended numerous bioengineering meetings over the years. I do recall the 1969 Chicago meeting where we witnessed the first lunar landing together with my "Uncle Bob and Aunt Alice."

I have followed Savio's life path for these seventy years and felt Happiness for his accomplishments, honors, and awards, e.g. an Olympic Medal, endowed chair, and the establishment of the Musculoskeletal Research Center at Pittsburgh. Savio is especially well known for his approach to joint mechanics in which he advocates that "motion is good", as well as his research on the ACL (with corresponding personalized license plate). It is also evident that Savio takes great pride in his students, now scattered around the world working in biomechanics and related areas.

Pam and I send our heartfelt congratulations to you, Savio - and also to Pattie and your family. We will always remember Savio's 70th birthday party in San Francisco. It was especially wonderful to meet the new Woo grandchildren, Zadie and Arden.

Savio, we continue to cherish your friendship and wish you, Pattie, and your growing family "all the very best" from "Simon boy", Pam, Fritz and Danielle, and Summer Simon.

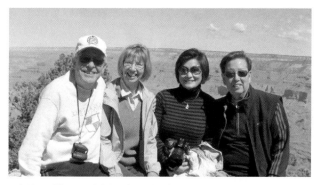

Bruce & Pam Simon with Pattie & Savio Woo; Grand Canyon, May 2011.

HAPPY 70TH BIRTHDAY, UNCLE SAVIO

Nancy, Irene, Helen and Kevin Chan
Delta, British Columbia, V4M-2T7, Canada
E-mail: yynancy@hotmail.com

Thank you for being an inspiration of our lives – not only think positive, BUT BE POSITIVE!!

You have shown us the love & commitment that you have placed in work,

The friendship that you have shared and treasured among everyone around you,

The bond of love and caring that you have shared with all of us... family.

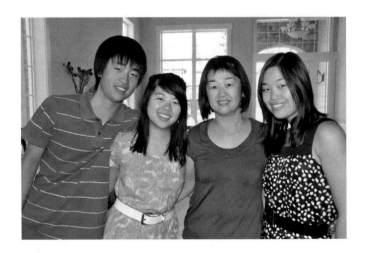

THE IMPORTANCE OF FAMILY

James Lai
Vancouver, British Columbia, V6L 1X5, Canada
E-mail: jklai@telus.net

I first heard about you when I was dating my dear wife Josephine way back in the mid-80s. I remember her constantly talking about her 3 uncles - #4, #5, and #6. But it was clear which one was her favorite because she beamed whenever she talked about you. Whether it was growing up as a young girl in Hong Kong or babysitting your kids in San Diego (including taking Kirstin to Vancouver), Mei Mei had so many good memories of you, Aunt Pattie and the kids. So it was so wonderful to finally meet you at our wedding in 1985 with Jon Jon and Wei Wei as our ring bearer and flower girl. From that day on, I gained a new Uncle who was not only a respected scientist and researcher (and soon to be world famous Olympic Gold Medal winner), but even more importantly, a great husband and father who also cared deeply for his extended family.

From our trip to San Diego a year after we got married, to the great Woo clan skiing gatherings in Vancouver at our place, your unexpected stop over on 9/11, Joshua's summer session at your lab, celebrating your 60th birthday bash in Pittsburgh, celebrating Kirstin's wedding, and the many other times we have crossed paths, you have enriched my life and taught me the importance of family.

My heartfelt congratulations on your 70th birthday, and many more happy returns to our number one Uncle Savio!

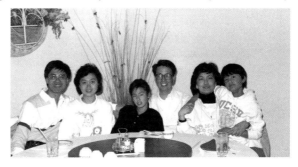

With much love and admiration,
James

AN UNFORGETTABLE EXPERIENCE

Joshua Lai

Vancouver, British Columbia, V6L 1X5, Canada
E-mail: josh_lai@telus.net

Dear Uncle Savio,

I cannot believe it has been nearly six years since I stayed with you and Auntie Pattie and shadowed in your lab! I still remember your outdoor BBQ steaks (still one of the best I have ever had), the morning drives to work, and your stories about our extended family. I was also lucky to share in the moment that Kirstin and Adam were engaged! Spending time in your home was so much fun, and an experience I will not forget.

Shadowing in your lab also turned out to be very formative for me – you inspired me to get involved in research early and for the past six years, I have had many wonderful experiences in various labs. I am just one of the many students you have mentored over the years, but it was wonderful to have someone in the family to look up to.

With love from,
Joshua

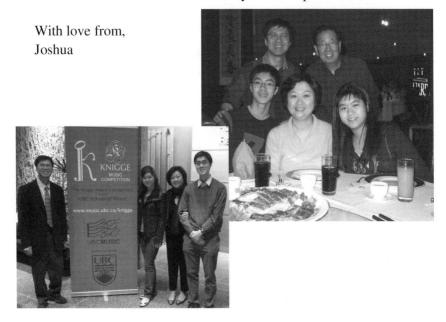

OUR TRIBUTE – A LIMERICK

Bob and Holly Frymoyer
Camp Hill, Pennsylvania, 17011-8355, U.S.A.
E-mail: mjhollyfrymoyer@yahoo.com, rcfrymoyer@aol.com

There once was a doctor from Pitt
Whose daughter had beauty and wit.
Our son became smitten
And soon he was sittin'
Seeking the right to commit.

The family was nervous as heck.
Would the good doctor wring our son's neck?
But soon we had smiles
As we prepared the aisles --
Adam had passed the inspect!

Six years have quickly passed by.
Our son is a lucky young guy.
Savio's Tochter
Is also a doctor.
Cheers for this man from Shanghai.

Our Savio is now 70 years old;
His accomplishments truly untold.
He is quite a fellow--
Increasingly mellow
And his life should be highly extolled.

This ditty must now soon be ended.
Our families have wonderfully blended.
Hooray for this birthday.
We certainly must say

This milestone could not be more splendid!

Happy Birthday!

Love from Bob and Holly

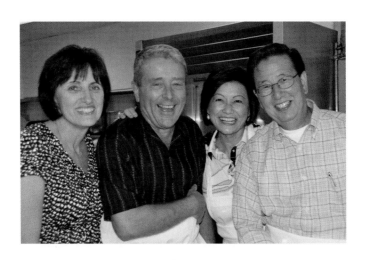

Chapter 2

Tributes

from

Students, Residents and Fellows

Affiliated With

the Orthopaedic Bioengineering Laboratory
Departments of Orthopaedics and Bioengineering
University of California, San Diego

SHOWING ME THE WAY

Cy Frank

*University of Calgary
Calgary, Alberta, Canada
E-mail: cfrank@ucalgary.ca*

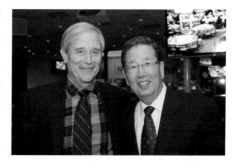

Right after I graduated in Orthopaedic Surgery in Canada, I moved to San Diego in January of 1981 with my young family (a 2 year old son and my pregnant wife, Joyce) and spent the next three years working with Dr. Woo as a Post-Doctoral Fellow in his lab and with the Biochemistry Laboratory of Dr. Amiel with the support of Dr. Wayne Akeson. Our second son, Tym, was born at Scripps Memorial in San Diego on July 4, 1981. I knew almost nothing about 'real research' when I arrived, so I literally learned all of the basics from Dr. Woo while I was there: how to review and cite the literature, how to design experiments, and how to actually test connective tissues biomechanically. Perhaps more importantly, Savio taught me (and all of the other students, residents and fellows passing through his lab), how to think critically about research. We had many interesting discussions about both philosophy and science, and he always encouraged us to be our own worst critics in what we were doing. He led by example, as he was always the first one into the office in the morning and the last one to leave at night. He also taught us how to present research results and how to write grants and papers; critical skills for success in my research career ever since then.

I made many research connections while I was in San Diego - meeting literally all of the giants in research at that time, mainly through Dr. Woo's connections. San Diego was 'on the circuit' at that time with all of the worlds connective tissue/knee/biomechanics experts passing through at one time or another. Those connections were transformative for me in research and in life, as many of those people became collaborators, friends, mentors and associates of mine over the years.

I remember many times at Savio and Pattie's house in Encinitas (as we were practically neighbors), with Jon-Jon and Kirstin being close in age to our kids - we had a lot in common! Pattie and my wife Joyce became great friends and spent a lot of time together at the park, beach, zoo and all the usual great places in San Diego. They even loaned us their pride and joy - a great car: a slightly sun-faded - but immaculately kept blue Volvo! I proceeded to lose the gas cap at a local service station - one of the most embarrassing things that happened while I was there. I replaced it with a chrome one, as I recall - but it was not quite the same. Savio let me off the hook, but I *still* feel guilty about it! The other story that I remember best is Savio and Pattie coming up to Joyce's parents golf course in Redlands for a visit - I think it was Easter. Anyway, it was typical of both of them to treat us all like family - showing an interest in us and our families and literally treating us like members of their own family. To this day, I am grateful for that support, love and affection – so very special.

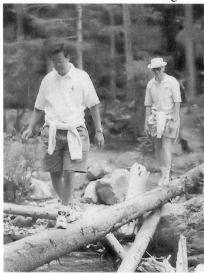

Savio showing me the way in ~1983

I would just like to say congratulations to Savio for another milestone birthday and thanks +++ to both Savio and to Pattie - for everything. They were (and are) role models of thoughtful, loving, caring and supportive friends and 'family'. It's been a real privilege to know them.

A TRIBUTE TO DR. WOO: A BIOENGINEERING PIONEER

Mark A. Gomez

Biomechanics Advanced and University of California, San Diego
Encinitas, California, 92024, U.S.A.
E-mail: drgomez@biomechanicsadvanced.com

My relationship with Dr. Woo began in 1977. I had just graduated from UCSD with a degree in Biology. The Biomechanics Lab was relatively new, but changes in personnel were afoot. Dr. Woo needed someone to help in the lab and specifically, to aid a yet-to-be appointed engineer who would run the lab. I met with Dr. Woo to inform him of my interest in the assistant position. Unfortunately, my background in Biology included no engineering. Of course, this gave Dr. Woo pause. I was extremely impressed by all that was going on in the lab and was somewhat disheartened about not being able to work there. I decided it was too good of an experience to pass up. I told Dr. Woo I would work for him for the next two weeks for free. At the end of that time, he was welcome to send me on my way or, once again, consider the possibility of offering me a job. Fortunately, he hired me.

The purpose of sharing this story is that it emphasizes the legacy that Dr. Woo has created for both his family and the research community. He has provided incredible opportunities for innumerable students, friends, faculty and peers. They have all achieved much success. In fact, if one pays tribute to any of these individuals, or acknowledges their respective degrees, awards, teaching and research activities, a tribute should also be given to Dr. Woo. His inspiration and willingness to support a "new" field of research cannot be ignored. Dr. Woo will always be considered a pioneer in the area of Bioengineering research.

Dr. Woo, I have always appreciated and benefited from our time together. It has provided me with a career, a way of taking care of my family, and most importantly, a special friendship that will always endure. I wish you and your entire family all the best and look forward to our future times together! - Mark

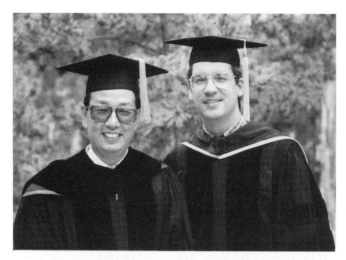

Dr. Woo with his first PhD student (1988)

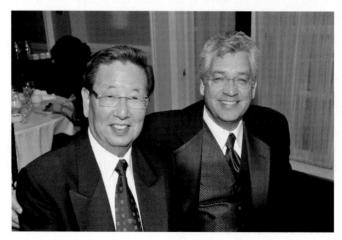

2011

DEMAND FOR EXCELLENCE

J. Marcus Hollis

*Blue Bay Research Inc.
Navarre, Florida, 32566, U.S.A.
E-mail: Marcus@bluebayres.com*

I worked in Professor Woo's biomechanics lab from Spring 1984 as a staff member and Doctoral student until the Fall of 1988.

Professor Woo is a very demanding leader and he expected high quality work from his students and staff. Professor Woo was able to help everyone to achieve their fullest potential. The friends that I made in Professor Woo's biomechanics lab in San Diego have been the closest and longest lasting of any of my friendships.

I would like to express my warmest congratulations to Professor Savio L-Y. Woo in celebration of his 70th birthday. Professor Woo has become the most successful orthopaedic researcher due to his ability to recognize the important issues and put together exemplary teams of researchers to pursue investigations in those areas. His demand for excellence and hard work has not only made him one of the most outstanding orthopaedic researchers, but has also left a legacy of successful students and colleagues that will continue his positive legacy far into the future.

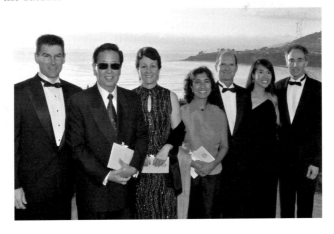

FROM STUDENT TO PROFESSIONAL: MOULDING YOUNG CAREERS

Jennifer S. Wayne

*Virginia Commonwealth University
Richmond, Virginia 23284-3067, U.S.A.
E-mail: jwayne@vcu.edu*

It does not seem possible that 27 years have passed since the ASME summer meeting where we met. It was my first scientific conference as a first year graduate student from Tulane University in 1984. I was already attracted to musculoskeletal research since my undergraduate years, and a torn ACL! Then, I heard you speak about your tendon and ligament research. Your passion and enthusiasm was contagious, and I immediately knew that I wanted to be part of your laboratory for my doctoral degree in the premier Bioengineering Department at UC San Diego.

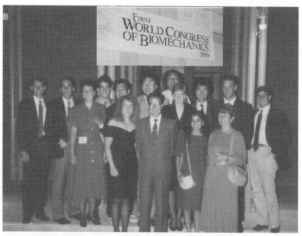

Dr. Woo's laboratory at the First World Congress of Biomechanics in La Jolla, California in 1990

I relished the years with you as my mentor at UCSD. You teach your students many vital lessons for their careers - the essence of quality scientific research, creating effective interdisciplinary research teams, the importance of giving back, and all the while loving what you do.

Allowing me and Deidre MacKenna to be integral organizers of the program committee for the very First World Congress of Biomechanics was an invaluable experience.

Your interest in the development of your students does not end with graduation. Just a few samples of so many - visits to the University of Pittsburgh, support of faculty promotions, encouragement of professional society service. I continue to value your advice in my career.

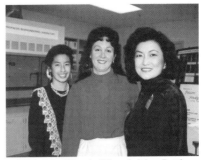

With Ms. Kirstin Woo & Mrs. Pattie Woo at Univ. of Pittsburgh MSRC

We celebrated your 60th birthday in Pittsburgh with "Bioengineering at the Dawn of the 21st Century". And we continue to celebrate your many contributions to musculoskeletal research and their translation to clinical practice.

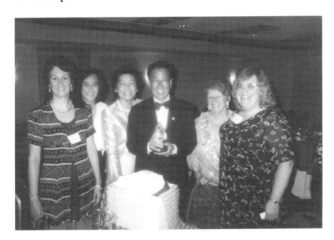

Dr. Jennifer Wayne, Ms. Caroline Wang, Mrs. Pattie Woo, Dr. Savio Woo, Ms. Lynnette Fleck, Ms. Karen Ohland celebrating Dr. Woo's 60th Birthday in Pittsburgh

It is with these many treasured memories that I am honored to wish you a Happy 70th Birthday and many more to come!

HAPPY BIRTHDAY, DR. WOO

Thay Q. Lee

VA Long Beach Healthcare System and University of California, Irvine
Long Beach, California, 90822, U.S.A.
Email: tqlee@med.va.gov; tqlee@uci.edu

I was a student of Dr. Woo from 1983 to 1986 at the University of California, San Diego. Much of the professional success I have been able to enjoy is the result of Dr. Woo's mentorship. Currently, I am a Senior Research Career Scientist for the Department of Veterans Affairs and a Professor in the Departments of Orthopaedic Surgery and Biomedical Engineering at the University of California, Irvine. I also serve as the Vice Chair for Research for the Orthopaedic Surgery Department. For the past 25 years, we have kept in close contact and served on many committees and boards together.

Happy 70th Birthday Dr. Woo. It is difficult to write a tribute for my mentor who has influenced my professional career in so many ways. It is without question that Professor Woo is an acknowledged leader in the biomechanics community in every aspect for over 40 years. He has contributed to orthopaedic research through his prolific writing and service, and received every possible award in our field. He is also recognized as one of the best thinkers in experimental science; always being ahead of his time. But more importantly, he has been the leader of many professional societies to direct the future of our field as well as mentoring countless number of students, residents and fellows. I am fortunate enough to be one of the beneficiaries. Happy Birthday, Dr. Woo.

Over four decades, Dr. Woo has advised a countless number of scientists and physician scientists who are in the forefront of orthopaedic research. My experience with Dr. Woo during my years as a student at the University of California, San Diego was challenging, but highlighted by him being an excellent teacher and a mentor. Dr. Woo is one of the friendliest persons you will ever meet. Everyone says, "What a nice guy!!!" after meeting him. However, in professional settings, he is both respected and feared, as he is always making constructive comments. This is the respect that he has earned with his work and accomplishments. He has always been ahead of his time as a thinker in our field and he is very effective in leading with those thoughts. I am proud to have learned some of those attributes. Happy Birthday, Dr. Woo.

Of note is that Dr. Woo really enjoys fine dining with good wine. This is one of many things that everyone can count on when you spend time with Dr. Woo. I always look forward to our next get-together for some great food and wine.

Happy, Happy Birthday Dr. Woo.

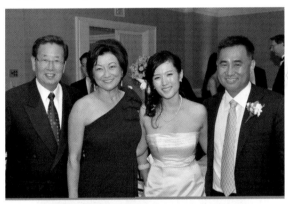

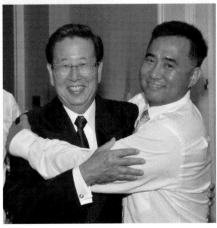

FOND MEMORIES

Lynnette Fleck
University of California, San Diego
San Diego, California, 92117, U.S.A.
E-mail: ljstax1y@yahoo.com

Dear Savio,

Just a note to help celebrate your birthday – although, I still remember June 3rd.

You have come a long way from our early days at UCSD. I thought I would note a few of my early memories...

I admired your organizational skills, as well as intelligence and warmth.

Through you, I got to meet a lot of incredible young people – (who worked very hard – they use to leave me voice mail messages at 2, 3, and 4 a.m.)

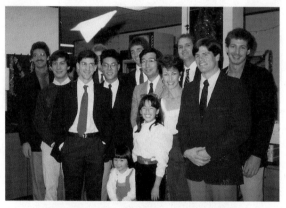

I do not know if it is possible in the current work environment, but it was nice that we took time for some social activities (birthday breakfasts, beach picnics, or going to Club Med as a group).

I always appreciated the way you acknowledged me, and understood that I did my best work when I looked and felt relaxed (you even once said that I was like a smooth basketball player).

I am also very honored that I still get a Christmas bonus after all these years – if I ever mention it, no one really believes it.

It is hard to believe how fast the years go. I wish for you and your family continued good health and happiness in all your endeavors – and I hope this collection of letters brings you joy.

Love,
Lynnette

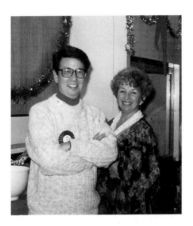

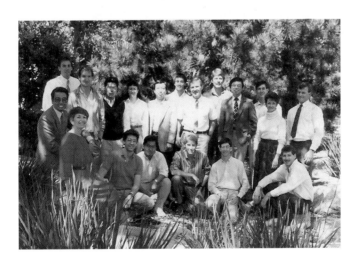

A GREAT MENTOR

Shuji Horibe

Osaka Prefecture University
Habikino, Osaka, 583-8555, Japan
E-mail: s-horibe@rehab.osakafu-u.ac.jp

Congratulations on the 70th anniversary (or Koki in Japanese)! I was a research fellow at UCSD from January 1987 to February 1989. I studied biomechanics of soft tissues and learned a lot from Dr. Woo. He is my great mentor.

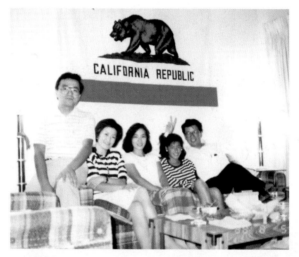

With Pattie, Masayo, Kirstin and Dr. Woo at our home (1988)

Masayo and I got married two weeks before starting our new life in the USA. San Diego life was like a honeymoon for us, but she sometimes felt lonely because she had never been abroad before. Dr. Woo treated us as members of his family and took us many places to cheer her up. Whenever we visited Dr. Woo's home, Kirstin played with Masayo like a real sister and Jonathan used to make me laugh. Thanks to Dr. Woo's family, we had a great time and we will never forget the wonderful life in San Diego.

We have two children. Yuki is 21 years old and a medical student at the same university that I graduated from. Pattie, do you remember what three-year-old Yuki said when you met him for the first time in Kyoto? He repeated to say "Give me a kiss" to you. Riho is 17 years old and a twelfth grader. I am afraid of her getting ACL injury because she is crazy about basketball. Masayo and I hope to see you and your family with our children in the near future.

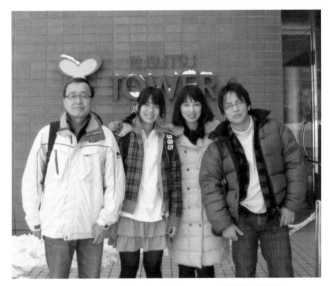

Our family: Shuji, Riho, Masayo and Yuki (2010)

MY SINCERE CONGRATULATIONS AND BEST WISHES ON THE OCCASION OF HIS 70TH BIRTHDAY

Shinro Takai

Nippon Medical School
Tokyo, 113-8602, Japan
E-mail: takai-snr@nms.ac.jp

I wish to express my sincere congratulations and best wishes to Dr. Woo on the occasion of his 70th birthday.

I had the great pleasure and honor to stay at UCSD to do research under Dr. Woo from 1989 to 1991. During my first six months there, having come directly from Japan, I had much difficulty in communicating with people in English. Dr. Woo always suggested that I speak English clearly and audibly, which proved to help me advance quickly. He always provided me with a chance to chat with him about not only my research progress, but about my family and whatever I wished to discuss at least once a week. That is, he always extended his warm hospitality to my family and me. We soon acclimated ourselves to the new surroundings under the protective support of Dr. Woo and the wonderful people in his laboratory.

I was doing research on flexor tendon and ACL biomechanics during my stay as a research fellow. Dr. Woo taught me a lot about how to do research biomechanically. I also learned from Dr. Woo how to advance a research project and how to nurture young people into research. But, his teaching was not limited only to academics, but to all aspects of life itself. He was truly a great mentor and role model to influence how I shaped my life.

While I was at UCSD, I got to know many of Dr. Woo's followers. At that time, Dr. John Xerogeanes was still a medical student, and Dr. Peter Newton was just a resident. Since then, John has been invited by the Japanese Knee Society to give a special lecture, and the Japanese Orthopedic Association has invited Peter to do so, as well. Their lectures in Japan were enthusiastically received. Dr. Thay Lee, who had just left

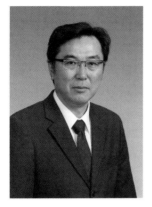
UCSD for UC Irvine shortly after I arrived, but who I got to know very well during my stay, has also been invited to lecture at several Japanese meetings. So, I am very proud of the fact that Japanese academic meetings are inviting my close friends from UCSD to lecture in Japan. I believe we all owe a great debt of gratitude to Dr. Woo for setting us onto the right course.

Today, I am Full Professor and the Chairman of the Orthopedic Department of Nippon Medical School in Tokyo. It is now my responsibility to do for the students and members of my department what Dr. Woo had done for me in the past. And, his example is always foremost in my mind as I carry out my duties.

This year, I have sent one of my staff as a post doctoral fellow to do research in Connecticut with Dr. Douglas Adams, with whom I had the pleasure of working with under Dr. Woo at UCSD, and I will be sending another promising orthopedic doctor to do research with Dr. Thay Lee at his laboratory in Irvine, CA. So, the line continues!

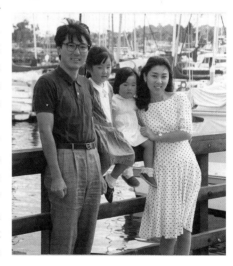

I wish to express my continued gratitude to Dr. Woo for all he has done to help make me what I have become today and to again congratulate him on his 70th birthday, with great wishes for many happy returns of the day.

LONG TIME MENTOR AND COLLABORATOR

Jack Winters

Marquette University
Milwaukee, Wisconsin, 53217, U.S.A.
E-mail: jack.winters@mu.edu

My relationship with Dr. Woo started in January of 1978, when I worked part-time in his Biomechanics Lab at the VA Medical Center near UCSD for over 17 months, until June of 1979. My primary job duties involved mechanically testing of medial and lateral collateral ligaments of rabbits, including both bone-to-bone and isolated samples, extracted from roughly 30 knees, about half of which were normal and most of the others had been immobilized (a few related to other studies). I also assisted with the preparation and testing of tendons, bones, and skin. We used, of course, the video dimensional analyzer, and among other skills, I got very good at painting lines of ink on tissue samples and obtaining biomechanical data. More importantly, I was introduced to research methodology, and to bringing classroom knowledge from Dr. Fung's courses, such viscoelastic tissue properties and remodeling, into practice. I also learned the value of research meetings, and experienced the joy of being a co-author on my first paper of any kind (an ASME proceedings paper that focused on the data I had collected, in 1979).

By the time I had been working in the lab for about a year, I felt that I was a pro, and knew rabbit ligaments and our elaborate testing protocols inside out. For this reason, I still distinctly remember the time I observed an unusually high load-extension relation, and with great excitement yelled to Mark Gomez, colleague and lab manager at the time (he would later get his Ph.D. working with Dr. Woo), to come over and check out this incredible tissue. Mark came over, observed the data, smiled, shook his head, and pointed to the temperature bath controller, which I had forgotten to turn on. Oops. Later on during our next meeting, Dr. Woo found it quite funny.

While a graduate student at UC Berkeley, I had a chance to give a talk at UCSD in 1984 and meet with Dr. Woo and his new students; I was impressed with the level of growth of the lab, as the number of students had more than doubled; Dr. Woo now had the aura of a senior faculty member.

In 1989, while I was an Assistant Professor at Arizona State University, our paths would cross in a more formal way, as Dr. Woo presented me with a unique opportunity that, to this day, I sincerely appreciate: he asked me to organized several tracks for the First World Congress of Biomechanics, which ended up growing into 15 sessions. In tandem, we decided to edit a book together that was loosely associated with these tracks. The result was *Multiple Muscle Systems: Biomechanics and Movement Organization* (Winters and Woo, eds.), Springer-Verlag, 1990, a 47-chapter book that proved to be pivotal to the field. It included collections of chapters on muscle and musculoskeletal modeling by recognized leaders of this field, and collections of chapters addressing principles underlying upper limb movements, spinal loading and postural stability, and propulsive and cyclic movements with lower-limb emphasis. It was a great professional experience for me.

Since this time, I have moved more into the area of rehabilitation engineering, as well as administration (e.g., Biomedical Engineering Departmental Chair at several institutions), but on occasion, I have had the pleasure of running into Dr. Woo – now Savio – at various meetings. One of the first of these meetings was right after his move from UCSD to the University of Pittsburgh, and I was taken away by the type of offer that Pittsburgh made to attract him away from UCSD. I knew then that he had achieved the level of pioneer and leader in his chosen field. I have also heard him give several keynote addresses, and at one of them, he presented a slide that included data from my research back in 1979, under his guidance. It brought back nice memories. I, like so many, have benefited from his mentorship, and wish to thank him for the opportunity to work for him, and with him.

ONE OF A KIND

Erin McGurk and Ron Dieck

PneumRx
Mountain View, California, 94043, U.S.A.
E-mail: erin@pneumrx.com
Magic Venture Capital
Palo Alto, California, 94301, U.S.A.
E-mail ron@magicvc.com

We want to wish you the best on your 70th birthday. We share so many happy memories and meaningful moments in our lives that we are sad that we cannot be with you in person to celebrate. However, we send our most sincere wishes for a wonderful celebration, continued by many more of the same. Savio, you are a man of great style and substance who has positively impacted more lives than you probably realize… including ours. We raise a glass to your 70 wonderful years and wish you many more – all joyful and surrounded by family and friends you are truly one of a kind. We deeply appreciate your friendship!!

"Oh to be 70 again!" – Oliver Wendell Holmes, Jr. (upon the occasion of his passing a pretty girl on the street… at the age of about 85 ☺)

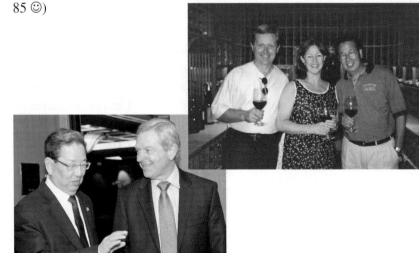

TRIBUTE TO DR. WOO

Robert A. Hart

Oregon Health & Science University
Portland, Oregon, 97201, U.S.A.
E-mail: hartro@ohsu.edu

It is an honor and a pleasure to contribute to this book commemorating Dr. Woo's contributions to the field of orthopaedic biomechanics as well as to the numerous students and residents whose lives he has touched over the years. I consider myself extremely fortunate to have had the opportunity to work with Dr. Woo as a medical student in San Diego from 1988-1991. Dr. Woo not only displayed a consummate mastery of the principles and techniques of biomechanical soft tissue analysis, he was an incredibly patient and balanced mentor to everyone around him.

Speaking strictly with respect to my own personal interactions with Dr. Woo, I can say that despite my relative lack of value to his research enterprise as a medical student, he never displayed any hesitation in making himself available to my questions or requests for advice. 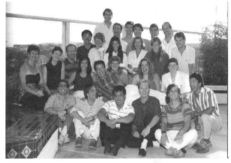 He was always warm and supportive in all interactions during that time, and indeed in subsequent years with respect to assistance in developing my own academic career.

While Dr. Woo's scientific contributions are without peer and need no introduction, it is his relationship with his students at all levels and his commitment to developing the careers of those around him that truly singles him out as not just a great scientist, but also a great man. I know from prior interactions with him that he indeed values these aspects of his own career above all others. With sincere appreciation and warm regards to both Dr. Woo & his family!

BIRTHDAY WISHES FOR DR. WOO

Caroline Wang

University of California, San Diego (M.S. 1989)
Menlo Park, California, 94025, U.S.A.
E-mail: carolinewang@alum.mit.edu

Although many years have passed since I graduated from UCSD, I have many fond memories of that time, and I thank you, Dr. Woo, for being such an influential part of that experience.

In your lab, we each worked hard, and we were rewarded with the knowledge that we had done our very best. But, we also worked together as a group and took time to have fun together. It was a dynamic and exciting place to be. I am proud and feel grateful to have been a part of that "family", to which your real family was always so warm and welcoming.

For your birthday, I wish you more of that same kind of experience: the rewarding feeling that comes with hard work, the joy of working with interesting people, and the time to have fun with your family. Happy Birthday, Dr. Woo!

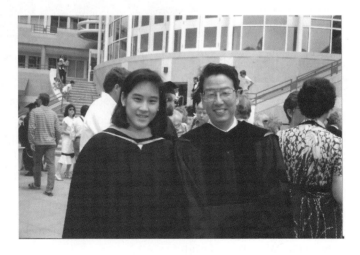

HAU`OLI LĀ HĀNAU TO DR. WOO!
WISHING YOU ALL THE BEST FOR MANY MORE WONDERFUL YEARS TO COME

Linda Kitabayashi

University of California, San Diego (1985-1995)
Kapaa, Kauai, Hawaii, 96746, U.S.A.
E-mail: LRK@hawaii.rr.com

It was a pleasure working for you as your Histologist at UCSD in the Department of Orthopaedics. I recall you telling me that it was very important for me to attend the Orthopaedic Research Society Annual Meeting to see how well-respected UCSD was. I was impressed and saw that the Department of Orthopaedics at UCSD was one of the top programs in the nation, if not the world. So, I knew that I had to do my job well to make it even better.

Hence, I worked hard to compliment Biomechanics/ Bioengineering, Biochemistry & Physiology. I believe we were the first to document the morphological difference between the MCL and ACL cells. We performed routine histology, transmission and scanning electron microscopy to show the differences. I was very pleased to be able to be at the cutting edge and also to enhance your research. I thank you for also choosing one of my MCL transmission electron micrographs as a cover for one of your publications. I will forever be grateful for that.

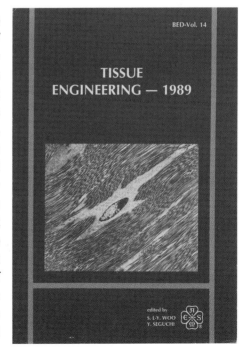

You have always been a calm & gracious person, always handling adversity with dignity and grace. As the younger generation would say: "You one cool dude!"

One regret I have is that I did not get to really know your wonderful wife, Pattie, as well as I would have liked. She, too, is such an elegant person. But, I am glad that we still continue to greet each other once a year during the holidays. You have such a wonderful family, and now with two grandchildren, life will be even more joyful.

So, here's wishing you many more birthdays.

A Hui Hou,
Linda

THANKS DR. WOO
FROM A MENTEE AT UCSD IN THE MID-1980s

David Hawkins

University of California, Davis
Davis, California, 95616, U.S.A.
E-mail: dahawkins@ucdavis.edu

Thank you, Dr. Woo for my start into the world of musculoskeletal biomechanics. Thank you for allowing me the opportunity to conduct my M.S. degree research in your lab during the mid-1980s and for all your mentoring during and after my M.S. degree. The mid-1980s were a productive time a UCSD. I thoroughly enjoyed the people working in your lab. They were all great colleagues. I learned a great deal studying rabbit MCLs and helping with a variety of other projects. I found the lab meetings stressful, but over the years I have appreciated the critical thinking skills that I developed during those meetings as I prepared my own presentations and listened to others present their project reports. I imagine you have influenced many young scientists, helping them to navigate the scientific method and hone their research skills. I wish you all the best. Happy 70th Birthday!

A SINCERE THANK YOU FROM ONE OF YOUR STUDENTS

Jeff Weiss

University of Utah
Salt Lake City, Utah, 84112, U.S.A.
E-mail: jeff.weiss@utah.edu

I met Dr. Woo during my sophomore year while I was an undergraduate in the Bioengineering Program at UC San Diego. I was looking for an opportunity to obtain some research experience as a volunteer. I continued to work in his laboratory as an undergraduate, and then subsequently as a Master's student in Bioengineering, from 1986 to 1990.

Dr. Woo had a profound influence on the direction of my career. I decided to pursue a M.S. and ultimately a Ph.D. based on my experiences in his laboratory and with him as a mentor. I will always be in debt to him for his tutelage and guidance.

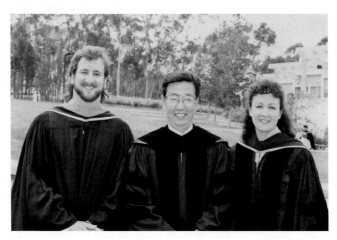

Congratulations, Dr. Woo on the occasion of your 70th birthday! I wish you the best for the future and I look forward to the next time that I will see you.

CONGRATULATIONS AND THANK YOU!

Edmond (Ned) Young

Kaiser Permanente
San Diego, California, 92020, U.S.A.
E-mail: Edmond.p.young@kp.org

Dr Woo,

It is remarkable and wonderful to realize that you are celebrating your 70th birthday when I can remember so clearly how young everyone seemed when I first met you in San Diego. There I was plugging away in bioengineering, trying to make sense of the subtleties and idiosyncrasies of capillary flow and rouleaux formation when along comes a guy named Savio Woo, giving a lecture about steel plates and bones and pulling things until they break. Now that was something I could relate too! Next thing I know, I am working in your lab, and I am hooked, not just on biomechanics, but also on the entire field of orthopaedic surgery.

I can honestly say that the time spent working in your lab, with amazing people like Thay Lee, Mark Gomez and Peter Newton, was one of the most formative and rewarding--not to mention enjoyable-- experiences of my professional career.

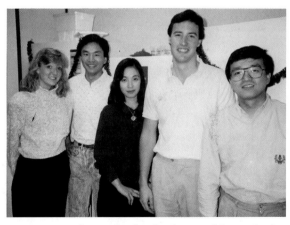

You have been a mentor to me from the beginning and have had a lasting impact, both professionally and personally. I wish you and your family the happiest of celebrations, and the enjoyment of so many years of life well-lived and so many yet to come.

THANK YOU!

Roger Lyon

Medical College of Wisconsin
Milwaukee, Wisconsin, 53201 U.S.A.
E-mail: rlyon@chw.org

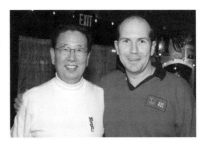

I worked with Dr. Woo from July 1986 to July 1988 as an orthopaedic surgery resident at the University of California, San Diego. I really enjoyed my time with Dr. Woo, his lab and his family. Contemporary of Mark Gomez, Jennifer Wayne, Marcus Hollis, Thay Lee, Karen Ohland, Jim Marcin, and Jeff Weiss, I made a lot of good friends and learned how good research should be done and presented. I want to personally thank Dr. Woo and Pattie, and the entire Woo family for making Rachel and I feel welcomed in the lab and in their home. It was a very special time for us. We are both extremely grateful to Dr. Woo.

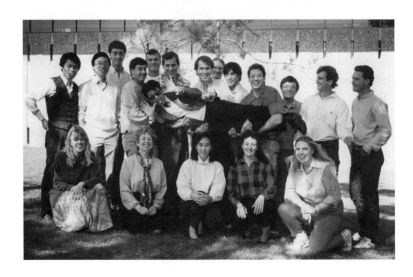

Chapter 3

Tributes

from

Students, Residents and Fellows

Affiliated With Both

the Orthopaedic Bioengineering Laboratory
Departments of Orthopaedics and Bioengineering
University of California, San Diego
and
the Musculoskeletal Research Center
Departments of Orthopaedic Surgery and
Bioengineering
University of Pittsburgh

"LIFE IS A JOURNEY, NOT A DESTINATION"
Ralph Waldo Emerson

Karen Ohland

The Metropolitan Museum of Art
Lyndhurst, New Jersey, 07071, U.S.A.
E-mail: ohlandk@asme.org

I was preparing to graduate from the University of Chicago with my M.S. in Anatomy and considering where I might begin my career journey. Dr. Jack Lewis recommended I contact Dr. Woo (then in San Diego) and see if there were any openings in his laboratory. My letter and resume arrived as Dr. Woo was searching for a laboratory manager. I flew out and interviewed and was thrilled when I was offered the position.

My journey working with Dr. Woo started in July of 1986 in the multiple laboratories in San Diego, CA – at the San Diego VA Medical Center, University of California, San Diego and the Malcolm & Dorothy Coutts Institute – where Dr. Woo's many research projects took place. So many wonderful memories – working with the graduate students, undergraduate students, residents, fellows and staff who joined the labs, excited to participate in the diverse research projects Dr. Woo oversaw.

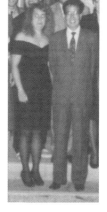

The journey continued as Dr. Woo accepted the position of Vice Chairman for Research in the Department of Orthopaedic Surgery at the University of Pittsburgh. I have many memories of the move to Pittsburgh – his confidence in his team to handle the transition of his research, including the associated equipment and paperwork; his persuading Lynnette Fleck and Jennifer Wayne to take up residence in Pittsburgh while they helped unpack many boxes in the laboratories in the Biomedical Science Tower. The next step in the journey involved recruiting faculty, staff and students - all wonderful choices by Dr. Woo to continue and expand his vision for orthopaedic research.

Dr. Woo provided me with the opportunity to make my first presentation at a meeting of the American Society of Mechanical Engineers (ASME); I remain involved with ASME, currently serving as an officer, and I still recall how Dr. Woo stressed the importance of preparing to present and of helping others prepare to present.

While my career journey has taken me many places since I started in San Diego, Dr. Woo has continued to be important to me. I was fortunate enough to be able to arrange my schedule to attend the celebration of his 60th birthday in Pittsburgh, and other special occasions including some of the International Symposia on Ligaments & Tendons.

I have always been impressed by Dr. Woo's ability to bring together so many wonderful people from all over the world, to inspire them to conduct high quality research, to prepare them to present and publish the results of the research, to continue to contribute to the field whether they were working in one of his laboratories or elsewhere, and build ongoing relationships with each other as well as himself. Dr. Woo supported the creation of the Orthopaedic Research Laboratory Alumni Council (ORLAC) and encouraged a spirit of camaraderie among those who worked in his laboratories; I treasure those friendships to this day.

Dr. Woo – Congratulations on your 70th birthday and on your achievements to date. I wish you additional successes as you continue on your journey.

WARM WORDS OF ENCOURAGEMENT

Hiromichi Fujie

Tokyo Metropolitan University
Tokyo, 191-0065, Japan
E-mail: fujie@sd.tmu.ac.jp

Mayo and I would like to send warm greetings on the 70th anniversary of Professor Woo's birth. Congratulations, Professor Woo and Mrs. Woo!

I joined Professor Woo's laboratory in San Diego in 1990, just before the First World Congress of Biomechanics held at UCSD. After spending 2 months in the laboratory in San Diego, we moved to Pittsburgh for another two years. Although many people joined or are currently working in his laboratory, I am one of the only 5 people who experienced his laboratories in both San Diego and Pittsburgh. The five people include, of course, Professor Woo, Karen Ohland, myself, Masahiko Noguchi, and Glen Livesay. I sometimes talk with my wife, Mayo, about how our 2-year experience in Professor Woo's laboratories was the best period in our lives. We have many good memories. Some of them are:

We had a son, Yuki, in Pittsburgh under the warm support by Professor and Mrs. Woo. Since Yuki spent 1 year in Pittsburgh and another year in Australia, his English is much better than ours.

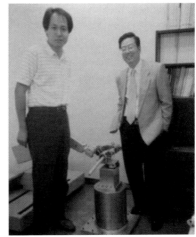

Professor Woo gave me a chance to work in the Robot/ACL research project when the project had just started. I really enjoyed the research on kinematic and kinetic analysis of the knee joint, and overall design of a robotic system for joint biomechanics study. The attached picture indicates Professor Woo and myself with the first robotic system developed by us (JBME 1993).

I worked so hard with Glen, one of my best friends, from early morning to late at night almost every day. When we experienced hard times in research, Professor Woo gave us warm words of encouragement. The following images are his hand-written notes given to me after I went back to Japan. They motivated me to meet the challenges in order to move to the next step.

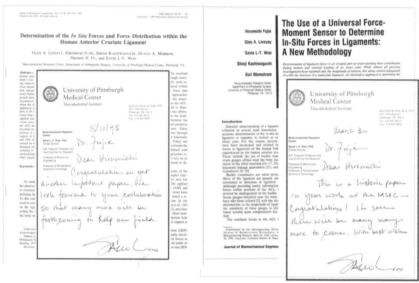

One of my dreams is to join Professor Woo's laboratory again. Mayo and I really want to come back to Pittsburgh where we have spent many wonderful days!

Professor Woo, please continue to guide us, because we would like to learn more and we certainly have more to learn from you.

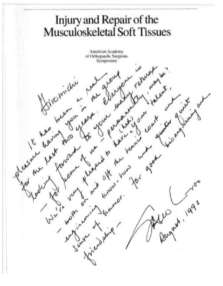

THE PAST ISN'T DEAD. IN FACT, IT'S NOT EVEN THE PAST. - WILLIAM FAULKNER

Glen Livesay

Rose-Hulman Institute of Technology
Terre Haute, Indiana, 47803, U.S.A.
E-mail: livesay@rose-hulman.edu

Dear Dr. Woo,

Greetings from the Midwest, and I hope you and Mrs. Woo are well! These remarks come from a lucky student of yours, who worked with you both in San Diego and then in Pittsburgh.

I would like to begin my congratulatory (and very thankful) remarks by noting a specific date – February 13, 1990. This was the day I scheduled a meeting with you (via Lynnette!) to say, "If you go to Pittsburgh, and you give me the opportunity to join you, I will go." Everyone came back from ORS 1990 with a rumor about you moving. And when you announced the possibility in Monday meeting, I made a decision. I never make snap judgments, but that day I did. I have never made a more important decision in my entire life.

Regarding the quote, while this may be a memory-driven tribute, you are never far from my thoughts, or my everyday life. You are right here, in my heart, in my teachings, and in the advice and support I give to young researchers I work with, everyday.

I have included two photos . . . one from a Summer party at your home (1997, I think) and one from the present (October 2011). I still wear MSRC tie-dye, and some of my best friends are from my lab days that I met because of you (like Fujie, *etc*.). As to being a part of my everyday life, the second photo is a great example. Fujie invited us to give a talk to young JSME researchers, and on this evening I met two former students of Professor Seguchi's and they were thrilled to learn that I was your student . . . they remember your time in Japan well.

Best wishes on this important birthday! And thank you for everything. As always, your student. Glen

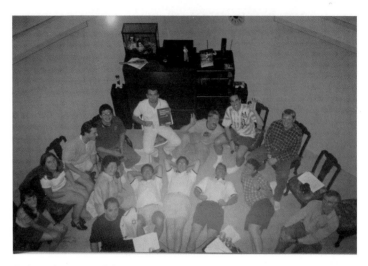

Fig. 1: A photo from one of the MSRC Summer parties at your home . . . and we host the annual, departmental party for students (a tie-dye party) at our home every Spring!

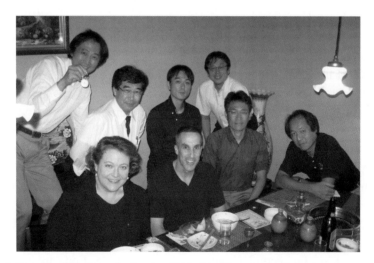

Fig. 2: Kay C and I in Japan in October 2011. You'll recognize Fujie, but you may also recognize Tanaka 先生 (2L in back, received 1st Seguchi Prize), and Wada 先生 (4L in back); both were Professor Seguchi's students and both work at Osaka University.

MY FRIEND, MY TEACHER
THANK YOU FOR THE "OPPORTUNITY"

John Xerogeanes

Emory Orthopaedics and Spine Center
Atlanta, Georgia, 30342, U.S.A.
E-mail: johnwx65@hotmail.com

Now that I am a father and a teacher, I find myself telling my kids and students that success is obtained by maximizing ones opportunities. Obviously that takes both hard work and perseverance, but luck or good fortune also plays a vital role. My story is simple. Through an introduction from a college friend in medical school I met Dr. Richard Riggins (this is the luck part). I told him I wanted to do research on the ACL. He said the top laboratory in the world was Dr. Woo's in San Diego. I wrote you and you offered me a summer internship in your lab (this is the opportunity part). The rest of my story is no different than any of my laboratory colleagues. We followed you to Pittsburgh where through your leadership and guidance, the MSRC was created. This was a truly special place where a pervasive culture of hard work, perfection and success was infused in each of us!

I spent the last week visiting with my close friend and research collaborator, Yasuyuki Ishibashi. While drinking wine on my back patio, we discussed your 70th birthday and our MSRC experience. Our thoughts follow.

A mentor is ultimately judged by the success of his students. It is truly a humbling experience to see that EVERY person with whom we shared our MSRC experience, has been very successful in their chosen field.

Thus, in my mind a picture of the MSRC team from 1994 validates your exemplary career more than any number of publications or NIH grants!

Thank you my friend, my teacher, for giving me an "opportunity" that truly changed my life's course!

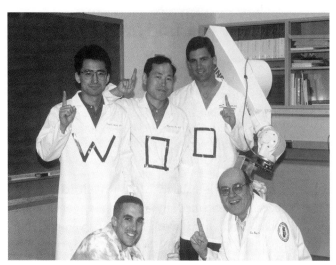

With (back row) Drs. Ishibashi and Kim,
(front row) Dr. Livesay and Mr. Ted Rudy (1994)

WARMTH

Meena Joshi
Vancouver, British Columbia, V6M2T8, Canada
E-mail: meenajoshi@mac.com

As an undergraduate student at the University of California, San Diego (UCSD), I worked in Dr. Woo's Orthopaedic Biomechanics Laboratory in 1989. Upon graduating from UCSD, I followed Dr. Woo to the University of Pittsburgh where Dr. Woo took me on as one of his Master's students at the Musculoskeletal Research Center (MSRC). Dr. Woo was my advisor until I completed my M.S. in Bioengineering in 1994.

There are many stories that come to mind when I think of my association with Dr. Woo. He was always intellectually inspiring, and encouraging of academic achievements. However, what I remember most is his warmth and kindness throughout my years with him. Dr. and Mrs. Woo hosted a lab party at their home in San Diego. All of the students and staff were invited to share a meal with the Woos. Being a student far from home, I was particularly overwhelmed by the welcoming nature of the Woos. I had a conversation with Dr. Woo similar to one I would have with my own father. Outside on the patio, I remember talking and laughing with Jonathan and Kirstin, who were young children then. It was a special night where Dr. Woo's hospitality allowed me to feel that I was truly part of another family -- the lab.

Dr. and Mrs. Woo attended my wedding in Sacramento 18 years ago. They traveled across the country and endured the tremendous heat of that day in order to be part of something that was of great personal importance to me. Dr. Savio Woo was never just my advisor.

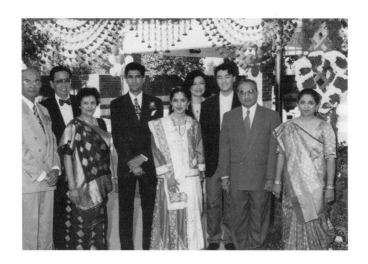

Happy 70th Birthday, Dr. Woo! You have achieved a tremendous amount in your lifetime already. Thank you for your guidance and faith in me all those years ago. I continue to follow your career with admiration and pride. I am wishing you warm, hearty congratulations with the hope that we will meet again soon.

Chapter 4

Tributes

from

Students, Residents and Fellows

Affiliated With

the Musculoskeletal Research Center
Departments of Orthopaedic Surgery and
Bioengineering
University of Pittsburgh

MY CAREER IN ORTHOPEDIC RESEARCH AND DR. SAVIO WOO

Patrick J. McMahon

McMahon Orthopedics & Rehabilitation
Pittsburgh, Pennsylvania, 15203, U.S.A.
E-mail: mcmahonp@upmc.edu

I first met Dr. Savio Woo in 1991 as a resident in orthopedic surgery at the University of Pittsburgh. But, the story behind that meeting goes back 3 years prior. I was accepted into the 8 person residency program as one of two individual for a 6 year stint that included a year of research. While doing my internship at New York University, I got a phone call from Dr. Ed Hanley, who was the interim chairman at that time. He surprised me in saying that one of the other 6 residents was having difficulties that prevented him from continuing with clinical work and would I be willing to give up my research year? I agreed to do so somewhat happily as it meant I could finish up my residency a year earlier. Two years later, Dr. James Herndon, who became the chairman of the department in early 1988, began speaking of his efforts to recruit the premier researcher in orthopedic biomechanics from the University of California, San Diego. I had already read some of Dr. Woo's research work, but as I read more, I began to regret having given up my research year. So early in 1990, I asked Dr. Herndon to restore my research year. He let me know that this was not possible since I was already 2 ½ years into my residency. Disappointed, I left his office thinking I had missed my opportunity to learn research from Dr. Woo. A few months later, I was called to Dr. Herndon's office and with a big smile, he let me know that he had arranged for me to begin a year of orthopedic research with Dr. Woo in July of 1991. I happily accepted.

I will not forget my impressions from those first few days working in Dr. Woo's lab. It was bustling with activity and people. Faculty members from the department were clamoring to work with him. There were great research projects from all of the orthopedic disciplines and there were engineers and orthopedic surgeons from all over the world including Japan, Germany and Korea. Dr. Woo, who had been in Pittsburgh for only a few months, was still setting up his lab, but managed it all, seemingly without effort and with great pleasure. Best of all was what I learned. Dr. Woo teamed me with an engineer and we dove into shoulder biomechanics research. Dr. Woo offered me to collaborate with him on the writing of a book chapter and over the next few months patiently taught me how to write a research manuscript, revising it again and again, more than twenty times until it was right. At the Monday morning meeting when it was my turn to present my proposed research project, he carefully suggested improvements. But more importantly, he gave me suggestions to improve my presentation style. He also taught me the proper way to evaluate journal articles. He took me to the Orthopaedic Research Society meeting for the first time. I sat next to him during the podium presentations and walked though the posters with him, learning how to present research findings. He introduced me to many of his associates, who, like Dr. Woo, were leading the way in musculoskeletal research. The learning was intense!

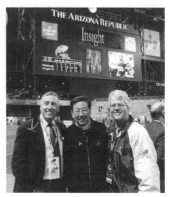

With Drs. Stone and Woo at the Insight Bowl

Other professors had said their office door was "always open", but with Dr. Woo, it was true. We spent hours in his office talking not only about my research, but he also wanted to know about me, my family, and aspirations. He took the lab --20 people, sometimes more-- out to lunch regularly. He expected only the best from me and let me know he really believed I could deliver. By the end of the year, the direction of my professional life had change. I would now read professional journals with a critical eye. And, more than 20 years later, I am still doing orthopedic research. Thank you Dr. Woo for sharing your expertise, advice, and insights!

DR. WOO, MY TEACHER AND MENTOR

Chih-Hwa Chen

Chang Gung Memorial Hospital - Keelung
Chang Gung University
Keelung, Taiwan
E-mail: afachen@doctor.com

Over the years, Dr. Woo has been my most respected teacher. My heart is full of gratitude and appreciation.

I met Professor Woo in 1995. At that time I was just a junior doctor from Taiwan Chang Gung Memorial Hospital pursuing clinical learning and research studies in orthopedics at the University of Pittsburgh. It has been 16 years since we started our teacher-student friendship.

Professor Woo is my first teacher of orthopedic research. Due to my interest in orthopedic basic research as I served as a clinical fellow at UPMC of the University of Pittsburgh, I was also participating in the MSRC as a research fellow in a biomechanical research program.

At the MSRC, I learned the concept of developing an orthopedic research program, the skill in planning and setting up a research organization, creating research ethics, writing research projects, and establishment of a research team and laboratory. These experiences were very precious and helpful when establishing my own research team and laboratory at Chang Gung Memorial Hospital. With Dr. Woo's encouragement and stimulation, I have been able to keep my enthusiasm and interest in orthopedics sports medicine until now. Dr. Woo is not only my academic supporter, he also encouraged me to participate in international organizations related to the orthopedic and sports medicine fields. I got the chance to learn and practice, from an international perspective, the latest trend and development of orthopedic sports medicine.

By participating in worldwide international conferences, I often have the opportunity to meet Dr. Woo. During the conferences, he always tries his best to find time to assemble together everyone in the group who were MSRC faculties and fellows. It is thanks to him that we, as international fellows from the MSRC, are able to maintain very good relationships.

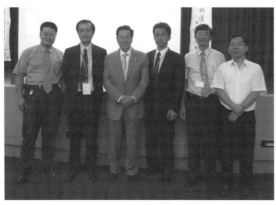

Although residing in the United States, Dr. Woo is currently serving as a member of Academia Sinica and the National Health Research Institutes in Taiwan. We have the chance to get together every year when he visits Taiwan. Dr. Woo always gives me lots of inspiration from his professionalism. What I admire most is his attitude towards research. Dr. Woo always brings out innovative ideas that apply well to clinical practice. His relentlessness motivates me to continuously search for excellence in the sports medicine field. He is my role model, my mentor, and my supporter forever. Although Dr. Woo has such great achievements, he and Pattie are very kind and warm.

Dear Dr. Woo, I would like to express my sincere appreciation and wish you all the best!

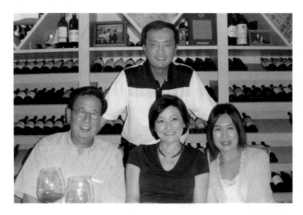

WOO-DAPEST, WOO-ASHINGTON DC

Christos D. Papageorgiou

Consultant in Orthopaedics
Ioannina, 45500, Greece
E-mail: chpapage@cc.uoi.gr

May 12th, 1996

After a preparation of two months, I was finally presenting my paper in English for the first time, at the conference of ESSKA for the carpal tunnel release. At the end, I asked my friend and colleague Haris how was the presentation. "You did 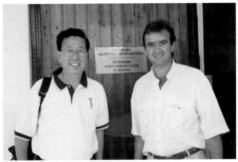 great," he responded. "You gave exact and scientific answers to the questions of the audience," he added. "I think the subject was very interesting," I said with a lot of confidence. "People kept coming during my presentation and the conference hall was full at the end of it." "Christos," Haris said with a smile on his face, "the hall was not full because of your presentation. The hall was full because everyone is expecting to see Dr. Savio L-Y. Woo, an invited lecturer at the conference." Seriously, I had no idea who Dr. Woo was at the time. Haris smiled once again and told me, "Are you serious my friend? You are not aware of the greatest biomechanic on sports' injuries alive?" After the lecture, I was totally stunned! I realized exactly why this person was considered as one of the most important scientists in the field of biomechanics.

At the end of the conference, we had a great discussion and we ended up inviting Dr. Woo to visit Greece and take part in a conference we were preparing at the time. I realized at once the quality of Dr. Woo as a scientist and also as an individual. I realized this even further during my two year fellowship at the MSRC and when I received the Albert Trillat Young Investigator's Award at ISAKOS in Washington, DC. Six months earlier, when I submitted my paper for the award, teacher Woo called me into his office and told me, "Christos, you have to know that when we submit our papers we do it only for the first placed!"

My Teacher, I would like to thank you for literally changing my life. You have taught me so many things that you made me "dangerous" for my own country.

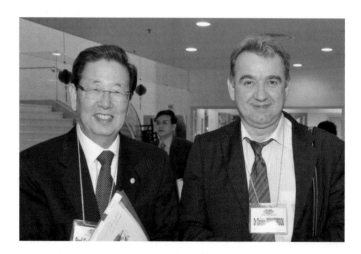

20+ YEARS AND COUNTING

Diann DeCenzo

University of Pittsburgh
Pittsburgh, Pennsylvania, 15219, U.S.A.
E-mail: ddecenzo@pitt.edu

I first met Dr. Woo when I interviewed for and subsequently received an accounting assistant position at the Musculoskeletal Research Center (MSRC) in 1991. After I had been working for Dr. Woo about 3 years, he called me to his office one day and asked me to be his executive assistant. I was both surprised and terrified. I was an accountant not a secretary. But Dr. Woo had faith in me, so I accepted the position and it turned out to be one of the best decisions I have ever made. It was a learning process, but even though it was not engineering, Dr. Woo was an excellent teacher. We developed such a good working relationship that we would always tease that I was his right hand and he was my left.

In 1997, Dr. Woo received the IOC Olympic Prize for Sports Science. He and Mrs. Woo generously donated the prize money to establish the Asian♦American Institute for Research & Education (ASIAM) to support the research and education of students and fellows. I received the honor of being appointed as Treasurer of this very important 501(c)(3) non-profit organization – this is a position which I still hold today.

Some of my fondest memories are of our occasional afternoon chats, where we have discussed a wide range of things, including the MSRC, our children, the economy, politics, or just life in general. No matter which subject, Dr. Woo provides much knowledge and wisdom.

Dr. Woo and Mrs. Woo are truly like family to me! We have shared many happy occasions together over the years, whether it was 4th of July picnics, Christmas Eve celebrations, and Dr. Woo's favorite, the Heritage Dinners. Each time they have been at my home they have made lasting impressions on my family and friends. And even though they have actually dined with royalty - the Princess of Thailand and

Presidents of Taiwan - they always treat people as if they are royalty. They are such gracious and fun people to be around.

Dr. Woo, I wish you a very Happy 70th Birthday and I look forward to many more afternoon chats, celebrations and picnics.

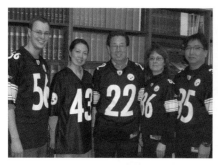

ISL&T-IX Planning Committee (2009)

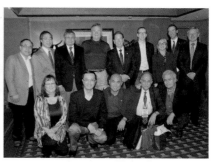

ASIAM Institute Board of Directors (2012)

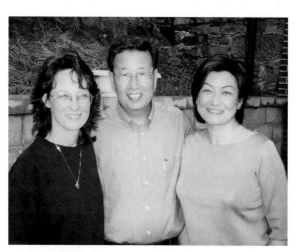

4th of July picnic at my home (2001)

TO DR. WOO, AN EXEMPLARY ENGINEER, THINKER AND TEACHER

Jorge E. Gil

ANSYS, Inc
Montigny-le-Bretonneux, 78180, France
E-mail: jorge.gil@ansys.com

I met Dr. Woo as a young undergraduate student in early 1995 and that encounter remains one of the most influential of my career. I had the unusual background of having attended medical school at the Central University of Venezuela (right after finishing high school!) and, when the MSRC took on the project of starting a full time undergraduate internship, I became one of the first to be selected. I was lucky for two reasons. The first was that most other internship recruiters were overlooking students in my relatively obscure academic program of Engineering Physics. The most important, though, was that I thus had the privilege of working with Dr. Woo.

Dr. Woo helped me at an especially critical junction in my career. Just before meeting him I was rounding out a troubled year that began to impact my studies at the University. He chose me as a student because he recognized that his guidance and the atmosphere of scholarship and excellence that he fostered at the MSRC could help me. I remain profoundly grateful that he did. In this environment I gained purpose as a student and was able to enjoy success and encouragement to carry me into my profession. Just the same, my peers at the time could point to this formative influence as a cornerstone in their careers. We, his students, remain examples of the power of education to enlighten and transform.

Dr. Woo taught me many important lessons. I want to recall two. The first was the importance of formulating specific questions and of distinguishing the better ones from the rest. I learned to see a question as an instrument and demonstration of thought and that, ultimately, the best are selfless generators of new knowledge. The second lesson may seem surprising but remains nevertheless important to me: I signed up to be an engineering student as an undergraduate without really knowing what engineers did! 'Engineering', in English, evokes engines. In Spanish, 'Ingeniero' evokes ingenuity. Thus, I had a rough sense of the subject: to work on ingenious engines! Dr. Woo taught me that the profession had these implications, of course, but also more significant dimensions. Engineers can help improve an engine, just as they can help doctors provide better care for their patients, or help public administrators deliver better services for their people. Our skills in critical and quantitative thinking, in asking excellent questions, are essential in producing goods for the national economy, in assuring safety for the public, or in steering the national debate. Engineers also have a wealth of social capital to share with their communities, as educators, parents and leaders. Thus, I am proud to be an engineer.

I thank Dr. Woo for these lessons and for being an exemplary engineer, thinker and teacher. I remain his student and friend. I thank him for his generosity and dedication to his students, that of his family and his colleagues at the MSRC, which I have been fortunate to partake. I congratulate Dr. Woo for a lifetime of accomplishment and wish him a wonderful 70th birthday.

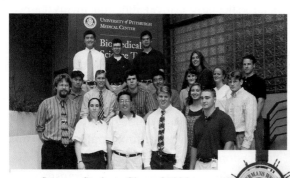

Summer Students Class of 1997

With Jen (Zeminski) Kanamori and
Dr. Woo in San Francisco (2000)

AN OPPORTUNITY FOR A YOUNG STUDENT, AN APPRECIATION FROM A LESS-YOUNG STUDENT

Duane Morrow

Mayo Clinic
Rochester, Minnesota, 55906, U.S.A.
E-mail: morrow.duane@mayo.edu

My relationship with Dr. Woo started over a year before I met him when I was still a senior at Penn-Trafford High School, 20 miles east of the University of Pittsburgh. In that time, I was trying to figure out what I would like to study and where I would like to study it when I went to college the following year. That was when I read an article in the paper about a biomechanical engineer who came to Pitt from the University of California at San Diego. When I finished the article, I knew what I would do, where I would do it, and with whom.

At the end of my freshman year at Pitt, as a recently declared Mechanical Engineering major, I saw an advertisement posted seeking students to work in Dr. Woo's Musculoskeletal Research Center. There was just one hitch: the posting was looking for junior and senior level students. Well, I never was one to let a technicality as seemingly trivial as "qualifications" be an obstacle, so I took the opportunity to get an interview and see if I could get my foot in the door. After an interview, in which I could only hope to show that I had enthusiasm inversely proportional to my lack of educational experience, Dr. Woo decided to take me under his wing. I still vividly recall being told by him, "I like you; you know nothing, I will teach you everything!"

I spent nearly four years in the MSRC; changing my course schedule (and graduation date) realizing that I was getting so much more of an education from my time in the MSRC than I could ever hope to get through coursework alone. There was more, however, than just the rigors of the academic learning I was exposed to: Dr. Woo had put together a wonderful team of passionate students, fellows, and research collaborators that made the MSRC a vibrant breeding ground for thought and development that spoke to my desire to do the kind of work that they were doing. I went forward from there knowing that the kinds of biomechanical questions Dr. Woo was trying to answer using engineering analyses were the only kinds of problems I would be satisfied working on.

I am now working at the Mayo Clinic in Rochester, MN, 20 years after first reading about Dr. Woo's arrival at Pitt. While my path has been a circuitous one, and I am at this time finishing writing my dissertation (focusing, naturally, on musculoskeletal questions), in a sense I have been guided continually by Dr. Woo. I will be forever grateful for the opportunity he gave a young man who did not know better than to wait his turn. I have cultivated this and tried to pay it forward with the young students who now come to my laboratory, similarly young and ready to have a world of ideas presented to them.

Dr. and Mrs. Woo have been so kind to me over the years and it is a genuine pleasure when our paths cross. No matter what I achieve, they are there with friendly reminders of the times of my youth (and crushes on local television news anchors) that should never be allowed to slip too far away. Congratulations, Dr. Woo, on a full and lasting career. While you have deservedly been awarded all of the titles worth earning in orthopedic biomechanics, the family of researchers that you have cultivated equally shows your profound impact.

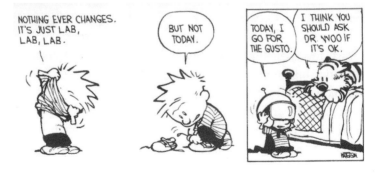

THANK YOU DR. WOO

Duy Tan Nguyen

Academic Medical Center
Amsterdam, The Netherlands
E-mail: nguyen2004@hotmail.com

Dear Dr. Woo,
In the spring of 2004, I was searching for a book at the medical library in Groningen. By chance, I came across a book that you wrote and I read it with great interest. Promptly, I wrote you a letter expressing my wish to come to the MSRC to learn more and to complete a thesis project. A week later, I was very glad to receive your warm and welcome email. This was my first encounter with your great generosity and hospitality. The MSRC was like a candy shop: too many interesting laboratories and too many interesting research projects. But most importantly, you have made the MSRC like a big family, consequently, help, guidance and laughter were always there. At the end of my research elective, you were very generous again by granting me a research fellowship for 2 years after my graduation from medical school. The fellowship and stay in Pittsburgh was a wonderful time and I still cherish those many moments. I have learned numerous lessons during my stay and it laid the foundation for my young research career. Describing those lessons would be too long for this tribute, however, two lessons I would like to share.

    The first lesson is obviously your great teachings. The wise saying: "Give a man a fish, and you feed him for a day. Teach a man to fish, and you feed him for life", would be very applicable. Though, you went even a step further: you also taught us how to craft our own fishing rod and fishing line, which, of course, had the proper biomechanical properties. Having the right fishing rod, you and other MSRCers taught me how to fish and to work seamlessly in a multidisciplinary team. For my current research projects, I also have made several collaborations. And recently, I also received a starting grant from the Annafonds | Netherlands Orthopedic Research and Education Fund Foundation.

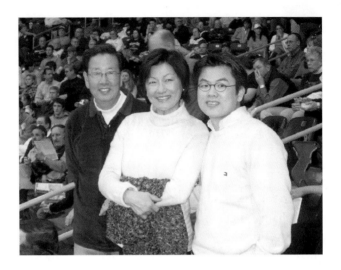

Another lesson that I learned is actually what you would least expect from your professor, namely: wooing. It is not exactly, what you teach us, but if one pays attention when Dr. Woo is around Mrs. Woo one will learn a great deal. For example, in 2007, we went to Florence for a conference. A very nice congress venue indeed, but also a very romantic one. During that meeting, Drs. Cerulli and Woo organized an ASIAM dinner at restaurant Da Il Latini for their friends & partners, the current MSRCers and the MSRC alumni. After the main course, three Italian musicians came into the room and they were playing music and singing. We all sang along and Dr. Woo was initiating a polonaise. At the end, he sang for Mrs. Woo! One could feel the love was in the air. Therefore, one can conclude: 1) Dr. Woo only needs two glasses of wine to be jolly and 2) Even decades after their marriage, Dr. Woo is still wooing Mrs. Woo.

Dear Dr. Woo, I feel very fortunate that I was your student and fellow and I am indebted for your teachings and the given opportunities to grow.

Happy 70th birthday!

A GREAT EDUCATOR IN THE FIELD OF BIOENGINEERING

Ryan Prantil

Weirton, West Virginia, 26062, U.S.A.
E-mail: rkp12@pitt.edu

I thank you, sir, for all of your kindness. I will never know how to repay you, but I will always be indebted to you for your expertise and guidance with regard to the advancement of my studies.

First of all, you have introduced me to the great field of bioengineering through your summer research program; you and your staff made every day a fruitful experience in research. Your guiding principles that I applied so early in my educational exodus remain valuable to this day. Furthermore, you have mentored my advisor who has, in turn, taught me throughout my graduate studies. Such an educational liaison has greatly benefited me. I also had the pleasure of working in your lab during the 2009-10 school years. Again, you provided me with ample opportunity to observe the inner-workings of your lab and included me as a contributing member. During these times, I enjoyed the opportunity to build relationships with you and your co-workers. Those esteemed relationships mean so much to me. And although, I cannot point to one specific memory, I do remember our individual meetings. I was always extremely nervous, but you could always recognize my temperament. And no matter how timid or nervous I may have appeared, you always made me feel at ease and more confident.

I have realized your help and inspiration as instrumental to my success in both my undergraduate and graduate endeavors. I have had the pleasure of meeting and getting to know you; and for that, I will always be thankful. Your strong work ethic and prolific list of accomplishments have made you a wonderful educator. Furthermore, you carry yourself with such humility and grace. Such characteristics make you an even more valuable and appreciated leader in education. Due to the goals of you and your MSRC colleagues, I have begun to realize the gravity of the principles of your lab's mission. Most of all, I thank you for everything you have done for me.

Finally, I consider myself very fortunate to have had the experience and the influence of such a great educator in the field of bioengineering.

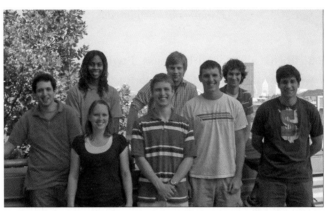

Summer Students Class of 2007

DR. WOO, A GREAT MAN I ALWAYS LOOK UP TO

Wei-Hsiu Hsu
*Chang Gung Memorial Hospital, Chia-Yi
Chia-Yi Hsien, 613, Taiwan
E-mail: 7572@cgmh.org.tw*

I first met Dr. Woo when I became an MSRC research fellow in January, 2003. Since I am from a subtropical region-Taiwan, Dr. Woo's warm 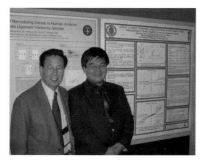 smile melted the greatest snows that I have ever seen in my life. In the following fifteen months I worked in the MSRC, I enjoyed the academic research on ligaments and tendons as well as harmonic friendship in the MSRC. In additional to the very important research training, Dr. Woo further inspired me in many ways.

Dr. Woo is always willing to guide me either in research or in life. For me, Dr. Woo is the greatest philosopher that I devote all my belief. Even though Dr. Woo has such great achievement in science and career, he is always very friendly to people. He taught me the importance of being humble that originated from humanism. By conquering drawbacks, Dr. Woo showed me leadership and courage. In devoting to science, he teaches me the insistence for truth and passion for discovery. He kindly shared his wisdom of life and eventually inspired many like me.

I am very lucky to be able to receive Dr. Woo's continuous education even after I left the MSRC in June 2004. Because of the Annual Meeting of Academia Sinica and National Health Research Institutes in Taiwan, Dr. Woo visits every year. He always squeezes his time for us, and gives his warm greetings to ensure everything was going well for his fellows.

Dear Dr. Woo, Thank you for your kindness in passing the pearls of philosophy to me. You are a lighthouse to me, encouraging me always to do the right thing. My sincere appreciation will last forever.

A GREAT SCIENTIST AND GLOBAL EDUCATOR

Rui Liang

Magee-Womens Research Institute
Pittsburgh, Pennsylvania, 15213, U.S.A.
E-mail: ruiliang07@gmail.com

Starting in the fall of 2003, I worked with Dr. Savio L-Y. Woo for almost seven years, at which time, he was already a famous scientist in the field of Bioengineering and Orthopaedics. In the beginning, I looked up to him as a glorious star far away on the unreachable horizon. However, the more I got to know him, especially during the last few years when I worked closely with him, the more I felt how real a role model he is. He took pains to teach me how to become a successful researcher - most importantly, how to do it correctly. He always said, "think more, ask more, and do more". This is actually educational for anyone who seeks to improve oneself, whatever their career.

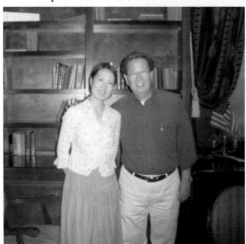

He has adopted western culture, yet remains committed to good Chinese tradition and philosophy. He wrote me a note of Chinese philosophy in fine Chinese calligraphy, which I hung over my desk where I could see it every day. It says: "Study broadly, investigate carefully, think discreetly, distinguish unambiguously, and do it practically". This is a philosophy that I will cherish all my life, and acts as a lighthouse to guide me whenever I am in the fog of puzzle.

Dr. Woo is a seeker of the truth and has always had enthusiasm to spread his knowledge around the world. He has been to many countries and has delivered countless lectures to surgeons and engineers, hoping that as many people as possible will benefit by what he has learned and investigated. What has impressed me the most is his consistent endeavor to help China - his home country - to advance in science and technology. He told me that education has always been his career goal.

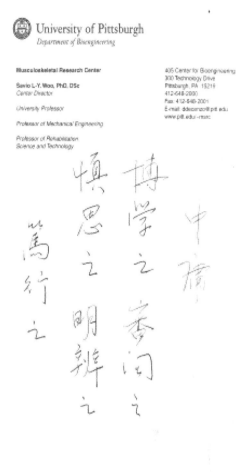

When he was not busy, he liked to have lunch with us in the library of the MSRC. He shares his stories with grace, humor, honesty and intelligence. I will always remember the period of time I spent in the MSRC and with Dr. Woo.

Happy 70th birthday!

LEADING ME INTO THE WONDERFUL RESEARCH WORLD

Yin-Chih Fu

Kaohsiung Medical University Hospital
Kaohsiung Medical University
Kaohsiung, Taiwan
E-mail: microfu@cc.kmu.edu.tw

Dr. Woo, my most respected teacher, led me into the wonderful field of research. My heart is still fulfilled with appreciation.

Before 2004, I was a faculty of the orthopaedic department without any research background. During that time, clinical work was my whole world. But, my life changed after I met Dr. Woo and after my research fellowship at the Musculoskeletal Research Center (MSRC) (2004-2005). Our last president of Kaohsiung Medical University, Dr. Guo-Jaw Wang, introduced me to Dr. Woo and wanted me to learn the research attitude from Dr. Woo. After one year of research training, I realized that without the basic research support, an orthopaedic doctor was just a high level technician without provision.

At the MSRC, Dr. Woo asked me to create a question that I wanted to know from my clinical work. After I raised a question, he did not tell me what the next step was. He wanted me to create my full proposal including how to establish the hypothesis, how to organize the research team, what were the research steps, and how to pursue the faculties permitted my project. That was a hard job for me without any basic research background before. But because of this first step, I learned the concept of developing orthopedic research, and the skill in planning and writing projects. That year experience changed my future. I also realized the real meaning of "from bench to bedside".

Dr. Woo gave me the opportunity to participate at the Orthopaedic Research Society meeting and opened my research vision in the orthopaedic field. By participating at the International Symposium on Ligaments and Tendons (ISL&T), I realized the beauty of research and it has inspired me a lot. Because of Dr. Woo's encouragement and stimulation, I keep my interest in orthopaedics research even now.

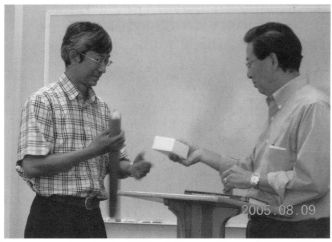

During my staying in the United States, Dr. and Mrs. Woo were so kind and warm that my family has a good memory of America. I remembered the day Dr. Woo invited me to see an American football game and taught me the rules of the game. I loved it!

After I came back to Taiwan, I really stepped into the research world. I still do research on bone scaffold. Although my projects are quite different from what I did at the MSRC, I knew how to plan the whole study. Also, the published research papers have given me the chance to be promoted to associate professor.

Dear Dr. Woo, I sincerely thank you for your teaching and inspiration and wish you all the best!

MENTORING TO PERFECTION: A TRIBUTE TO DR. SAVIO L-Y. WOO ON THE OCCASION OF HIS 70TH BIRTHDAY

Matthew Fisher

University of Pennsylvania
Philadelphia, Pennsylvania, 19104, U.S.A.
E-mail: fmatt@mail.med.upenn.edu

It is my honor to extend my warmest congratulations to Dr. Savio L-Y. Woo on his 70th birthday. I was lucky enough to join the Musculoskeletal Research Center (MSRC) in the summer of 2005 as a Ph.D. student, and graduated in 2010, making me Dr. Woo's tenth, and most recent, Ph.D. student.

Those five years were some of the most challenging of my life. Training under Dr. Woo is very demanding. I still remember the shock of friends in graduate school when discussing the rigors of working at the MSRC. All experiments must be performed correctly. All data must be explained. All presentations must be precise. In sum, all details must be thoughtfully considered.

In fact, one of the most gratifying things as a student was when Dr. Woo said that a paper was ready to be submitted after numerous revisions (sometimes six or seven drafts), since you are aware of how much work went into it. I suspect many scientists would have deemed the paper "publication-ready" many revisions before; however, Dr. Woo strives to make sure every sentence has purpose and clarity and is presented logically.

While having a small breakfast at a conference in Las Vegas, Dr. Woo revealed his mentoring style to me in simple terms. After discussing how I could improve upon my presentation from the previous day, he finished by stating that his goal was to make his students "perfect." Not average, not good, not even top tier, but perfect. Needless to say, this places an enormous pressure on the students, as this goal is not readily achievable, and yet, it is the standard.

However, when spending some time with Dr. Woo, one begins to understand why perfection is the standard. He demands perfection of himself. Even today, he works long, tiring days, and I have been amazed with the stamina and spirit he can still muster to remain highly productive. He is well-known for being a great presenter, and I can say this is only from the many hours of work he puts into them. Thus, in mentoring his students, he simply tries to pass this exquisite quality on to them.

Despite being a challenging environment, one major perk of working at the MSRC is that your co-workers really become a family. In fact, many of my closest friendships are a result of the MSRC. Additionally, you have the opportunity to spend time with Dr. Woo outside of the MSRC. Dr. Woo is an avid and knowledgeable sports fan, and I was lucky enough to watch many important Pitt football and basketball games with him. We also had many delicious meals together, and I am grateful to have had these opportunities.

In closing, Dr. Woo, thank you for forcing the best out of your students and congratulations on your 70th birthday! As I sit in amazement of your accomplishments in your first 70 years, I wish you many perfect years to come!

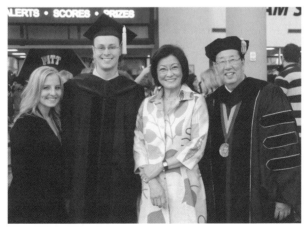

With Dr. and Mrs. Woo and my wife, Lisa (2010).
A perfect day for me.
(Photo courtesy of Mrs. Pattie Woo)

MY FOND MEMORIES OF DR. WOO - HIS MENTORSHIP, UNCANNY INSIGHTS, AND MY GOOD FORTUNE

Todd Doehring

Drexel University
Philadelphia, Pennsylvania, 19104, U.S.A.
E-mail: tcdoe@drexel.edu

I have so many fond memories of Dr. Woo and my 10 years working at the Musculoskeletal Research Center (MSRC) that I could probably write a short novel, but here I am very happy to share some highlights.

A long, long time ago, I was working in the ME department of the UPitt as a master's student, but I was not really very happy. I was working on a project to model bone-implant interfaces, and I was stuck. I did not really have enthusiasm for my project, and there was no 'bioengineering' department – thus, I did not have a community to encourage me. In fact, I was kind-of disillusioned and was thinking of 'giving up'.

Then, something happened that changed my life. I was told that a new faculty member had joined UPitt and was developing a bioengineering program! I had the opportunity to meet with this person (a certain Professor Savio L-Y. Woo), and I immediately became very excited. In just this first meeting, Dr. Woo showed me a whole new world of opportunities. I remember that I shared some of my ideas about my work (bone-implant interfaces) and immediately, Prof. Woo had some startlingly accurate insights for me. That meeting left me with a huge impression. For the first time, here was a person who understood. After applying, I was accepted as a member of his new team, and the MSRC. Thus began an incredible 10 years of work at the MSRC, my Ph.D. and great relationships with all my colleagues and advisors (Drs. Harry Rubash and Lars Gilbertson, in particular).

One of the greatest things that I learned from Dr. Woo is his amazing capability to ask questions (both during our lab meetings and conferences) that open up new ideas. I cannot really describe it. Often the question/comment would seem to come out of nowhere, but after two seconds of thinking about it, "wait... that's obvious now, that's a great question! Why didn't I think of that??" In this way, with each question, Dr. Woo has helped uncountable numbers of students and researchers with their work.

I wish I had more space to share some great stories, but here I will share one in particular. I am always amazed at Prof. Woo's talent for the 'mixed metaphor'. We were sitting at a big conference together, and the presenter was asked a pretty simple and somewhat critical question. The presenter proceeded with a 3 minute rambling answer... during that, Prof. Woo leaned over, nudged me and said, "You see, Todd... give him enough rope, and he'll dig his own grave." It was perfect.

Prof. Woo created an amazing environment at the MSRC: a place where people worked, played, learned, and lived together almost like a family. Sometimes he was tough, but most times sensitive and caring. He helped me through a lot of tough times with great advice, support, and motivation. He and Pattie invited us into their home, and made us feel at home. I am eternally grateful. So, this is congratulations to you Grandpa Woo, and to Pattie, Jon, and Kirstin, and everyone in your family. Also, my very best regards to all those from the MSRC... far too many friends to list here. It was my Good Fortune, thanks to Dr. Woo, to have been a part of the MSRC.

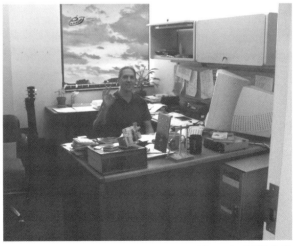

Thanks for everything Dr. Woo, and to all from the MSRC ☺

TEACHER, MENTOR AND GUIDE

Serena Chan Saw
Fuquay Varina, North Carolina, 27526, U.S.A.
E-mail: ssaw19@gmail.com

Dr. Woo has been my guide and role model throughout my career in bioengineering. From the time that I began as a summer student in 1992, until I moved from Pittsburgh in May 2005, I had the privilege of working and being mentored by Dr. Woo.

My first and last job interview came in the spring of 1992 when I interviewed to be a summer student at the MSRC between my junior and senior years at Carnegie Mellon University. From summer student, I moved on to being an undergraduate student during the school year, graduate student, research engineer, laboratory supervisor and finally part-time assistant (if there is such a title…). I have pretty much held any position that did not require an M.D. or Ph.D.

First, I want to express my appreciation to Dr. Woo, because he gave me a chance and accepted me as a graduate student when my grades may not have necessarily been the best of the bunch. Later on, Dr. Woo was also extremely supportive of allowing me to work part-time so that I could spend time with my children. Finally, I still have the privilege of helping Dr. Woo out remotely from North Carolina. Thank you, Dr. Woo.

I have many wonderful memories of my time at the MSRC in addition to the great research we were doing; eating lunch in the hallway, picnics at Schenley Park and the annual summer party at Dr. and Mrs. Woo's home. I spent so much time with fellow MSRC'ers it was like a second family. But, there is one story that sticks in my mind about Dr. Woo that demonstrates he is first and foremost, a teacher. Back when I was a graduate student, I was struggling in my classes and just could not quite get one of the concepts; it turns out I am a visual learner. Dr. Woo was able to explain the concepts (I think it was Bernoulli's principal) in such a way that I finally understood it.

Dr. Woo, I wish you a very happy 70th birthday. It is indeed a great achievement. As Dorothy Thompson, the "First Lady of American Journalism" once said, "Age is not measured by years. Nature does not equally distribute energy. Some people are born old and tired while others are going strong at seventy." Dr. Woo, you are most certainly still going strong as you continue to travel the world and share your knowledge with others. My best wishes to you and congratulations on all your accomplishments.

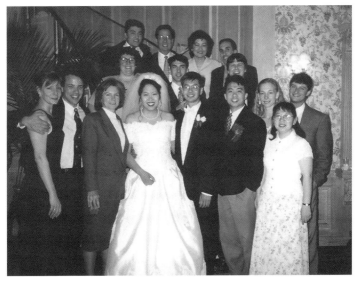

Dr. & Mrs. Woo and MSRC friends at my wedding to Kyi (1997)

AN INSPIRATION TO GENERATIONS OF ENGINEERS, SCIENTISTS, AND PHYSICIANS

Kristen L. Moffat

Columbia University
New York, New York, 10027, U.S.A.
E-mail: kristen.moffat@gmail.com

I first met Dr. Woo in 2002 as a summer student in the Musculoskeletal Research Center at the University of Pittsburgh. I had been pursuing a degree in Materials Engineering & Biomedical Engineering at Carnegie Mellon University and up until that time had only performed electronic materials research. Through the Pittsburgh Tissue Engineering Initiative Internship program I was able to secure a research position in the Summer Undergraduate Research Program at the MSRC and was ecstatic to be working at one of the world's preeminent bioengineering/ biomechanics research centers.

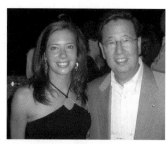

ASME Summer BioE Conference Awards Ceremony Vail, CO (2005)

My first day at the MSRC began with a morning meeting – the first for the new summer students – in which Steve Abramowitch, Dr. Woo's doctoral candidate and my student mentor at the time, was presenting his latest research on ligament mechanics and QLV theory. The meeting guest of honor was Dr. Van C. Mow. After introductions concluded, Steve launched into his research presentation – which was both elegant and inspiring, especially for an aspiring biomedical engineer. What an honor it was to have begun my biomedical research career in the presence of two legendary biomechanics gurus who have shaped the way we understand, design, and test orthopaedic tissues and procedures.

That summer in the MSRC truly changed my life and career. I gained such a strong appreciation and a love for the field of bioengineering. The MSRC was a functional unit of scientists, engineers, and physicians diligently working to understand and solve orthopaedic-related problems with a passion that was contagious. Dr. Woo understood that creating such a synergistic environment comprised of people with diverse backgrounds and research interests would lead to better orthopedic solutions. He also understood that it was important to share those experiences with undergraduate students, the next generation of researchers and medical professionals. Despite a busy summer schedule filled with ORS abstract submissions, guest lectures, and manuscript and grant preparation, he found time to attend each and every summer student's final research presentation and celebrate the work we had done.

From that point forward, I knew that pursuing a Ph.D. in biomedical engineering was exactly what my future held. Little did I know, however, was how much Dr. Woo would continue to be an important part of my academic life. After graduating in 2003, I headed to Columbia University to work with Dr. Helen H. Lu in the Department of Biomedical Engineering. My first conference presentation as a doctoral candidate was at the International Symposium on Ligaments and Tendons (ISL&T-V) in 2005 in Washington, D.C. Upon arrival, I received a warm greeting from Dr. Woo, which certainly helped to calm my nerves. After my presentation, during the Q&A session, I looked out into the crowd and who were the first two people to rise to the microphone? None other than Dr. Woo and Dr. Mow. I could only smile and think back to my first day at the MSRC.

Dr. Woo, you planted a seed in my heart for an area of research that has touched my soul, which has grown to be an incredibly important part of my life. It is challenging to describe how extraordinarily grateful I am to you for opening up your lab to a group of summer students and providing us an unparalleled opportunity. Your leadership and vision has influenced generations of scientists, engineers and physicians and I hope to keep your spirit alive throughout my career.

A PROVIDENT DECISION

Kwang Kim

University of Pittsburgh
Pittsburgh, Pennsylvania, 15219, U.S.A.
E-mail: kek68@pitt.edu

Three years ago, having freshly graduated from the University of Washington, where Dr. Woo is also an alumnus, it was unbeknownst to me how my decisions at the time would lead me to one of the most important encounters of my life. My choice was between a guaranteed full stipend from a 5 year NIH R01 at the University of Utah and late admission to the University of Pittsburgh where I had no clear research plan yet. Many people might tell me that turning down a funded NIH R01 in this difficult time when funding opportunities are scarce and unpredictable was not such a smart decision. However, the past 3 years have proven the opposite. Under Dr. Woo's mentorship, I have learned many aspects of conducting research that an ordinary graduate curriculum does not usually touch upon - such as grant writing, organizing workshops and seminars, mentoring students, working closely with clinicians, and collaborating with multiple research groups from multiple institutions, just to name a few. Instead of instant gratification of a ready-made thesis project, I have acquired the indispensible skills to independently carry on a research project and learned the ins and outs of being a scientific researcher. I cannot thank Dr. Woo enough for these.

Personally, I really enjoy going to a Pitt basketball game or some other sporting events in Pittsburgh with Dr. Woo. Sharing the excitement of the game with thousands of other fans has been a really great experience. It was also amazing to see how Dr. Woo could foresee every single move that our coach Dixon makes in the Pitt basketball games. He could see how some of the players were not playing well at that particular moment and would predict that a substitution is coming, which unmistakably came soon after. He also shared many inside stories about the Pitt basketball team and other sports teams. His insights into sports not only helped me understand the game that I was watching, but also made a lasting impression on how the principles of sports are applicable to our life and research.

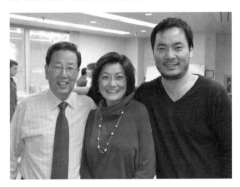

I do not think I can write a tribute to Dr. Woo without a paragraph about Mrs. Woo, as they are literally inseparable. First off, the best meals I have had in Pittsburgh were undisputedly those cooked by Mrs. Woo. All the fancy restaurants I went to in Pittsburgh served nothing comparable to what I had at the Woos' home. Besides the culinary delights, Mrs. Woo's support for Dr. Woo and vice versa has been something to admire. I have personally witnessed how deeply they care about each other when I saw Dr. Woo go without shaving and combing for few days (which is outrageous if you really know Dr. Woo) while Mrs. Woo was at the hospital for a checkup.

I am really thankful that the decisions that I made unknowingly at the time of graduation led me to meet Dr. and Mrs. Woo and gave me an even greater opportunity to study under Dr. Woo. I wish Dr. and Mrs. Woo many more happy decades with Zadie and Arden and look forward to learning more from them, contributing to Dr. Woo's legacy, and just simply having a good time with them for many more years.

HAPPY BIRTHDAY DR. WOO

Maria Apreleva-Scheffler and Sven Scheffler

*Topsfield Medical GmbH, COPV - Chirurgisch-Orthopädischer PraxisVerbund,
Charite University Medicine Berlin
Berlin, 10717, Germany
E-mail: maria.apreleva@gmx.net, sven.scheffler@gmx.com*

Once upon a time, Maria Apreleva, originally from St. Petersburg, Russia, started working at the MSRC in Pittsburgh in 1995 as a Ph.D. student in Bioengineering under Dr. Woo's guidance. Coincidentally, two years later another European, a medical student from Germany, Sven Scheffler, joined the lab on a one-year scholarship. Little did they know that 13 years later they still continue sharing not only their interest in orthopaedic biomechanics, but their life and two children in Berlin, Germany.

Dr. Woo has influenced our lives well beyond our time at the MSRC. Put aside our private life, our professional careers as a bioengineer and orthopedic surgeon would not have been where they are today without the teaching, support and help of Dr. Woo and the members of the MSRC "community". He shared with us not only the fundamentals of biomechanics and research, but also his philosophy of teaching, working together and leadership.

We would like to congratulate Dr. Woo on this special day and wish you many more years of health, happiness, and life filled with new challenges and adventures. May your family, your children and grandchildren be a source of your strength, inspiration and joy.

With warmest wishes,
Maria & Sven Scheffler

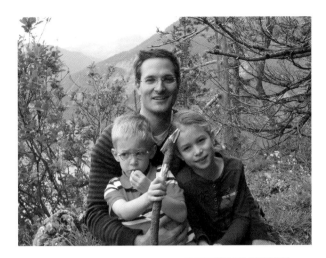
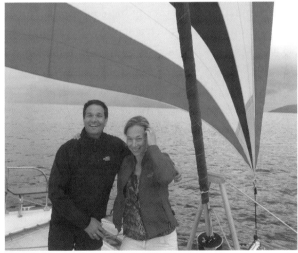

MAKING SOMETHING OUT OF NOTHING

Steven Abramowitch

University of Pittsburgh
Pittsburgh, Pennsylvania, 15219, U.S.A.
E-mail: sdast9@pitt.edu

I met Dr. Woo when I interviewed for graduate school in 1998. What impressed me most about that meeting was that we actually talked very little about science; instead, the primary focus was on philosophy. It did not take me long to realize that the philosophy he was preaching was very much congruent with my own, so my decision to become his student was pretty much decided during the course of that meeting. It is a good thing that we did not talk much science, because to say that I was a little green as an incoming graduate student was an understatement. Here I was agreeing to work under one of the world leaders in the field of biomechanics, and I had no idea what a free-body diagram was or how to even define strain—they did not teach math majors such things as undergrads. However, just 5 short years later, the mentorship of Dr. Woo and the environment of the Musculoskeletal Research Center (MSRC) allowed me to obtain my Ph.D. Not only that, but I was able to finish my degree with 14 publications and a wealth of experience that rivaled most post-docs in the field. This experience put me in a position to move directly into a faculty position after graduation and onto the tenure track 3 years later. Even though I experienced all of this first-hand, I still find it impossible to believe and I am convinced that it would not have happened if I had chosen to work with anyone else.

I often hear that imitation is the sincerest form of flattery, but I would like to replace "flattery" with the word "respect." When I transitioned from graduate student to faculty, I emailed Dr. Woo that I wanted to do for the field of Urogyncology (a field that I am now in thanks to Dr. Woo) what Dr. Woo had done for Orthopaedics. Of course, this goal is nearly impossible to achieve; but, being as naïve in the transition from grad student to faculty as I was in the transition from undergrad to grad student, I thought that I might just have a chance. Now, a couple of rejected grants later, I am more realistic. However, I am still choosing to investigate the same research questions about the impact of mechanical loading on connective tissue remodeling in the context of pelvic organ support that Dr. Woo answered so elegantly in the 80's in the context of knee immobilization. I hope that Dr. Woo realizes it, but I am choosing to imitate his science because of the deep respect that I have for his contribution to the field!

I have learned more from Dr. Woo than anyone outside of my immediate family and I will forever be appreciative of what he has done for me. May your 70th birthday be happier than the sum of the 69 before it, Dr. Woo!

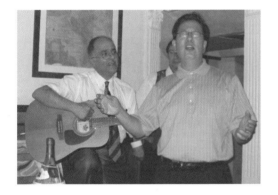

My favorite picture of Dr. Woo, singing in Italy with Dr. Doral playing guitar. Note the empty bottle of wine next to them.

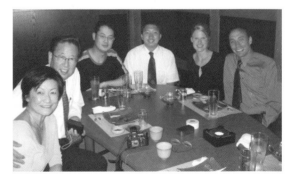

This is a picture from one of the best meals I have ever had in Nara, Japan. Seated left to right includes: Mrs. Woo, Dr. Woo, Dr. Takakura, Dr. Moon, Sarah Abramowitch, and myself.

THE IMPORTANCE OF AN ADVISOR

Akihiro and Jennifer Kanamori
University of Tsukuba
Tsukuba, Ibaraki, Japan
E-mail: jazst15@hotmail.com

Akihiro Kanamori was a research fellow at the Musculoskeletal Research Center (MSRC) from 1997-2000. Jennifer Zeminski started at the MSRC as a summer student in 1997 and continued on as a graduate student until 2001. Akihiro's area of research was focused on the ligaments of the knee joint, including the ACL and PCL. He was awarded the Fellows Award for Basic Science Research from the Arthroscopy Association of North America for his research entitled, "The Effects of Axial Torque on Grading the Pivot Shift Test: A Biomechanical Analysis". In 2001, Jennifer received her master's degree for her research entitled, "Development of a Combined Analytical and Experimental Approach to Reproduce Knee Kinematics for the Evaluation of ACL Function". During this time, both Aki and Jen were under the direction of Dr. Savio L-Y. Woo as their primary advisor.

It can be said that when choosing a college for an undergraduate degree the reputation of the school is most important. However, when deciding on a graduate school it is the advisor that is the determining factor. For Aki and Jen, no one could have known how much this choice would affect the rest of their lives. Without Dr. Woo and the MSRC, Aki and Jen would never have met, gotten married, started their life together in Japan, or had their two beautiful boys, Noah and Owen. Dr. Woo can count their life together and the lives of their children on the list of his many accomplishments. For this, they are and will forever be grateful.

Dr. and Mrs. Woo are forever present in their story; at their first date, celebrating their wedding, visiting them in Japan where they went to Onsen and sightseeing at Nikko, and for the birth of their eldest son.

Tributes from Students, Residents and Fellows Affiliated with the MSRC 113

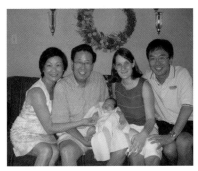

Mrs. and Dr. Woo, baby Noah, Jen and Aki at Jen's parent's home when Noah was just three days old.

Dr. Woo has taught Aki and Jen many valuable academic lessons, as well as showcasing his excellent leadership through dedication and pride. It is the warm feeling of family and friendship that they remember most when they think of Dr. Woo. They are happy to have the opportunity to congratulate Dr. Woo on the most prestigious event of the seventieth anniversary of his birth. May he relax and enjoy looking back through those years and celebrating all of his accomplishments. Best wishes to him and his family always!

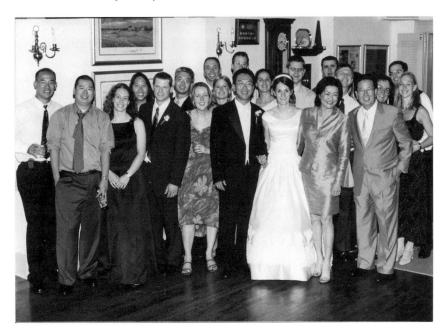

BRINGING US TOGETHER

Alejandro Almarza and Sabrina Noorani
University of Pittsburgh
Pittsburgh, Pennsylvania, 15261, U.S.A.
E-mail: aja19@pitt.edu

Dr. Woo was my mentor for my postdoctoral fellowship at the MSRC, and he was also the advisor for Sabrina's Master thesis. When I first arrived in Pittsburgh, Adam had just proposed to Kirstin and Dr. Woo did not hesitate to share with us his happiness. This made me feel welcomed right away. At the MSRC, I was trained on how to lead a team of researchers, write grants thoroughly, and to not only work hard, but to work smart. Dr. Woo taught me to be proactive and tackle research hurdles head-on. Furthermore, Sabrina was lucky to have such a unique research experience with the use of the robots and human cadaveric knees. Sabrina also truly enjoyed her interaction with the surgeons. The friendships we made at the MSRC will last us a lifetime, and for that we are truly thankful to Dr. Woo.

More importantly, my wife Sabrina and I met at the MSRC. It was quite a day when I met with Dr. Woo to inform him that not only was I dating Sabrina, I had also asked her to marry me. To this declaration he said, "Boy, I am always the last one to hear about things around here". Dr. Woo then stood up, hugged me, and said "Congratulations!" One year later, Dr. Woo and Pattie were in China at a conference being held in Dr. Woo's honor. They left the conference early to come to our wedding. We truly appreciated having Dr. Woo and Pattie there, as it made our 2 day wedding even more special.

Dear Dr. Woo, thank you very much for being a great mentor during my postdoctoral fellowship. This opportunity not only allowed me to grow as a researcher, but it also brought me to my beautiful wife, Sabrina. We truly appreciate everything you have done for us, and it was amazing when the next MSRC baby arrived in August 2011 and changed our lives. This is partly your fault!

We joined the MSRC shortly after your 60th birthday and we will enjoy your 80th, with as many kids as Sabrina allows us to have.

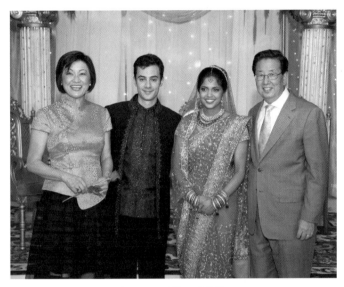

At our wedding (2008)

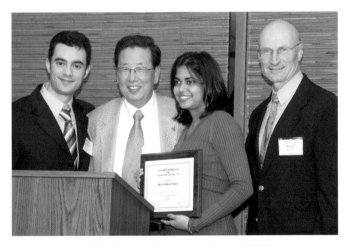

ISL&T Best Student Paper Award (2007)

MARRIAGES AND LIFELONG FRIENDSHIPS

Carrie (Voycheck) Rainis
University of Pittsburgh
Pittsburgh, Pennsylvania, 15219, U.S.A.
E-mail: cav23@pitt.edu

I came to the MSRC as a doctoral student in August of 2006. Before arriving I had heard great things about Dr. Woo's research center but it was not until recently, as I was finishing my degree and starting to look towards my future, that I realized what a remarkable education I had received. Although I did not study directly under Dr. Woo, he has bestowed upon me a wealth of knowledge that extends far beyond the field of biomechanics through his reflections and life lessons, and for that I am extremely grateful.

After spending about a week at the MSRC I learned of something called the "MSRC curse". To my knowledge, this curse, which is particularly applicable to graduate students and post-docs, states that if you are in a committed relationship when you arrive, after spending some time at the MSRC, you will eventually suffer a break-up and end up with another member of the MSRC family. While I will leave out the details, I will say that I swore up and down that this "curse" would not happen to me...

Five years later, Eric and I were married. Dr. Woo takes great pride in the fact that many marriages have developed at the MSRC and in some cases may even have tried to do a little match-making. However, it is not just marriages that the MSRC fosters, but lifelong friendships. In establishing the MSRC, Dr. Woo has not only developed an outstanding educational research facility, but a community of friends and colleagues who are forever connected. My time spent at the MSRC has not only earned me a Ph.D. but left me with lifelong friendships and the love of my life. Dr. Woo, I cannot thank you enough for allowing me to be a part of such a wonderful family.

The strong relationships that develop at the MSRC are undoubtedly a result of the family environment Dr. Woo has created. In his own life he cherishes family and values friends more than anything else in this world and has always taught us to do the same. If I had to pick the one thing that I admire most about Dr. Woo it would be his love for and devotion to Mrs. Woo. He has shared countless memories with us about how he and Mrs. Woo met and fell in love. All these years later, she still brings a smile to his face every time he thinks of her, just as she did the first day he saw her. Anyone who has ever seen the two of them together can see just how much he loves her and that he would do anything for her. Very few people in this world are able to experience this kind of happiness and it is truly inspiring.

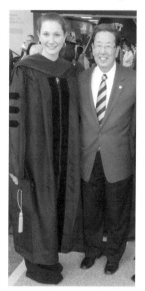

Dr. Woo – I can never thank you enough for everything you have taught me about biomechanics, research, and life in general. The opportunities you have given me have influenced the rest of my life. Congratulations on 70 wonderful years and may you be happy and healthy for many more! Eric and I wish you, Mrs. Woo and the rest of your family all the best in the years to come!

COMING FULL CIRCLE:
DR. WOO AS A MENTOR AND A COLLEAGUE

Mininder S. Kocher

Children's Hospital Boston
Harvard Medical School
Boston, Massachusetts, 02030, U.S.A.
E-mail: mininder.kocher@childrens.harvard.edu

I spent a year in the Musculoskeletal Research Center at the University of Pittsburgh with Dr. Woo in 1991-1992. At the time, I was a third year medical student at the Duke University School of Medicine where we spend a year doing research. I spent my research time learning orthopaedic biomechanics and studying shoulder kinematics and proprioception. This led to my first scientific publications and presentations, and fostered my career in academic orthopaedic surgery.

I am an academic orthopaedic surgeon at Children's Hospital Boston and Harvard Medical School. My clinical practice focuses on pediatric sports medicine. I direct an applied clinical epidemiology research unit. My clinical research focuses on comparative effectiveness research, outcomes assessment, randomized clinical trials, and health services research. I have published over 150 peer reviewed scientific articles, received the Kappa Delta clinical research award, and have been on the board of directors of the Pediatric Orthopaedic Society of North America and the American Orthopaedic Society for Sports Medicine. I am currently on the board of directors of the American Academy of Orthopaedic Surgeons.

Dr. Woo had a major influence in my career decision to go into orthopaedics and to be actively engaged in research. Although I do not do basic science biomechanics research, the lessons that I learned from him regarding the scientific method, controlling for confounding, scientific integrity, academic excellence, and respectful collaboration still resonate.

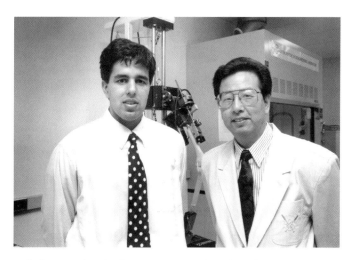

Beyond the academic lessons, Dr. Woo has been a personal friend and mentor. He and Pattie are close friends with my wife and her parents. They have provided mentorship, support, and friendship to me and to our family over the last 20 years.

I now have the opportunity to work with Dr. Woo as a colleague on the Scientific Advisory Committee for the Steadman Philippon Research Institute. His insight into running a research program of excellence remains profound.

Dr. Woo - Thank you!

贺胡流源教授70岁生日

Guoan Li

*Massachusetts General Hospital and Harvard Medical School
Boston, Massachusetts, 02114, U.S.A.
E-mail: guoanli12@partners.org*

值此胡流源教授70岁生日之际，谨祝教授生活之树常绿，生命之水长流！

自95年有幸结识教授并在教授指导下工作2年多，使我能初窥运动医学中的生物力学问题。至今它仍为我研究工作的重要部分。记的第一次和教授在匹次堡大学见面的时候，教授谈起机器人在生物力学研究中的运用，引领我进入了一个广阔自由的天地，使我98年离开匹次堡大学到波士顿后，能把机器人技术运用于骨外科生物力学的不同领域。教授于我不仅是学术上得导师，

更是作为生活中挚友。值此教授70岁生日之际，与您分享一些岁月的脚印，祝您生日快乐！

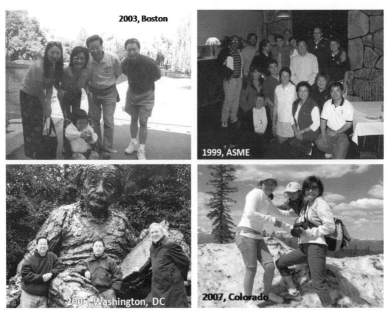

THE CONFUCIUS OF BIOMECHANICS

Daniel K. Moon

*Moss Rehab Hospital & Temple University Hospital
Philadelphia, Pennsylvania, 19129, U.S.A.
E-mail: danielkmoon@gmail.com*

Confucius once said, "By three methods we may learn wisdom: First, by reflection, which is noblest; second, by imitation, which is easiest; and third by experience, which is the bitterest." I am pretty sure anyone who has been under Dr. Woo's mentorship will agree that this quotation captures his style of teaching perfectly.

From 2002 to 2005, I was a graduate student at the Musculoskeletal Research Center (MSRC). Those three years were some of the most challenging yet productive years of my life. In the first month, I was not only given a project to lead, but also assisted other researchers in their investigations. I learned a great deal from working with senior research fellows and graduate students. I found it odd that I would meet with my advisor once every couple of months and he left a lot of the decision making up to me, but in retrospect, I realize that the autonomy is what allowed me to grow the most during graduate school. Most importantly, Dr. Woo allowed me to make mistakes and learn to overcome them. This experience was definitely rough in the beginning and at times bitter as Confucius pointed out, but it strengthened my resolve and decision making skills. Even to this day, I continue to apply what I learned at the MSRC under Dr. Woo to my daily practice at the hospital.

Happy 70th Birthday, Dr. Woo! Thank you for advising me during graduate school and also for sharing your wisdom and philosophy with us. I wish you and Pattie the best and hope you have many more active and productive years.

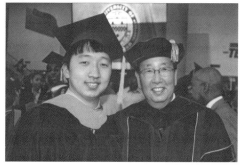

STRIVE FOR EXCELLENCE

Thomas W. Gilbert

University of Pittsburgh
Pittsburgh, Pennsylvania, 15221, U.S.A.
E-mail: gilberttw@upmc.edu

Dr. Woo was my PhD advisor at Pitt from July 2000 through May 2003. My time at the Musculoskeletal Research Center meant a great deal to me. It was a time of great personal and intellectual growth. Dr. Woo pushed us all to strive for excellence and to help those around us to do the same. The environment was one that could be well described as intense, but the result was productivity and close, meaningful relationships. It was during that time, that I first developed a love for research that redirected my intended path from industry to the academic pursuits in which I am now engaged.

I certainly did not fully appreciate it then, but I am now very grateful that Dr. Woo set high standards for himself and for those that worked for him. I remember my first graduate student seminar when I barely made it through 15 slides in an hour as I was asked to explain and re-explain what I was trying to say. I remember the month of late nights in the lab working on an R01 submission for Dr. Woo for the first time in my career. These experiences trained me to think and to clearly communicate my ideas to others, and have been immensely helpful experiences as I present and write my ideas frequently now.

Unfortunately, my time in the MSRC ended abruptly after a period of disagreement between myself and Dr. Woo. Despite this disagreement, I always respected Dr. Woo and did my best to follow through on the commitments that I made. During the next few years of my PhD, I felt that I matured as a graduate student and was able to assemble a very respectable CV in the process. I credit this success to the time that I spent in the MSRC. I took great pride in the fact that Dr. Woo was still willing to serve on my PhD committee and that we have rebuilt our relationship thanks in part to our mutual participation in the NSF Engineering Research Center for Revolutionizing Metallic Biomaterials.

Now that I have my own lab, I have recognized more fully the wisdom of many of Dr. Woo's initiatives. I have begun to institute Graduate Student Seminars for my students so that they get the benefit of the experience, including responding to criticism and defending their ideas. I have also instituted lab gatherings throughout the year to help build a stronger community amongst the members of my lab.

Dr. Woo, I congratulate you on your accomplishments throughout your career, and am grateful to be counted among them.

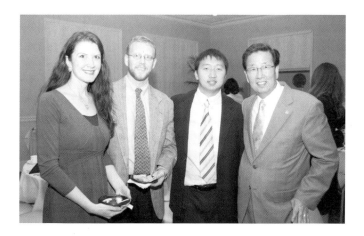

WE ARE GETTING MATURE

Yoshitsugu Takeda

Tokushima Red Cross Hospital
Komatsushima, Tokushima, 773-8502, Japan
E-mail: ytakeda@tokushima-med.jrc.or.jp

I was at the MSRC as a research fellow from October 1992 to March 1994, and I did research on the ACL under Dr. Woo. Although I had some experience on basic research before coming to Pittsburgh, I really learned what research and science is from Dr. Woo for the first time. I believe that I gained my scientific way of thinking during my time in his laboratory in Pittsburgh, and since then, it has been working not only for conducting clinical research, but also for my clinical work as an orthopaedic surgeon.

More than 17 years have passed since I left Pittsburgh, but now I feel much closer to Dr. Woo than before. After leaving Pittsburgh, I would see Dr. Woo at many international conferences all over the world. Every time I saw him, it felt like seeing my elementary school teacher, and I would feel excited. I have enjoyed his lunch and dinner parties with many good friends and famous people. I still remember the wonderful breakfast with Dr. and Mrs. Woo at the old hotel in Nara, which is the oldest capital of Japan. We talked about basic research and orthopaedics, family, life and so on.

Four years ago, Dr. Woo and I were in Florence for the ISAKOS Congress. At that time, I was a little bit tired with my busy work, and was losing a little bit of interest for clinical research, so I said, "I recently feel that I am getting old." Dr. Woo told me "Yoshi, we are not getting old, we are getting mature." I was encouraged by his words which got me back on track. I found that it is very important to have a great mentor. Yes, we do not have to feel limited by age. Dr. Woo, please keep getting mature. I will follow you.

Tributes from Students, Residents and Fellows Affiliated with the MSRC 125

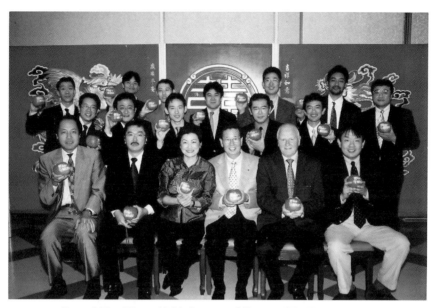

Dr. and Mrs. Woo with his Japanese fellows and Dr. Lars Peterson
Hirosaki (2002)

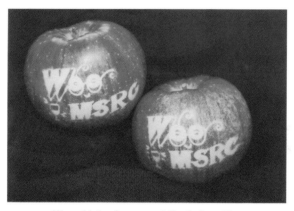

Hirosaki Apples – specially designed by
Mrs. Mitsuko Tsuda

祝古稀

Masataka Sakane

University of Tsukuba
Tsukuba, Ibaraki, 305-8575, Japan
E-mail: sakane.masataka@gmail.com

I joined Dr. Woo's circle in 1995 as a research fellow at the MSRC. At that time, we were so excited that experiments using human cadaveric knees had just begun. I worked hard for two years with Ted Rudy, Glen Livesay, Tom Runco, Christy Allen, and Guoan Li under the supervision of Dr. Woo.

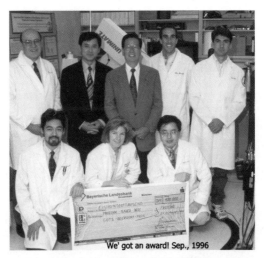

Fig. 1: The ACL group in 1996.

I, my wife Michiko, and my daughters Natsumi and Tomoha enjoyed life in Pittsburgh. Kennywood Park, Idlewild Park, Pittsburgh Zoo, and Monroeville Mall were especially memorable. Our youngest daughter, Mafuyu was born in 1996 at Magee-Women's Hospital. In 2011, she visited her hometown.

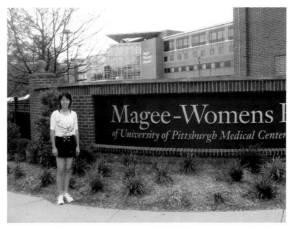

Fig. 2: Mafuyu visited her birth place. (August, 2011)

Time goes by so quickly. However, my fundamental attitude for research and collaboration is the same as what Dr. Woo taught me during my Pitt days. I learned much from Dr. Woo and friends at MSRC.

In China and Japan, the 60th and 70th birthdays are special. Our family had the chance to attend Dr. Woo's 60th birthday celebration.

We call the 70th anniversary, "a KoKi cerebration", which means "Rare case" from old saying in China. Congratulations and Happy Birthday! We all wish you happiness and good health.

Masataka and Michiko Sakane

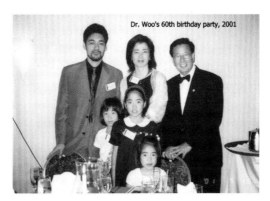

Fig. 3: Family picture at Dr. Woo's 60th birthday party.

NICE TO MEET YOU

Yukihisa Fukuda

Fukuda Orthopaedic Clinic
Izumo, Shimane, 693-0012, Japan
E-mail: fukuda@i.softbank.jp

Needless to say, Dr. Woo is obviously very famous in the world as a scientist and has been invited to give his lecture to the Japanese orthopaedic congress many times, however, I first met him in his office. Although he was so busy, he was kind enough to meet me. He welcomed me and talked to me with a smile, but I could not understand all of them because of my poor English. I just understood "Nice to meet you". My Japanese mentor, Dr. Shinro Takai, recommended me to conduct research in the U.S. 13 years ago.

After I had succeeded Nobuyoshi Watanabe as a researcher for 6 months and had acquired his apartment and car, I went back to Japan to have a wedding ceremony with Sachiko. Unbeknownst to me, Dr. Takai had arranged a special video letter from Dr. Woo for Sachiko and I and showed it at the wedding party. This surprised me since old Japanese style wedding ceremony party did not have surprises.

One bright, sunny day, Dr. Woo invited Masayoshi Yagi and I to San Francisco and cooked a special crab cuisine in his home. The crab was as big as the smile on his face. I was so impressed that the professor served us a homemade dish that was so delicious. I would like to take this opportunity to express my appreciation to Dr. Woo.

My dad is now 78 years old and hard of hearing, however, he has been vigorously working. I wish Dr. Woo many more years of research and passing his knowledge to young researchers.

When I lived in Pittsburgh, we embedded a cherry tree at Dr. Woo's home ten years ago. I think the cherry blossom will be getting prettier in every April year after year.

Tributes from Students, Residents and Fellows Affiliated with the MSRC

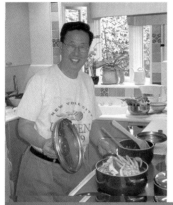
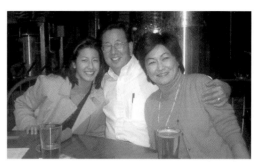
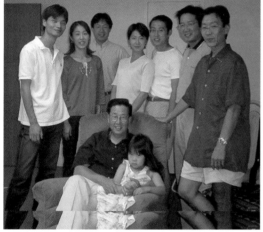
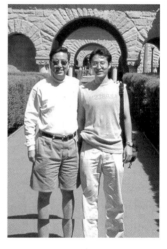

CONGRATULATIONS FOR DR. WOO'S 70 YEARS YOUNG BIRTHDAY FROM A JAPANESE FELLOW

Kazutomo Miura

Mutsu General Hospital
Mutsu, Aomori, 035-8601, Japan
E-mail: miurak0993@aol.jp

I congratulate Dr. Woo on his 70th memorial birthday. It is my pleasure to praise his long and successful career in the field of bioengineering research. I also thank him for all of his kindness and friendship to my family.

I am the 6th research fellow from the Dept. of Orthopaedic Surgery in Hirosaki University from Japan. Five doctors: Dr. Aizawa, Dr. Ishibashi, Dr. Tsuda, Dr. Sasaki, and Dr. Yamamoto spent their research life at the MSRC in Pittsburgh under Dr. Woo's direction in earlier years. I had a fruitful and great time in Pittsburgh from May 2004 to September 2005, the same as they did.

I first met Dr. and Mrs. Woo in Switzerland while attending the ISAKOS meeting in 2001, which was my first participation in an international conference. Dr. Woo was a mentor of the symposium in which I presented my paper. Although I could not communicate well, he kindly directed me and made suggestions.

The second time I met Dr. Woo was when he came to Japan to give the keynote presentation at the annual meeting of the Japanese Orthopaedic Basic Research Society in 2002. I was allowed to participate in the dinner party where more than 20 doctors who were Dr. Woo's Japanese fellows attended. I was so amazed to hear all the fellows give a self-introduction in English so well. I gradually became motivated to do research at the MSRC in the near future, for which I wrote an English paper.

Finally, I was able to go to Pittsburgh as a research fellow and become a member of the MSRC after Dr. Yamamoto in 2004, just after my first English paper was published. During my one and half years at the MSRC, I completed a project to find the optimal knee flexion angles at the time of graft fixation in double bundle ACL reconstruction under the direction of Dr. Woo. I was so surprised to find out how long time it takes to prepare presentations and how many times it takes to correct papers. However, it was so precious an experience for me to write papers later.

Although I was not familiar with English, new environment, and knowledge of bioengineering, Dr. Woo kindly taught me research as well as how to enjoy our life in Pittsburgh. My wife, Maki and my daughter, Kirara, also enjoyed parties at Dr. Woo's house several times. We could not forget a special dinner cooked by Mrs. Woo. Dr. Woo gave us many great days and memories in Pittsburgh. I hope Dr. Woo is healthy and lives a long and wonderful life from now on, and we will see you again soon in Japan or USA.

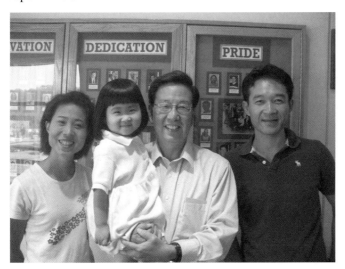

In the laboratory (2005)

A GREAT MENTOR

Sinan Karaoglu

Orthopaedic Surgeon
Kayseri, 38004, Turkey
E-mail: sinankaraoglu@hotmail.com

I first met Dr. Woo in Ankara, Turkey where he told me that I had a chance to work at the MSRC. I was so excited. It was really important for me to hear such a thing from Dr. Woo. I gave up my career in Turkey for two years to work with a great team and a great mentor.

The two years that I spent at the MSRC was very instructive for me. Dr. Woo has a wide spectrum perspective, well rounded scientific thought, and great experience in the field. I learned a lot from him and from his team. There were many kinds of people from different countries at the MSRC and it was a really good chance for me to get to know them. Dr. Woo gave me the opportunity to work in a good place that has everything for making new projects. Even though I left my hometown, and my life in Turkey, the years that I spent at the MSRC with Dr. Woo and his team was worth it. Projects that I worked on at in MSRC were the climax for my career and I owe a thank you to him.

He is a supporting mentor and a very successful scientist. Besides this, he has a great personality and a social life. He hosts his guests in a great generosity with Mrs. Woo, I always enjoyed their parties. He is not like a boss, on the contrary, he is very friendly. After I came back to Turkey, Dr. and Mrs. Woo came to visit us and I was delighted to have them in my hometown.

After all we have been through what we have in our hands is a good and strong friendship. It has been a pleasure working with someone who knows the secret to a being a good mentor, being a good person.

The first forty years of our life give the text, the next thirty furnish the commentary upon it, which enables us rightly to understand the true meaning and connection of the text with its moral and its beauties. Happy 70th birthday!

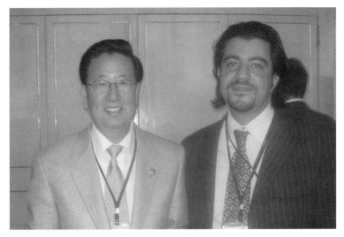

3rd Congress of Asia-Pacific Knee Society, Ankara (2004)

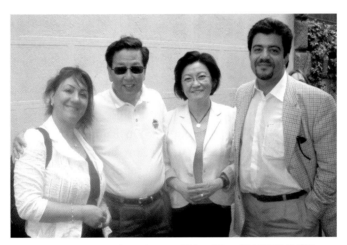

With Sema, my wife and Dr. and Mrs. Woo, ISAKOS (2010)

....YOU ARE MY TEACHER
YOU ARE MY FAMILY...

Fabio Vercillo

University of Perugia
Perugia, 06127, Italy
E-mail: fabio.vercillo@gmail.com

I have only few words, but plenty of true affection I would like to express for Dr. and Mrs. Woo. Since the first time I met Dr. Woo in Italy, I was impressed by his capability for teaching young students. He was able to make me really love the research aspect of my job and he gave to me a great motivation that I have kept with me. But that was only the beginning of a wonderful experience that continued a short time later. When I flew to Pittsburgh, I was scared. My English was not good enough to start the experience, and sometimes, I thought to turn right around and fly back to Italy.

During the first few days that I worked at the MSRC, Dr. and Mrs. Woo did their best to make me comfortable, probably because they understood my fears. We went out for lunch and dinner many times. They would talk to me about my family, my country and my problems. Within a few days, they became my new family in Pittsburgh, so thanks to them, I started to be more confident in what I was doing. Dr. Woo used to pay attention to how I was conducting my research study at the MSRC, and he was really able to motivate me without pressuring me. By just talking and observing me, he was able to make me understand what I was doing bad or well. I remember during a group meeting he taught to me how to fight for my research, how to think about my research and how to work together as a good team with the ACL group. From that time on I really started putting a lot of effort into my research so that it was completely done and published a short while later.

But what I would like to say is that the effort and the intensity on my job that Dr Woo gave to me was the most important gift I got from him, because that will to fight in my job I have also applied to my life. He was able to improve my relationship with people; he was able to make me able to connect with people from many different countries; he gave to me the desire to discover new things in my work and in my life.

So far, I have been talking about Dr. Woo as a teacher, as a guide, and together with Mrs. Woo as a family, but now I would like to spend a few more words about Dr. and Mrs. Woo as friends. With them, during the time that I was in Pittsburgh, I shared memorable moments like parties at their house, Dr. Woo's birthday at the tennis club, a nice lunch at the Italian restaurant named (I cannot forget the name!!) "la bruschetta", the Steelers winning the Super Bowl and as Italian I was honored to share with them the Italian team winning the soccer World Championship.

For all of these things, and many others that I keep in my heart, I would like to say to you two, Dr. Woo and Mrs. Woo,

Thanks,

....you are my Teacher

you are my Family...

Sincerely,
    Fabio

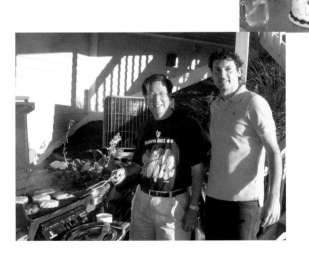

QUICKLY LEARN TO USE CHOPSTICKS

Louis E. DeFrate

Duke University Medical Center
Durham, North Carolina, 27710, U.S.A.
E-mail: lou.defrate@duke.edu

I first met Dr. Woo after my freshman year at the University of Pittsburgh, when I began work as a summer student at the Musculoskeletal Research Center (MSRC). After completing a summer internship in the lab, I was excited to continue my research experience, so I worked in the lab as a cooperative education student until graduating from Pitt in 1999. I am extremely grateful to have had the opportunity to work with Dr. Woo and everyone in the MSRC, who taught me so much about research. The experience of working with such an outstanding research team has helped me throughout my career.

In addition to learning how to do research, I have many fond memories of my time in the lab. In particular, I remember many of Dr. Woo's great sayings. For example, after we run into difficulties with a study in my own laboratory, I frequently quote Dr. Woo to my students and staff. I tell them that if we always got our work right on the first time, it would be called "search" and not "research". I also remember going to lunch at the Orient Kitchen, where I had to quickly learn to use chopsticks to keep up with all the delicious food served to us.

I am extremely grateful to Dr. Woo for helping me to get started in research, and for all of his great advice throughout my career. I wish him the best on his 70th birthday.

AN INCREDIBLE INSPIRATION

Mara Schenker

University of Pennsylvania
Philadelphia, Pennsylvania, 19104, U.S.A.
E-mail: mara.schenker@uphs.upenn.edu

Congratulations on your 70th birthday and best wishes for many healthy and happy decades to come! I attribute my career choice to the passion that you instilled in me for orthopaedic research, and I owe you many thanks for that.

I first met you as an excited (and very green) undergraduate summer student in your lab in 2002. I was a pre-med neuroscience major, and was looking for something to do while I recovered from hip surgery. Up until that point in my life, I had one major focus: competing in taekwondo. The hip injury was a huge set-back to me at the time, but little did I know how pivotal this moment would be in establishing my career. In the year and a half that I spent in your lab, I learned the definition of "modulus"; I acquired the skill of suturing; I began to appreciate the value of academic debate in lab meetings; I ate my first chicken foot; and, with the help of my many friends that I met, I probably made more noise than any previous or subsequent group of students in your lab. Also, during this time, I cut back on my strict taekwondo schedule, and for the first time, I found something else I could be passionate about – orthopaedic research. Now, I am a 4th year orthopaedic surgery resident at the University of Pennsylvania, and I am planning to pursue a career in orthopaedic traumatology. In my future career (which is quickly creeping up on me), I plan to have 50% dedicated academic time, and intend to have my own basic science laboratory. Without the discovery period that I experienced in your lab, I most certainly would not be where I am and would not be headed where I am headed.

You are an incredible inspiration to the many students who have worked with you. Your ability to answer clinically relevant orthopaedic issues with elegantly simple methods is truly unmatched. On occasion, I reference your words of wisdom that I picked up and subconsciously stored away. For example, I am quick to pounce on people when they begin speaking or writing with the line, "this is the FIRST study that showed...", because you never *really* know this, right?

I look forward to seeing you at the orthopaedic research meetings, and truly appreciate that you have always been there when I have needed advice. I wish you the happiest of birthdays, and best wishes for many more to come!

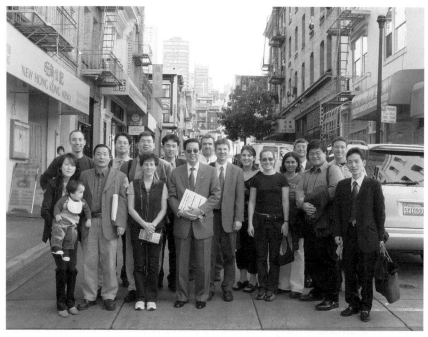

Dr. Woo and MSRC at ORS, San Francisco, CA (2004)

CHINESE FOOD AND DR. WOO

Noah Papas

Ethicon Inc. (Johnson and Johnson)
Bridgewater, New Jersey, 08807, U.S.A.
E-mail: npapas03@gmail.com

Growing up, I was a very picky eater, and the dinner table was a war zone. On the one side, my parents would plead with me to eat, on the other, I stubbornly refused. By the time I was working towards a Masters degree in Bioengineering as Dr. Woo's graduate student at the MSRC (2005-2007), I enjoyed a much larger variety of foods. This was a glorious and wonderful thing, because the MSRC, like a family, communicated around lunches, dinners and picnics. I can recall the amazing Chinese food that always seemed to be present at MSRC functions including the standard lunch orders from Yen's Gourmet and the special dinners where Dr. Woo would utter a few sentences in Chinese and order a plethora of what I could only presume to be more authentic Chinese dishes. Nonetheless, students, fellows and professors alike always had full bellies while dining with Dr. Woo.

Some special memories are tied to Chinese food as well. For example, as a prospective student, I distinctly remember hearing Dr. Woo state, "If you are accepted to the MSRC you must learn how to use chopsticks in 3 months." Of the prospective students at that lunch, three of us joined the lab, and you better believe we made sure our chopstick skills were honed before our start dates. There was also the time after finishing a grant that we all gathered at Dr. Woo's house and made dumplings. I also still have the apropos fortune I received from lunch the day I defended my thesis, which foretold, "All your hard work will soon pay off."

Despite these many wonderful memories, there was one meal which was not as pleasant. As I stated, I was a very picky eater growing up. As I aged, my palate did expand, but there are still three things I don't enjoy: mushrooms, salad and eggs. If I do not want to eat something, no one can force me. There have been two exceptions to this hard line rule: 1) the Metropolitan of Karditsa, Greece once told me to eat salad (as an Orthodox Christian you are obedient to the Bishop) and 2) Dr. Woo. At a lab lunch at the Rose Tea Room, Dr. Woo told me to eat a soy pickled egg. Without question, but maybe slight hesitation, I obediently ate the cold, funny tasting, brown, salty sustenance. This is an example of the respect that I and other students had and have for Dr. Woo. Thank you for everything that you have done for me in my career and life as a whole (even introducing me to the pickled egg). Congratulations on your 70th birthday and blessings for years to come!

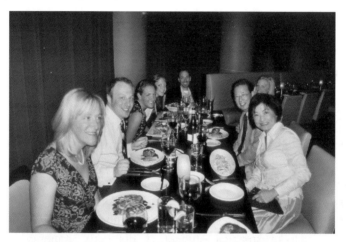

Dinner with Dr. and Mrs. Woo and my family after graduation

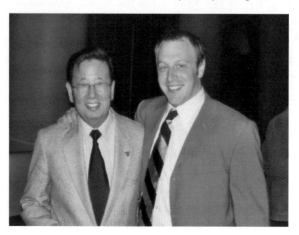

YOU DON'T HAVE TO BE AN EINSTEIN ...

Xia Guo

The Hong Kong Polytechnic University
Hong Kong SAR, China
E-mail: rsguoxia@inet.polyu.edu.hk

Albert Einstein said *"Try not to become a man of success, but rather try to become a man of value"*. Dr. Woo proves Einstein wrong. He is a man of both success and value!

Happy 70th Birthday to Dr. Woo!

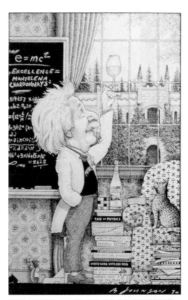 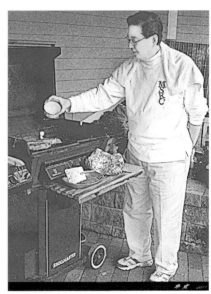

YOU DON'T HAVE TO BE AN EINSTEIN...   YOU ARE A MAN OF BOTH SUCCESS AND VALUE

I have known of Dr. Savio Woo for around 20 years as a famous professor and the author of the book **"Injury and Repair of the Musculoskeletal Soft Tissues"**.

I got to know Dr. Woo personally during my sabbatical at the MSRC four years ago. I do not remember the exact date I arrived at the MSRC, but I do remember that when I did, I loved the MSRC immediately. It felt just like a big family with such a friendly atmosphere. Every colleague got along well with the others and it was easy to make friends.

The longer I stayed, the more I discovered that the MSRC is a remarkable institute which provides researchers a high-quality, but relaxed and pleasant research environment. There were frequent research seminars for presenting new findings of each project. Almost all seminars were kicked off with pizza, Chinese food, or cake. I have learned that stress is not necessarily a requirement in high academic achievement.

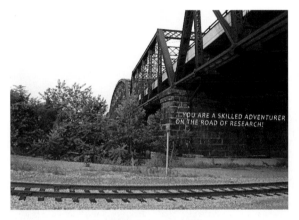

There is a railroad behind the MSRC. MSRC is just like a train rolling on the road. For 20 years Dr. Woo has been driving the MSRC train and has picked up many passengers, including me (I feel lucky :D), along the way.

Dear Dr. Woo, happy 70th birthday!
You are still young,
Fuel up your mind,
And fire up your heart,
And drive on, drive on... ... drive on

MY ETERNAL PROFESSOR!

Greg Carlin

McKeon, Meunier, Carlin, & Curfman, LLC
Atlanta, Georgia, 30308, U.S.A.
E-mail: gregorycarlin@yahoo.com

Dr. Woo has always been my eternal professor, long after I have forgotten about other teachers. I think if I were to make a toast, I would say: "As my father will always be my father, Dr. Woo will always be my professor. They have both taught me things that have made me what I am today."

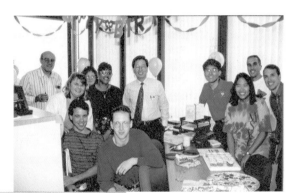

MSRC celebrating Dr. Woo's birthday (1995)

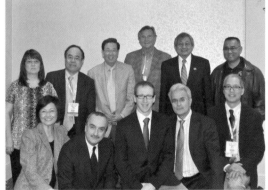

ASIAM Institute Board Meeting (2011)

HAPPY BIRTHDAY, DR. WOO

Guoguang Yang

Pittsburgh, Pennsylvania, 15227, U.S.A.
E-mail: yangguoguang@hotmail.com

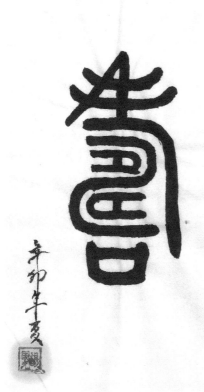

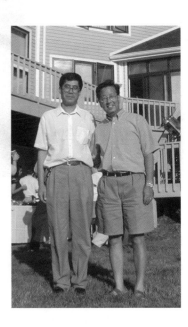

Longevity

AN EDUCATION AND EXPERIENCE OF A LIFETIME

Richard Debski

University of Pittsburgh
Pittsburgh, Pennsylvania, 15219, U.S.A.
E-mail: genesis1@pitt.edu

Over twenty years ago, I entered an office on the second floor of Scaife Hall at the University of Pittsburgh looking for an opportunity to continue my education in graduate school while performing exciting research. Little did I know that a meeting with Dr. Woo at his "small round table" would lead to a lifetime of opportunities and an educational experience that cannot be rivaled. He was willing to take a chance on a mechanical engineer with little research experience and eventually convinced me to stay for a PhD. The first few years were difficult. However, as the philosophy and rigor of the training sunk-in, I was able to become a productive researcher and take advantage of the many research tools and collaborations within the Musculoskeletal Research Center (MSRC).

Throughout my training as a graduate student researcher, post-doctoral fellow, and assistant professor, I was quite fortunate to have Dr. Woo as an advisor, mentor and friend. The wealth of knowledge and experiences that were bestowed upon me was "unbelievable" and continue to guide my research efforts to this day. It is hard to believe that I have been with the MSRC for half of my life. There have been so many great moments, but the most memorable was my graduation and hooding ceremony at the completion of my doctoral training.

On his 70th birthday, I would like to thank Dr. Woo for all of the wonderful contributions that he has made to my life. May each and every passing year bring you more wisdom, peace and cheer. Happy Birthday!

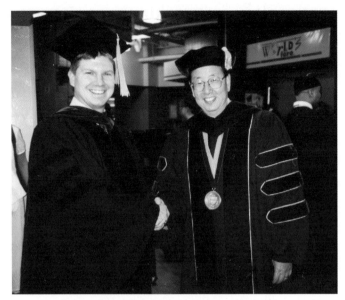

Dr. Woo and I following graduation and hooding ceremony at the University of Pittsburgh (1998)

MILESTONE AND TESTAMENT

Kevin Hildebrand

University of Calgary
Calgary, Alberta, T3Z 2B9, Canada
E-mail: hildebrk@ucalgary.ca

I was a fellow at the Musculoskeletal Research Center in Pittsburgh from August 1995 to June 1997. I worked on the MCL project.

My time at the MSRC was critical in my development as a surgeon-scientist. I learned about biomechanics, experimental design, data analysis, grantsmanship, manuscript writing and reviewing articles. We were provided many life lessons and excellent opportunities to present our research and network with the orthopaedic research community. I met many interesting people during my time in Pittsburgh. This part in my training was critical for me to develop my independent research laboratory studying post-traumatic contractures and link this to my clinical practice treating elbow disorders. It was ironic to discover after my time at the MSRC that Dr. Woo also did research on joint contractures in the past!!

Congratulations on reaching this milestone, your 70th birthday. It is a testament that you continue to contribute to musculoskeletal knowledge in many areas of biomechanics. This milestone is also a testament to your family. It is an outstanding example for the generations that preceded you and that follow. Your legacy will continue with your nuclear family and the extended MSRC family.

Kevin, Kathy, Kurt and Karys Hildebrand

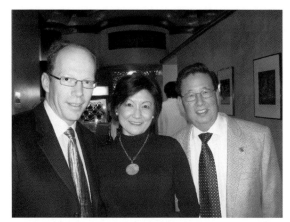

Fig. 1: Kevin, Mrs. Woo, and Dr. Woo in San Francisco (2008)

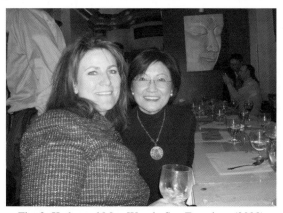

Fig. 2: Kathy and Mrs. Woo in San Francisco (2008)

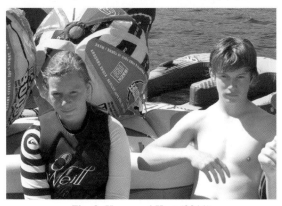

Fig. 3: Karys and Kurt (2011)

A REAL LEADER

Dimosthenis Alaseirlis

Consultant in Orthopaedic Surgery
Thessaloniki, Greece
E-mail: iraridim@hotmail.com

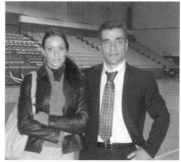

I will always feel grateful to you because I had the opportunity to work under your direction on MSRC projects. I can easily remember the standards and values that you were inspiring to all of your colleagues: deep knowledge, focusing on target, proceeding step by step, co-operation and hard-work.

I think that all of your colleagues (current and past) will keep very strong feelings about the unforgettable "Monday Mornings" at the MSRC.

I also feel honored that I was once invited at your home during "Thanksgiving", having the opportunity to meet the members of your excellent family; I can say that I can still feel the warmth of the hospitality.

You are acknowledged worldwide as one of the most important Professors in the academic society, leading the MSRC to produce an enormous number of high-quality publications that contributed to remarkable progress in the understanding of the musculoskeletal system, its pathology and new horizons of treatment.

Someone who has worked near you can easily understand that knowledge and hard work should be associated with wisdom, kindness and high ethical standards for a man to become a real leader.

REFLECTIONS ON MY TIME AT THE MSRC WITH DR. WOO

Ken Fischer

*University of Kansas
Lawrence, Kansas, 66054, U.S.A.
E-mail: fischer@ku.edu*

I owe a lot to you, Dr. Woo, personally and professionally. You gave me my first post-doctoral job in the MSRC! Not long after, my bride Sandie joined me in Pittsburgh, and you and Pattie welcomed her, as well. And I learned a lot about how to perform quality research from my time at the MSRC with you—for instance, the importance of staying on top of publications, which I learned through the dreaded publication reviews. It showed me well that internal deadlines help keep things moving!

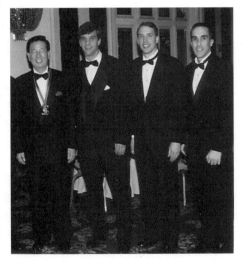

Of course, the highlights of my time at the MSRC revolve around the celebrations... the summer parties at your home, the lab dinners with incredible Chinese food, a couple of Superbowl parties, and, of course, your Olympic Gold medal ceremony!

Sandie and I want to extend our heartfelt congratulations to you, Dr. Woo, on your 70th birthday! May you enjoy many more to come!

Tributes from Students, Residents and Fellows Affiliated with the MSRC 151

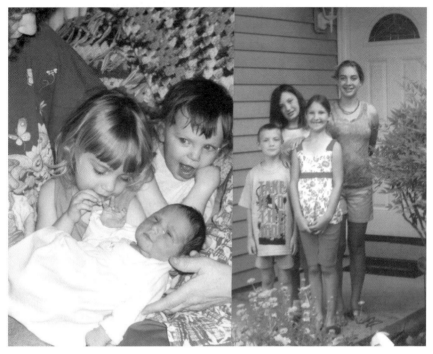

The Fischer children in 2000 and in 2011

Happy Birthday,
From Ken and Sandie Fischer

TRIBUTE TO SAVIO L-Y. WOO ON HIS 70TH BIRTHDAY

Christopher Schmidt

Allegheny General Hospital
Pittsburgh, Pennsylvania, 15212, U.S.A.
E-mail: cschmidthand@comcast.net

Dr. Woo, I need to thank you for not only fostering in me a love for basic science research, but also, teaching me the tools for successfully designing a study, and completing and publishing the findings.

One of the greatest lessons taught was the ability to distill a complex clinical dilemma into a simple anatomy question. For example, over the years of clinical practice, I observed that my patients, despite a distal biceps repair, had supination weakness with the forearm in supination. We went back and studied the repair site and realized that my repairs were anterior to the native insertion site. Well, that concept has led to 2 basic science publications, a graduate student thesis, a Charles S. Neer nominee, possible clinical paper in JBJS, and an on-going prospective clinical series.

By the way, I run the research lab with a Tuesday morning lab meeting. Sounds familiar doesn't it.

I think one of the funniest moments of the lab year was when Don McCarthy failed to return to Pittsburgh after the ORS in San Francisco. He took the scenic route back to the Burg. We did have a great group of guys in the lab: John X, Pappas, Smith, Hung, and Jim. I have all fond memories. It was a great year!

Despite having a great lab year, I must of learned something because I scored in the 99th percentile in basic science on the ABOS exam.

I wish you another 70 years of health and prosperity!

Sincerely,
Chris

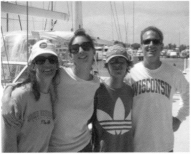

Happy Birthday from Camille, Corrine, Dan and Chris!

DR. SAVIO WOO – THE RESEARCHER, TEACHER AND OLYMPIC MEDALIST

C. Benjamin Ma

University of California, San Francisco
San Francisco, California, 94122, U.S.A.
E-mail: maben@orthosurg.ucsf.edu

I joined the Musculoskeletal Research Center in 1997 when I completed my one-year research experience during my orthopaedic residency. I did not expect that year to have such an impact on my development, but looking back at my training, it surely had been my turning point into academic medicine.

My year at the MSRC was a memorable one. There were projects after projects and the 'robot' was busy every day. It was amazing how many 'smart' people there were in the laboratory. We had experts in ligament research, cartilage research, spine and shoulder investigations. The breath of research was amazing. Moreover, the group was quite productive and it was rare that a meeting goes by without one of the laboratory members or studies being recognized. However, my most lasting experience of the laboratory was my first laboratory meeting. As a brand new resident researcher coming out from general surgery internship, I have no idea how to present my study. I can tell you that a scientific presentation is very different than presenting vital signs and laboratory values during morning ward rounds. I could not articulate a sound hypothesis, nor did I understand the difference between the definition of mechanical properties and structural properties. After the presentation, I remember Dr. Woo teaching me and my fellow research resident on how to present in front of a group and how to present a scientific study. I still use these tools on my own presentations and also my students now.

The highlight of the laboratory during that year was Dr. Woo's award of the first Olympic Gold Medal for the 1998 Winter Olympic Games. The laboratory was full of joy and it was great to be part of the celebration. It was a great year for the MSRC. My laboratory 'year' did not end in 1998. I am fortunate to be part of the MSRC family and the knowledge that I gained, mentorship that I received, and friendship that I developed will last forever.

Dr. Woo, thank you for all your teaching and guidance over the years and happy 70th birthday!

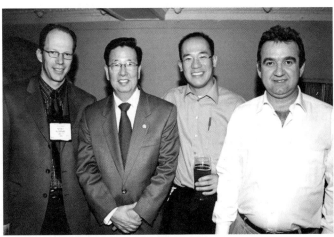

With Dr. Kevin Hildebrand, Dr. Woo and Dr. Christos Papageorgiou

DISCIPLINE & INSPIRATION
A BRIEF STORY OF GOOD MENTORSHIP

Christopher A. Carruthers

University of Pittsburgh
Pittsburgh, Pennsylvania, 15218, U.S.A.
E-mail: chc86@pitt.edu

Dr. Woo has been both a mentor and a friend to me. I first met Dr. Woo during the summer of 2006 through the Pittsburgh Tissue Engineering Initiative. Dr. Woo graciously hosted seven undergraduate student researchers at the renowned Musculoskeletal Research Center (MSRC). Working at the MSRC in multi-disciplinary research with the support and guidance of extraordinary researchers gave me valuable insight into the scientific process, applied engineering, and clinically relevant research. Dr. Woo gave all of us the opportunity to participate in the weekly lab meetings where we developed the ability to critically evaluate our peers' research. At the conclusion of the summer internship we all participated in an undergraduate symposium, where each undergraduate presented the culmination of their work to the entire center. The time, the guidance, and the education that I received gave me valuable encouragement.

From this experience I found a passion in the field of biomechanics in regenerative medicine. I decided to pursue a doctoral degree at the University of Pittsburgh and Dr. Woo has supported me throughout this process. Be it meeting with me to give me advice on how to be successful, or inviting me to dinner at one of his favorite restaurants, Dr. Woo's support has been unrelenting. I thank Dr. Woo for both inspiring me, and helping me to attain my own aspirations. Congratulations Dr. Woo on turning 70 years young, and for not only your success, but the lasting impact that you have made on the field of biomechanics both through your research and your mentorship.

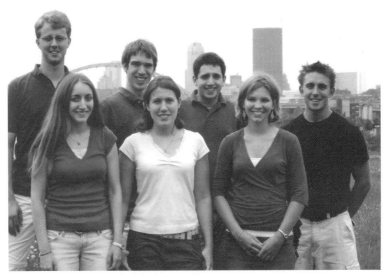

MSRC Summer Students Class of 2006

LUNCHTIME IN THE LIBRARY: THE TALENTED STORYTELLER

Katie Farraro

University of Pittsburgh
Pittsburgh, Pennsylvania, 15206, U.S.A.
E-mail: kfarraro@gmail.com

As a graduate student in Dr. Woo's lab beginning in the fall of 2010, I have had the privilege of getting to know Dr. Woo over the past year. I clearly remember my first meeting with him as a prospective graduate student, where I was quickly able to tell that he cared deeply for his students on both a professional and personal level. In addition to describing his lab and his work in biomechanics, he asked me many questions about myself and my career goals over a tasty lunch at a local Chinese restaurant, and despite his prestige, I found him to be very welcoming and easy to talk to. I left the meeting with the feeling that this lab was definitely a place where I would fit in.

A year later, this first instinct has certainly proven to be true, and I have immensely enjoyed my time so far as a student in Dr. Woo's lab. I think the best way to describe Dr. Woo's group is that everyone works hard, but also knows how to have a good time. Clearly, his body of work reflects the impressive research his lab has produced over the years, but he and Mrs. Woo have also been kind enough to invite his group to many socials at their home, and Dr. Woo also often treats students to Pittsburgh sporting events or to meals out at Panera Bread and other local restaurants. In fact, weekday lunches in the lab library have become one of the group's greatest traditions, when everyone gathers together around the table to eat and chat for the lunch hour. Not only is this a pleasant mid-day break from the laboratory or computer, but it really creates a strong sense of camaraderie within the group. There is never a quiet or dull moment at the table, with diverse topics of conversation including the latest news in politics, childhood stories, and even "Dancing with the Stars"! Dr. Woo is also quite the talented storyteller, and always has an entertaining story to share about his recent travels, the latest in Pitt sports, or his adorable grandchildren in California, Zadie and Arden. As I am a native of the San Francisco Bay Area, we have also found a special connection in our love of this region, often discussing landmarks, local cuisine, and the beautiful sunny weather.

As we reflect back on Dr. Woo's career on his 70th birthday, I would like to congratulate him on all of his achievements thus far. I feel very fortunate to have the opportunity to learn from the wisdom and experience he has gained over such a successful career, and I am grateful to him for sharing advice and lessons with me that I can carry with me as a graduate student and in my future career. I have learned so much in just this past year and look forward to continuing my studies under Dr. Woo and enjoying many more library lunches in the coming year and beyond!

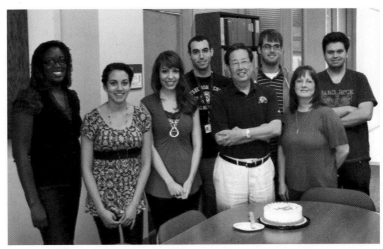

Dr. Woo's birthday celebration at the MSRC, June 2011

DR. WOO'S 70TH BIRTHDAY TRIBUTE
TIES IN PITTSBURGH AND TOKYO

Takatoshi Shimomura

Otsu Municipal Hospital
Otsu, Shiga, 520-0804, Japan
E-mail: t.shimomura@municipal-hospital.otsu.shiga.jp

I was the fourth Japanese fellow from the Orthopaedic Surgery Department of Kobe University. Prof. Mizuno introduced me to Dr. Woo in July 2000. I worked with Dr. Fengyan Jia in antisense gene therapy in an injured MCL model. During my time at the MSRC, I met many faculty, international fellows, residents and students. That precious memory, which Dr. Woo provided, is still my fortune.

When I was to move to Pittsburgh, Dr. Woo encouraged me to bring Kazumi (my spouse), because she was pregnant. Reika (my daughter) was born in Pittsburgh December 3, 2000 in Magee Women's Hospital. Not only I, but our family could enjoy the 2-year fellowship in Pittsburgh.

Happy 70th birthday Dr. Woo! I wish Dr. and Mrs. Woo health and happiness.

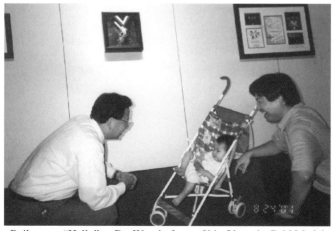

Reika says "Hello" to Dr. Woo in front of his Olympic Gold Medal.

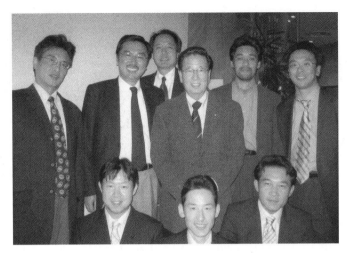

Myself (front row, left) and previous Japanese fellows attended the first ISL&T meeting in Tokyo, hosted by Prof. Takai (back row, second from left).
I recognized the strong ties between Dr. Woo and Japanese fellows even in Tokyo.

COMMITMENT, DEDICATION AND PRIDE

Andrew Feola

University of Pittsburgh
Pittsburgh, Pennsylvania, 15219, U.S.A.
E-mail: ajf12@pitt.edu

During the relatively early stages of my academic career, I have had the unique opportunity and good fortune of being part of the Musculoskeletal Research Center headed by Dr. Woo. Even though I was not a doctorate student of Dr. Woo, he always treated me as a member of his laboratory and regarded me with the same high expectations he held for his own graduate students. I am grateful Dr. Woo held me to these higher standards because it helped me become a better researcher and presenter. At the beginning of my graduate career, I contributed to a review article in honor of Dr. Y.C. Fung, which was overseen by Dr. Woo. It was my first experience writing a journal article and became my first publication. The lessons I learned throughout this experience will help me continue to publish high-quality journal articles for the rest of my time in academics.

Dr. Woo often stresses the importance of good work ethic and quality research, but aside from this serious side of Dr. Woo, he still understands the need to relax and enjoy each other's company. Dr. Woo, who is a season ticket holder to Pitt's football and basketball teams and often can get his hands on a few coveted Penguin tickets, has always been kind enough to invite several students to attend the games with him or give the tickets away to students to allow for some much needed time together outside of the work environment. Dr. Woo and I have frequently discussed at great lengths the Pittsburgh Penguins. Our conversations have included the current trades, roster moves, upcoming prospects, injury reports, and overall performance of the players. Ironically, the MSRC philosophy of commitment, dedication, and pride was quite applicable to following the Penguins during hockey season. Although I am positive that my use of this philosophy is not how it was originally intended, it is a motto I referred to each day as we discussed the recent games and hope for the future. As a fortuitous result of our shared passion for the game, Dr. Woo has been kind enough to invite me to several hockey games over the past five years and together we often enjoyed good food, a good game, and great company.

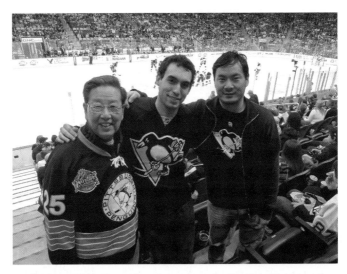

Dr. Woo (left) attending the Penguins victory over the Devils with his graduate student Kwang Kim (right) and myself (middle)

These experiences with Dr. Woo - in and outside the laboratory - have been both educational and gratifying. I have learned a great deal from him, ranging from how to run a successful laboratory to how to conduct oneself in both professional and personal situations. I would like to take this opportunity to wish Dr. Woo a happy 70th birthday. May you have many more, and I look forward to more good times together - and more playoff hockey!

THANK YOU FROM NORTHEASTERN JAPAN

Yasuyuki Ishibashi

Hirosaki University
Hirosaki, Aomori, 036-8562, Japan
E-mail: yasuyuki@cc.hirosaki-u.ac.jp

We, at the Department of Orthopaedic Surgery, Hirosaki University Graduate School of Medicine, are deeply grateful for Professor Woo's help and generosity while we were doing our research fellowships at the University of Pittsburgh, both professionally and personally. His encouragement, support, and thoughtful suggestions while doing biomechanics research at his lab was of great value and our experience in the US was of tremendous help when we returned to Japan. I strongly believe that our research experience at the MSRC has made a difference in providing our patients with superior orthopaedic care.

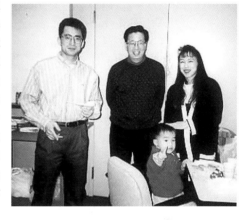

During my stay in Pittsburgh, Professor & Mrs. Woo extended their hospitality to my family when my daughter, Hikaru, was born. Financial assistance was also given to us through the MSRC and we were also able to use the insurance provided by the University of Pittsburgh. The staff at the MSRC threw a birthday party to commemorate the birth of my daughter, one which I remember to this day.

Congratulations on your 70th birthday and may the partnership of our institutions thrive as we continue our efforts to provide the highest quality patient-centered care through research.

A FANTASTIC LEADER

Stefano Zaffagnini

Istituti Ortopedici Rizzoli
Bologna, 40136, Italy
E-mail: s.zaffagnini@biomec.ior.it

Dear Savio,
I have had the pleasure to be one of your foreign post-doctoral fellows and probably the first Italian one.

When I arrived in Pittsburgh on the 21st of August in 1993, I did not know what was expected of me from the scientific and social point of view and I was a little bit scared about it.

However, on Monday morning when I had the pleasure to start my fellowship by participating in the Lab Meeting, I immediately realize what fortune I had to be involved in a group with such a fantastic leader.

The six months I spend with you in the lab, has formed and created my scientific background and I learned the approach on how to perform a good research project.

The enthusiasm, the time, and effort spent to create and develop new projects have inspired me so significantly that, now, I could not only be a simple orthopedic surgeon, but I need to produce research to improve knowledge in our scientific field.

I believe that what I have reached in the years after my fellowship from research viewpoint is definitely related to inspiration obtained during the fantastic time spent with you.

From the social point of view, it was again extremely positive.

You know that I could not forget my stay in Pittsburgh because Giulia was born there. I really want to thank you for the warmth and attention that you gave to my family in this important and beautiful time. It was extremely helpful and you and Pattie helped us so much that we really did not feel the sadness of being far from home during this precious moment.

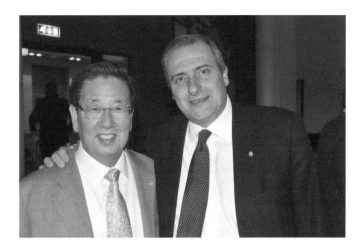

Therefore, I want to say thank you for your help in letting me grow. I am sure that without this time with you, I could never have become who I am now. I am very proud to have been one of your fellows and I hope you will continue to inspire thousands of others.

Happy, Happy Birthday Savio!
With all my Best Greetings,
Stefano Zaffagnini

ALMOST LIKE A FATHER

Masayoshi Yagi

Kobe, Japan
E-mail: mayagi@yagi-seikeigeka.jp

I would like to offer my sincere congratulations to Dr. Woo on his 70th birthday.

How times flies! It has been 12 years since I studied at MSRC. From 1998 to 2000, I was given the opportunity to study under the direction of Dr. Woo thanks to a recommendation by Professor Kosaku Mizuno of Kobe University, Japan.

When I first started my new life in Pittsburgh, I struggled to adjust. I kept facing all sorts of problems; not just academically, but also in terms of personal growth. Fortunately, Dr. Woo was always there to give me his kind advice; he was almost like a father to me. I was able to learn so many things that I could not have known in Japan. For all he has done, I really do not know how to express my deep appreciation. From the bottom of my heart, I thank him for his kindness. And wish him many happy returns of the day!

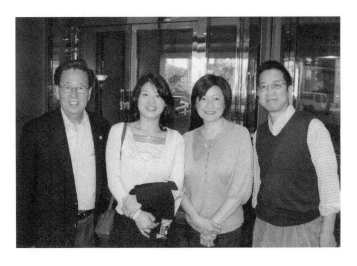

CELEBRATING WITH FAMILY AND FRIENDS

Becky (Levine) Leibowitz
*ETHICON, a Johnson & Johnson Company
Scotch Plains, New Jersey, 07076, U.S.A.
E-mail: bec_lei@comcast.net*

I was a graduate student at the University of Pittsburgh from 1991-1996 and spent most of those years conducting doctoral research at the MSRC with other students, staff, research fellows, and residents. We were a close-knit bunch and Dr. Woo encouraged team work and instilled a sense of family in us. We heard stories about and looked forward to meeting "older siblings" – students who had come before us. New family members arrived each year and others graduated or returned to their home countries. Each year, the new family would grow close as we ran our experiments in the lab, sat on the carpet in the hallway eating lunch, and taught each other new languages (or accents - I tried to no avail to teach a Japanese research fellow to speak English with a New York accent, but did pick up a pretty good Sapporo accent). Dr. Woo encouraged us to celebrate with each other and each other's families, inviting everyone to his house for a summertime picnic or to the Carnegie Museum for the annual Holiday party. This photo shows me with Dr. and Mrs. Woo in 1993; we traveled all the way from Pittsburgh to northern California to celebrate a student's wedding. So for a milestone such as this, I am honored to be among the family and friends paying tribute and congratulating Dr. Woo on his 70th birthday. Enjoy the celebrations and best wishes!

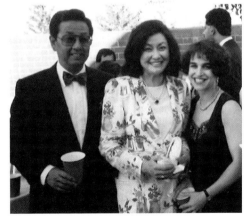

DR. WOO: MY MENTOR FOREVER

Yuhua Song

*University of Alabama at Birmingham
Birmingham, Alabama, 35294, U.S.A.
E-mail: yhsong@uab.edu*

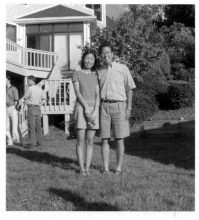

Ten years ago (2001), I joined Dr. Woo's Musculoskeletal Research Center (MSRC) as a postdoctoral research fellow to develop a computational model of knee joint and a subject-specific anterior cruciate ligament (ACL) model. The nearly two year post-doctoral training with Dr. Woo as my mentor was a life-long beneficial experience for me. I not only learned from Dr. Woo how to perform serious research, but Dr. Woo also served as my role model for being a great educator and mentor. The open and active research environment at the MSRC led by Dr. Woo opened a window for me to understand the importance of integrating the knowledge of engineering and biology for studying biomechanics, tissue engineering and regenerative medicine. This drove me to want to learn more biology, biophysics and biochemistry beyond my engineering education. Ultimately, this led to my post-doctoral training at the Department of Biochemistry and Molecular Biophysics at Washington University in St. Louis, and further as an Assistant Professor in the Department of Biomedical Engineering at The University of Alabama at Birmingham. My education and training with Dr. Woo laid a solid foundation for my pursuit of an academic career. My research group is currently using integrated multi-scale computational modeling and biochemical and biological experimental approaches to investigate the fundamental structural and functional mechanisms of the biomolecular interactions underlying the apoptosis and cell adhesion signaling pathways.

I was fortunate to get a chance to celebrate Dr. Woo's 60th birthday in 2001. I would like to join together with all Dr. Woo's students and trainees to congratulate Dr. Woo on his 70th birthday. I send my best and most sincere wishes for Dr. and Mrs. Woo for a continued happy and healthy life. I look forward to celebrating Dr. Woo's 80th birthday.

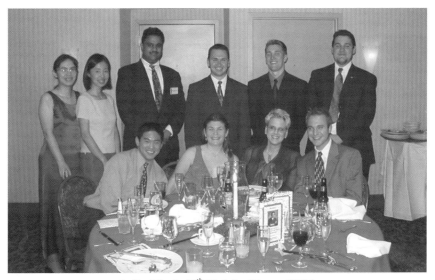

At Dr. Woo's 60th Birthday Dinner (2001)

TO MY LIFETIME MENTOR ON HIS SEVENTIETH BIRTHDAY

Fengyan Jia

Allegheny General Hospital
Pittsburgh, Pennsylvania, 15212, U.S.A.
E-mail: fyjia@hotmail.com

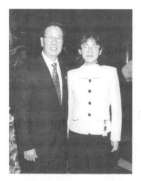

As a fellow and staff working at the Musculoskeletal Research Center (MSRC) from 1999 to 2005, I am honored to have had the chance to work with you on various research projects. I learned almost every aspect about life from you, and it will stay with me forever.

I still remember the day I interviewed for the job opening at the MSRC, you told me to not only work hard, but also to work smart. Later, you led our research center, taught us how to work smart for high quality research, and how to present in front of a big audience. All the training I received from the MSRC helped me later in my training program and new job. How could I forget all the parties at your house, my kids are still talking about the good time they had there.

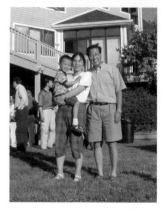

It is your birthday and my whole family wants to congratulate you on your successful life – all those countless awards. More important, we want to let you know our appreciation. Your teaching rooted so deep, it forever changed our life. Happy birthday!

THE DAYS OF OUR YEARS
- A TRIBUTE TO DR. WOO ON HIS 70TH BIRTHDAY

Changfu Wu

Food and Drug Administration
Silver Spring, Maryland, 20993, U.S.A.
E-mail: cwu70@yahoo.com

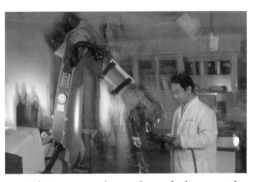

I completed my postdoctoral training with Dr. Woo at the MSRC in 2006 and 2007. I was the leader for the ACL Laboratory.

While working on my doctoral dissertation on mechanical heart valves, I became interested in the field of bioengineering and wanted to expand my knowledge on the "bio" side of bioengineering. Right after the New Year of 2006, I had the fortune to come to the MSRC whose motto is "education through research." In the nearly two years that followed, like over 100 other MSRC alumni, from undergraduates to graduates, to post-doctoral and clinical fellows, I was deeply immersed in a research environment that seamlessly integrated research at the molecular/cellular level, tissue level, joint level, and computational level. Outside the lab, Dr. Woo joined us at the Steelers' Super Bowl XL parade on a freezing February morning and took us to Pitt basketball games. Today, my son and I remain Steelers fans in the land of the Ravens. By the time I completed my training, I found that I had stepped from the outside to the inside of the gate of biomedical engineering. For this, I am always indebted to Dr. Woo and the MSRC.

"The days of our years are threescore years and ten" (Psalm 90:10). A great Chinese poet in the Tang Dynasty, Du Pu (杜甫), also said, "人生七十古来稀." Congratulations on achieving another milestone in your life, Dr. Woo!

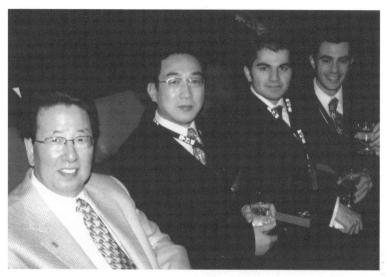

Dr. Woo, myself, Ozgur Dede, and Alex Almarza
at the Carnegie Science Center 2006 Awards for Excellence Ceremony
where Dr. Woo received the "Life Sciences Award"

THE BEST TEACHER

Sarita Maheedhara
Seattle, Washington, 98021, U.S.A.
E-mail: maheedhara_s@yahoo.com

I was Dr. Woo's graduate student from 2004-2006. Dr. Woo influenced my life to a great extent. He was - and still is - the best teacher from whom I have learned not just academically, but also on a personal front. Dr. & Mrs. Woo are very compassionate and always made me feel at home, even though I was just a graduate student. Dr. Woo and the MSRC are very near & dear to my heart and I will never forget my experiences with them.

Dear Dr. Woo - hearty congratulations to you on this very special occasion and for all of your lifetime achievements!

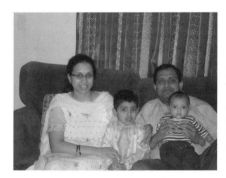

With my husband, Sree and sons, Nishanth, & Arjun

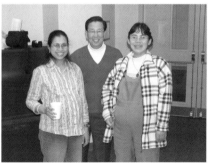

With Dr. Woo and Dr. Fengyan Jia

COMPASSIONATE INSTRUCTIONS

Yuji Yamamoto

Hirosaki University Graduate School of Medicine
Hirosaki, Aomori, 036-8562, Japan
E-mail: yuji1112@aol.com

I was a post-doctoral research fellow at the MSRC from September, 2002 to March, 2004. Under Dr. Woo's direction, I performed ACL biomechanical research with Drs. Wei-Hsiu Hsu and Yoshi Takakura, Andy Van Scyoc, Jesse Fisk, and other members of the ACL group. During my stay in Pittsburgh, Dr. Woo taught me many things, such as how to plan a research project and implement it, as well as how to write a scientific paper and review it. I would like to thank Dr. Woo for his compassionate instructions.

I took my family to Pittsburgh when my son, Reo was just 1 month old. Dr. and Mrs. Woo were always very kind to my family. A picture of my son, which Mrs. Woo took, is still displayed in my home. He is now 9 years old and in 4th grade of elementary school. In fact, he is now a big brother to a sister who is 8 years younger than him.

Many congratulations and much happiness on your birthday!

Thank you again for everything you have done for us.

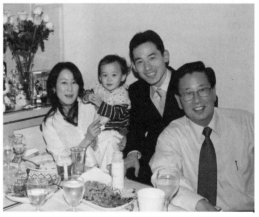

My family and Dr. Woo at ORS San Francisco (2004)

A WISE MENTOR

Ben Rothrauff

University of Pittsburgh
Pittsburgh, Pennsylvania, 15217, U.S.A.
E-mail: Ben.Rothrauff@gmail.com

I had the good fortune of working in the MSRC in the summer of 2010 as an incoming student in the MD/PhD program at the University of Pittsburgh. As an aspiring orthopaedic surgeon-scientist, I was drawn to Pitt due to its breadth and excellence in orthopaedic research, most notably that of Dr. Woo and his work on ACL regeneration. But having limited undergraduate exposure to biomechanics and tissue engineering, I had doubts regarding my ability to assimilate into a new field.

Within minutes of meeting, Dr. Woo allayed my concerns as he explained his philosophy on research and educating scientists. My feeling of incompetence was transformed into excitement about the opportunity to learn and grow. In time, Dr. Woo helped me appreciate scientific investigation as a process, where sheer will and the dedication to discovery can overcome any initial ignorance. Though I only spent a short time with Dr. Woo, I consider him one of my most influential mentors.

With that, I offer the sincerest of thanks to Dr. Woo for his commitment to education and his innumerable contributions to orthopaedic research. Congratulations on 70 years of a wonderful life, and warm wishes for many more to come!

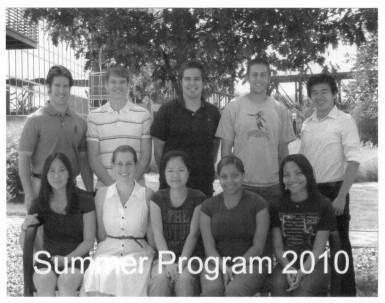

Front Row (L-R): Elizabeth Chen, Nicole Scarbrough, Fei Yan Lin, Shannon Prentiss, Tavia Binger
Back Row (L-R): myself, Dan Browe, Josh Mealy, Brad Edelman, Kelvin Luu

THE LAST "REAL" TEACHER

Matteo Maria Tei

University of Perugia
Perugia, 06127, Italy
E-mail: matteotei@gmail.com

I had the opportunity to attend the Musculoskeletal Research Center (MSRC) directed by Dr. Woo in 2010-2011, the year of his 70th birthday. Now it is an honor for me to contribute to his tribute book. It was a pleasure and an incredible opportunity to have had the chance to work with Dr. Woo as an Orthopaedic Fellow at the MSRC in Pittsburgh. Dr. Woo is a distinguished professor and a pioneer in the bioengineering field, but I consider him most of all a great man and a close friend. Dr. Woo is one of the last "real" teachers, he loves to teach, not just about biomechanics, he was for me a mentor of life. I learned in his laboratory more than ever in my life, and Dr. Woo taught me the basics for my future career. I miss eating with him at Chinese restaurants and going to watch Pitt Panthers basketball games. In a year, I became one of the best Italian guys to eat with chopsticks.

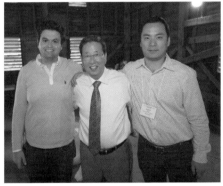

With Dr. Savio Woo and Kwang Kim (2011)

With cordial gratitude and best regards to Dr. Woo, Mrs. Woo and all their family!

A PRIVILEDGE TO MEET DR. WOO
AS A PERSON AND AS A PROFESSIONAL

Gustavo Miguel Azcona Arteaga

Regional Military Hospital in Sonora, Mexico
Col. Loma Linda, Hermosillo, Son, Mexico
E-mail: gusyena@netscape.net

I had the opportunity to work with Dr. Woo during the period of July 1999 to August 2000, at the entrance of the new century.

As a Fellow visitor at UPMC, I had the idea of investigating some new advances in the Musculoskeletal Research Center (MSRC). I interviewed with Dr. Savio Woo, and he accepted me as part of the group studying the MCL, where I learned all the current techniques in tissue repairs.

It was a great privilege to meet him as a professional and as a family person. We were invited to spend Thanksgiving dinner with his family at his beautiful home in Pittsburgh; memories that my wife and I cherish with joy and happiness since they treated us like family and made us feel at home. My children felt comfortable enough that they started dancing and having fun with Dr. Woo's teenage children. That night he spoke about his recent trip to California, and I recall him telling how he enjoyed walking down to the park watching and observing the wonderful trees around him. My thought at that moment was "Wow, how can a successful man as Dr. Woo still be as sensible that he can enjoy simple things as the smell of the trees......?!" I hope I can be like him, when I get to his age. To me he is a role model to follow.

As his student and friend, I send my very best wishes to him and his dear wife Mrs. Woo, hoping for health and keeping that brilliant research career for many years to come. We look forward to celebrating his 80th birthday.

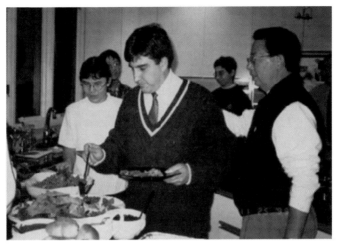

Dr. Woo giving us some tips on good food.

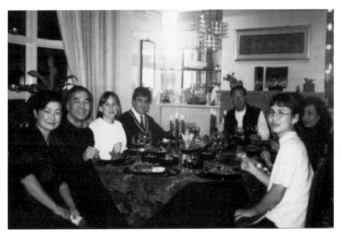

Thanksgiving dinner at Dr. and Mrs. Woo's home
A night to remember.

HAPPY 70TH BIRTHDAY DR. WOO!

Eiichi Tsuda

Hirosaki University Graduate School of Medicine
Hirosaki, Aomori, 036-8562, Japan
E-mail: eiichi@cc.hirosaki-u.ac.jp

I was a research fellow at the MSRC from October 1999 to September, 2001. My research consisted of performing biomechanical analysis of the ACL under Dr. Woo's supervision. While doing research at the MRSC, I was fortunate enough to attend Dr. Woo's 60th birthday celebration. It was very busy organizing such as large party, but I was glad be a part of such a special occasion and I remember it very fondly.

My experience in Pittsburgh had a very positive effect on my family also. My daughter is considering studying at a university in the United States because she had such a great experience there. Her English grades are excellent, even though 10 years have passed. My wife and son also remember their time in Pittsburgh and retain some American customs. Every year for the last 10 years, they still celebrate their favorite holiday, Halloween - by inviting 100 neighbors and guests. I would like to take this opportunity to thank Dr. Woo and his family, and all the staff at MRSC for welcoming my family 10 years ago. Happy 70th Birthday, Dr. Woo.

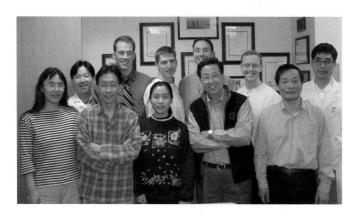

HEARTIEST CONGRATULATIONS

Rajesh Jari

Spine Medicine and Rehabilitation Therapies
Westminster, Maryland, 21157, U.S.A.
E-mail: rjari1@gmail.com

Heartiest Congratulations to Dr. Woo on this grand occasion and on so many remarkable achievements. You have been an incredible mentor to so many students, and fellows, helping them achieve great academic accomplishments.

I recall how I met you while at a Wimbledon Tennis Tournament and Conference where you were a keynote speaker in 2000. Subsequently through your efforts, I joined the MSRC as a research fellow.

I particularly remember Dr. Woo organizing breakfast get-togethers for the soccer world cup games. This was very memorable indeed. Shama (my wife) and I still remember coming to your beautiful home and enjoying your kind hospitality.

After my research fellowship at the MSRC, I joined Johns Hopkins University/Hospital for a 4-year research fellowship and then went on to complete my residency still at Johns Hopkins. I then completed an interventional spine/pain fellowship at Temple University and am now in private practice in Baltimore.

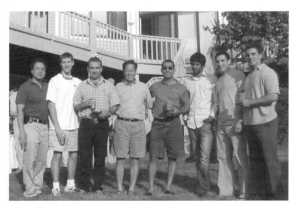

Again, congratulations and I thank you.

TRIBUTE TO DR. WOO FROM THE STEHLE'S

Jens Stehle

Clinic for Sports Medicine Ravensburg
Weingarten, Germany
E-mail: stehles@gmx.de

We first met Dr. Woo at the MSRC in Pittsburgh 2001 when we visited the US to find the best place for me to study biomechanics. After all my grants were funded, we came in 2003 to the MSRC and I worked until 2005 in the shoulder group with Drs. Debski and McMahon. We had the time of our life in Pittsburgh and our first son, Noah, was born there in 2004. Dr. Woo invited us to several parties at his home, made it possible for us to visit conferences, meet numerous people, and find friends from all over the world. After we left Pittsburgh, we were able to visit Pittsburgh several times as well as have met each other on numerous occasions. Dr. Woo even accepted an invitation to come to Wuerzburg in 2006 for a conference where the picture below was taken. In the meantime, we proliferated and since 2011, we are five Stehles (after Noah came Marah and lately Micah)

We want to thank Dr. Woo for the great times we had in Pittsburgh and all the possibilities he offered to us.

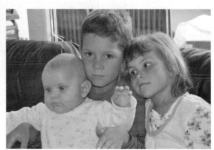

Micah, Noah and Marah

"UNCLE SAVIO"

Chee-Hahn Hung

*Greater Metropolitan Orthopaedic Institute
Clinton, Maryland, 20735, U.S.A.
E-mail: cheehung@gmail.com*

"Uncle Savio", as he was known in our house, with his sports car, wine cellar, and various skiing photos, was more colorful than the typical Chinese engineering immigrant in Pittsburgh, and was like a kindred spirit with my Dad. Little did I know, that when Uncle Savio got me a summer job at the MSRC, a position I was woefully unqualified for, that was something designed to keep me occupied for the summer and be a notch on my resume, would become such a memorable experience. Years later, I would become a musculoskeletal doctor and manage patients with the same titanium hip implants that I had studied that summer. For that, I will be always grateful.

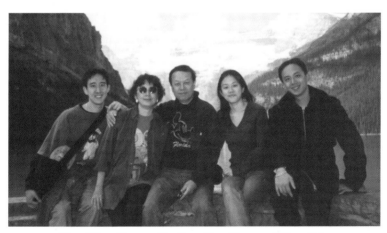

Chee-Ming, Shunan, Tin-Kan, Chee-Yuen and Chee-Hahn

HAPPY BIRTHDAY DR. WOO!

David Provenzano

Ohio Valley General Hospital
McKees Rocks, Pennsylvania, 15136, U.S.A.
E-mail: davidprovenzano@hotmail.com

For periods of time from 1993-1996, I worked as an Intern and Research Assistant at the Musculoskeletal Research Center (MSRC). This time period occurred during my summer breaks from college and medical school. I truly value the time that I spent in the research lab. I was exposed to both basic and clinical science projects. Projects included studying the interosseus membrane and flexor tendon repairs. Dr. Woo and the rest of the team were extremely generous with their time and guidance. In addition, I always remember how they valued input from every individual of the research group. The time spent at the MSRC helped cultivate my interest in research and advancing the field of medicine. It was truly an honor to be part of a first-class research department at a young age. Dr. Woo created and promoted a productive family atmosphere. I still remember going to his home for the summer gatherings.

Thank you Dr. Woo! You have accomplished so much and cultivated the future research careers of many individuals. I am ever grateful for the opportunities that you and your team provided me.

MY TRIBUTE TO DR. WOO

Eric Wong

DFine, Inc.
San Jose, California, 95134, U.S.A.
E-mail: ewong@alumni.duke.edu

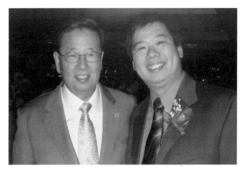

I have known Dr. Woo since I was a summer student in 1993 at the Musculoskeletal Research Center (MSRC). I returned home to Pittsburgh and the MSRC for the next few summers and finally became a graduate student after I finished my undergraduate degree at Duke. After completing my Masters degree with Dr. Woo as my advisor, I moved to the San Francisco Bay Area in 2001 to start my career as a Biomedical Engineer, which I still am to this day. The foundation for everything that I do at work is from what I learned at the MSRC from Dr. Woo.

I wish to congratulate Dr. and Mrs. Woo for having such a great family: nuclear, extended, and academic (both in San Diego and Pittsburgh). The relationships I have developed through the MSRC are very dear to me, and I appreciate all the advice and wisdom Dr. Woo has passed on to me over the years. I look forward to seeing him every time I go home to Pittsburgh for Christmas. I also cherish his visits to the Bay Area, which luckily are occurring more often with Kirstin, Jonathan and the grandkids so close to where I live now.

Jean and I would like to wish you a Happy 70th Birthday and here is to many, many more.

Chapter 5

Tributes

from

Colleagues and Friends

A TOAST TO SAVIO

Y. C. and Luna Fung
University of California, San Diego
La Jolla, California, 92093, U.S.A.
E-mail: cfung@earthlink.net

To Dear Savio,

It has been such a joy to be your friend and colleague for such a long time – a combined 82 years if we count in both directions – and to see your career and family blossom.

Our scientific discoveries during our long collaboration, and your pioneering work in the years since, have accumulated to an extraordinary contribution to humanity. Each discovery, and each interaction, has been personally satisfying.

The personal connection is most precious. How rare is the chance to combine work and friendship, so deeply, and for so long! We have been blessed with more than our share of harmony and opportunities. Living close by for 20 years enabled our families to become fast friends, and bioengineering conference organizers pick such great venues that our community has remained close for decades since.

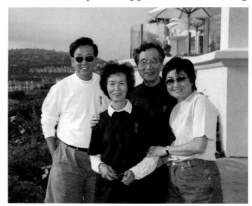

We remember celebrating your and Pattie's 30th anniversary on Laguna Beach, and the lesson of the beautiful day.

A Lesson at Laguna Beach, 1999 (revisited)

The sky and the sea had the same shades of blue.
The white crests of the waves sparkled over the sea
    like frolicsome gulls.
The sun was warm, and the breeze was cool.
We backed up the hill from the water's edge,
with our eyes looking at the ocean,
and using muscles I normally do not use.
Our vista increased with our steps,
Our well being melted into the grandeur of the Pacific.

Savio, on this wonderful occasion of your 70th birthday, we toast you and Pattie, Jonathan, and Kirstin and her family, wishing you many, many happy returns and the best of health to you forever!

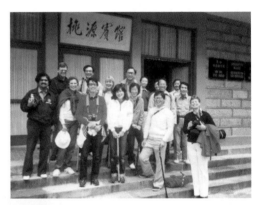

The Group for the Yellow Mountain Climb (1983)

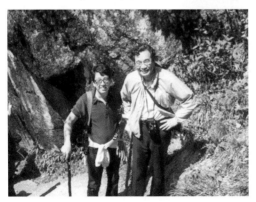

Two Pioneers on Yellow Mountain (1983)

HAPPY 70TH BIRTHDAY, DEAR SAVIO!

Shu Chien
University of California, San Diego
La Jolla, California, 92093-0427, U.S.A.
E-mail: shuchien@ucsd.edu

Warmest wishes for a Happy 70th Birthday!!

I had the pleasure of meeting you during the Biomechanics meeting in La Jolla in 1971; it is surprising that forty years have gone by, as it seemed like yesterday. I was very fortunate to come to the University of California, San Diego (UCSD) Bioengineering in 1988 when you were still here in Orthopaedic Surgery and Bioengineering. We had wonderful times together. I was very sorry to see you move to Pittsburgh. That was a big loss for UCSD, but it is great to see you developing to even greater heights by establishing the outstanding Musculoskeletal Research Center (MSRC), which is the world's leading Center in this field. I am very pleased and impressed to see your remarkable accomplishments in research and education. Your over 300 superb papers in tissue mechanics, robotics, computational modeling, and functional tissue engineering have set the standard and led the progress in these important fields of research in orthopaedic engineering. Your training of over 400 first-rate scientists, physicians and engineers will generate great impact for generations to come. You have received all the top awards and honors in your field. Besides being a member of the National Academy of Engineering and the Institute of Medicine of the National Academy of Sciences, it is a tremendous honor to be bestowed the Olympic Gold Medal at the 1998 Winter Olympic Games in Nagano.

You have been passionate and dedicated to the promotion of science and engineering in the United States and in other countries. I enjoy very much working with you at the annual meetings in Taiwan to review the grant applications submitted to the National Health Research Institutes (NHRI). I am always impressed by your marvelous ability to lead the review sessions as Chair of the Bioengineering Study Section. It clearly shows your profound knowledge, broad perspectives, fair judgment, and superb leadership, as well as your care for the advancement of scientific research in Taiwan.

Dear Savio, K.C. joins me in wishing you a Very Happy 70th Birthday and all the best to you and Pattie with many happy returns!

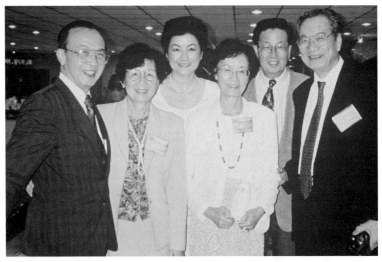

Shu Chien, K.C. Chien, Pattie Woo, Luna Fung, Savio Woo, Y.C. Fung

CONGRATULATIONS SAVIO ON YOUR 70TH BIRTHDAY!!

Albert and Betty Kobayashi
University of Washington
Seattle, Washington, 98195, U.S.A.
E-mail: ask@uw.edu

As I mentioned previously, progress is made only by the student exceeding his/her teacher. You have exceeded your teacher many times over for which I salute you.

In your recent invited lecture at the University of Washington, you looked almost the same as you did 27 years ago in the attached pictures taken in San Antonio. What is your secret for the fountain of youth?

Betty and I wish you and Pattie many happy and healthful years ahead and keep up the good work.

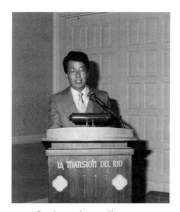

Savio at the podium

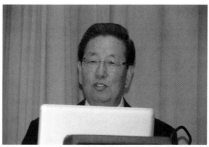

In Seattle (2011)

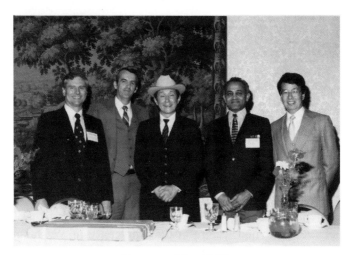

The gang of four PhD's

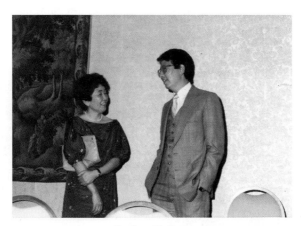

Savio with Betty

IN THE PRESENCE OF GREATNESS

Chancellor Michael Lovell

University of Wisconsin-Milwaukee
Milwaukee, Wisconsin, 53211, U.S.A.
E-mail: mlovell@uwm.edu

Every once in a great while you are given the opportunity to brush against greatness. These are times in your life when you meet and interact with an individual who exhibits a level of skill and ability that so far surpasses their peers that you remember them forever. I have been very fortunate to have had the opportunity to meet a handful of these individuals in my life.

First, there was playing basketball against Doug West in a PIAA playoff game in high school. Even though I only guarded Doug for a short few minutes, I knew that I had never played against anyone else like him before (or after). Doug went on to be a star at Villanova University and in the NBA for the Minnesota Timberwolves. Then there was Dr. John Swanson, my mentor and boss during my first job out of college at ANSYS Inc. John was the most intelligent person that I had ever met. Working with him was amazing - even after having hundreds of employees developing hundreds of thousands of lines of code with him for 25 years, John still personally knew every subroutine in ANSYS. He had the answer to any question that I ever had and would recall specific lines of code when I had questions. Finally, there was Savio Woo, the person we are honoring for his 70th birthday. A person like Doug West and John Swanson, Dr. Woo has awed me with his shear greatness for being innovative and for performing cutting-edge research.

Few people in my academic career have transcended time, but Savio has clearly been one of those individuals for me. I first encountered Savio as a graduate student at Pitt, when I attended his interview seminar back in 1989. He gave the most incredible talk on work that he had been doing on beagle osteochondral allografts. His work was so far ahead of the bioengineering field that I knew I was witnessing greatness. I was truly amazed and inspired by his research that, on the very day I attended his talk, I decided to pursue my PhD at Pittsburgh. As my career progressed and I got to work with Savio personally on a number of research proposals, my opinion of his abilities continued to expand. I can honestly state that he is the best researcher that I have personally interacted with in my career, which includes hundreds of highly talented individuals. I do not believe that we would have gotten the NSF Engineering Research Center grant without Savio being associated with it, his name carries that much weight in the scientific community. I am still inspired on how his work continues to improve the lives of others and literally change the world. All of the accolades and awards that he has received are well-deserved and serve to recognize his greatness.

There are several things that I miss about Savio now that I am in Milwaukee. The thing that I might miss the most is his Christmas parties. Savio has always had an extremely large research group, with individuals from all over the world. Each year Savio would host a party and all of the students and researchers would bring food to share from their native cultures. As an invited guest, I always looked forward to the parties and I took great pleasure in meeting the researchers and enjoying the holiday food and festivities from around the world. I was also so impressed by the camaraderie and civility exhibited at the party among those working in Savio's research lab. He truly was not just a great researcher, but a great mentor who was improving the career and lives of dozens of future academic and scientific leaders for decades to come.

For all that Savio has given to so many, I am very grateful to be able to provide a short message for Savio on his 70th birthday. He is a person that has exhibited greatness in all that he has done and he has been instrumental in transforming so many people's lives, including my own.

O! WHAT A BEAUTIFUL DAY

President H.K. Chang
*City University of Hong Kong
Kowloon, Hong Kong SAR
E-mail: hkchang@cityu.edu.hk*

That Dr. Savio L-Y. Woo is a scientist of the first rank is indisputable. But that alone could not account for my enthusiasm to write, while traveling in Kazakhstan, a few paragraphs in celebration of his 70th birthday. Indeed, when I think about what my long-time friend Savio is, I think of much more than a talented researcher and a caring teacher. He is, in my view, also a skilled organizer, a consummate diplomat and a brilliant strategist, in addition to being a loyal friend, if he thinks you deserve his friendship and a formidable adversary, if you make him one.

Let me explain. I had known Savio Woo by reputation for quite some time when we first met in 1983. I was immediately impressed by not only his accomplishments, but also his energy and enthusiasm. Later, I tried my best to recruit him to the Department of Biomedical Engineering at the University of Southern California. He and I went through a fairly long period of "romance", but to my chagrin, he eventually chose Pitt over USC and possibly others.

Little did I know at the time, that I would myself leave Los Angeles for Hong Kong a few years later and then became a candidate for deanship of the School of Engineering at Pitt. Even less would I have ever guessed, that Savio would serve on the Search Committee. He must have displayed his superior judgment in the selection process, for I was invited to join the Engineering School at Pitt!

After my arrival at Pitt in 1994, Savio and I worked together closely to enhance the already considerable strengths in Biomedical Engineering. These efforts, under the encouragement and guidance of Chancellor Mark Nordenberg, Dr. Tom Detre and Provost Jim Maher, led to very satisfactory and tangible results. It was in this period that I began to realize the qualities of Savio Woo which I mentioned above.

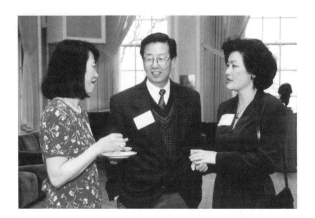

Fifteen years have gone by since I left Pitt for Hong Kong again. I occasionally get to see Savio in Hong Kong or Pittsburgh and also receive news about him and his wonderful family.

Now that my good friend Savio is celebrating his 70th birthday, I regret that I cannot be on hand to help celebrate this wonderful day with his family and other friends, but I would like to sing with my keyboard the line that I learned many years ago from the Broadway musical Oklahoma: "O! What a beautiful day!"

A TRIBUTE TO PROFESSOR SAVIO L-Y. WOO ON THE OCCASION OF HIS 70TH BIRTHDAY

Provost Emeritus James V. Maher

University of Pittsburgh
Pittsburgh, Pennsylvania, 15260, U.S.A.
E-mail: jvmaher@pitt.edu

Most members of sophisticated modern societies take research universities for granted, not realizing that they depend on those universities for: 1. the education of virtually all of society's leaders, including all of its scientists, engineers, and health professionals, along with the more visible leaders in government and business; 2. significant economic development in the environs of the university as the substantial research performed at the university drives local employment and more general prosperity; and 3. societal progress as the fruits of university research soften the harshness of the human condition both by alleviating hunger and suffering and by fostering humane approaches to social problems and the development of cultural life.

At the core of any good research university stands a faculty who educate the students, design the research programs, and generally drive the societal contributions of the university. If the faculty of the university do not include truly outstanding individuals, the university will not succeed. Professor Savio Woo stands out even in the company of the very best faculty. Over the years of his distinguished career, he has consistently performed research that has led to many improvements in the treatment of human injuries, and he has used both his laboratory and the classrooms in which he has taught to educate many of the world's best biomedical engineers. He also treats his faculty colleagues generously, contributing by his encouragement and example to the success of many of us.

All of us at the University of Pittsburgh deeply appreciate Professor Woo's important contributions to our success as a university and to the betterment of society in general. I am proud to be able to offer him this tribute on his 70th birthday, and I look forward to seeing him have many more productive years.

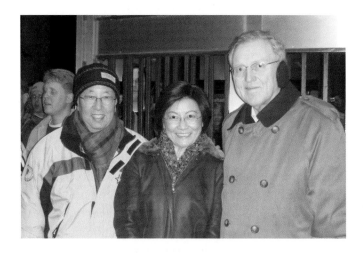

A MOST ACCOMPLISHED SCHOLAR, FAMILY MAN AND FRIEND

Dean Gerald Holder

University of Pittsburgh
Pittsburgh, Pennsylvania, 15261, U.S.A.
E-mail: holder@engr.pitt.edu

On the occasion of his 70th birthday, I can reflect on the impact that Dr. Savio Woo has had on the Swanson School of Engineering and me. He is arguably the most accomplished scholar ever to hold a faculty position in the Swanson School of Engineering. I would place him alongside Reginald Fessenden, the "father of radio" in the impact that his work has had on the world. His election to three national academies and his receipt of the Olympic Gold Medal in Sports Medicine are unique in the history of the school and something that every faculty member in the school can take pride in.

I really came to know Dr. Woo when we were applying for the first Whitaker Grant. Along with Jerry Schultz, he took a leading role in the successful application and deserves enormous credit for the birth of bioengineering at Pitt and for the rise of this program to the top of the national rankings. We worked more closely when he decided that his proper home was in the Bioengineering Department and that the MSRC should move to the Center for Bioengineering where it remains today. Soon after, Dr. Woo was selected for appointment as Distinguished University Professor which is the highest rank possible at the University of Pittsburgh. I still remember the ten page "summary" of his many accomplishments which itself might be a record. In this process, I got to more fully embrace the scope of Dr. Woo's worldwide impact and the deep respect for his scholarly work in biomechanics.

I also was fortunate to come to know Pattie and attend some of the gracious social events that she and Savio held at their home in Fox Chapel. It was at these events where I came to understand their love of and pride in their family, especially their children, Jonathan and Kirstin.

The Swanson School has been fortunate to have Dr. Woo as one of its leading scholars and international ambassadors. Today, at the young age of 70, he continues to provide leadership and serve as an outstanding example to our faculty.

Congratulations on your 70th birthday. May there be many more.

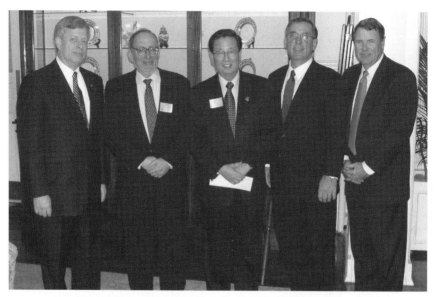

2005-2006 Swanson School of Engineering Board of Visitors
Faculty Award Recipient -- Dr. Savio L-Y. Woo
Chancellor Mark Nordenberg, Professor Harvey Borovetz, Dean Gerald Holder, and Tom Usher, Chairman of U.S. Steel and SSOE Board of Visitors

ESTEEMED FRIEND AND COLLEAGUE

Dean Cliff Brubaker
University of Pittsburgh
Pittsburgh, Pennsylvania, 15260, U.S.A.
E-mail: cliffb@pitt.edu

I had been aware of Savio Woo and his extensive scientific and scholarly contributions well in advance of our first meeting. This occurred in the fall of 1989 when a steering committee sponsored by the National Science Foundation was convened with the charge to form an organization that could speak authoritatively for the field of Bioengineering. Over the course of the next three years, this committee formulated and founded what is now the American Institute for Medical and Biological Engineering (AIMBE). At the outset of this effort, Savio was a Professor of Surgery (Orthopedics) at UC San Diego, and I was a Professor in the Department of Biomedical Engineering and Director of a Rehabilitation Engineering Research Center at the University of Virginia. By July 1991, we had both moved to the University of Pittsburgh – Savio to Orthopedics in the School of Medicine and later to Bioengineering. I have served as Dean of the School of Health and Rehabilitation Sciences (SHRS) since my arrival at Pitt in 1991. I take pride in noting that Savio has held a secondary appointment as Professor in SHRS over this period. I am both pleased and honored to acknowledge Savio L-Y. Woo as both an esteemed colleague and friend of more than 20 years.

I was privileged to attend Dr. Woo's induction to the Institute of Medicine in 1991 and to the National Academy of Engineering in 1994. I have had the pleasure of nominating him for the Chancellor's Distinguished Research Award, which he received in 1999. I also participated in his nomination to the rank of Distinguished University Professor in Bioengineering to which he was appointed in 2007. He has been at the forefront of discovery and innovation over the course of his remarkable career with seminal contributions to knowledge and to the development of new technologies. Notable among these has been his seminal research in the determination of the function of ligaments in the control and constraint of motions of joints, which he elucidated through a progression of studies based on robotic manipulations and computational simulations. This research has provided a basis for predictive models and led to both prophylactic measures for prevention of ligament injuries and also to the development of innovative procedures for surgical repair for restoration of function following severe injuries. He was particularly instrumental in providing evidence to support joint movement and early weight bearing in lieu of immobilization following surgical repair. The importance of this and other research to technological innovation for repair, healing and restoration of function is manifest in the remarkable array of awards and other forms of recognition that Dr. Woo has been accorded by national and international societies and organizations. Even with the remarkable number of seminal contributions Dr. Woo has made to the fields of bioengineering, biomechanics, orthopedics and rehabilitation, perhaps his greatest and most enduring legacy is evident in generations of scholars he has mentored who have also gone on to make seminal contributions to these disciplines.

It is indeed a pleasure for me to recognize and acknowledge the distinguished career of my esteemed friend and colleague, Dr. Savio L-Y. Woo, Distinguished University Professor of Bioengineering in the Swanson School of Engineering of the University of Pittsburgh, Member, Institute of Medicine and National Academy of Engineering, and consummate scholar and teacher. His contributions have been both extensive and exceptional. I consider my friendship and association with Dr. Woo a privilege and a highlight of my professional life.

FOR CELEBRATION OF THE SEVENTIETH ANNIVERSARY OF DR. SAVIO L-Y. WOO

Theodore Wu

Caltech
Pasadena, California, 91125, U.S.A.
E-mail: tywu@caltech.edu

The international academic collaborations on biomechanics began culminating from the 1984 Special Symposium so fittingly entitled "Frontiers in Biomechanics." Dr. Savio Woo is one of the Chief Editors working with Geert Schmid-Schönbein and Ben Zweifach in many talents to produce an innovative and provocative volume in honor of the 65th birthday of Professor Bert Yuan-Cheng Fung, now renowned worldwide as the Father of Biomechanics. Dr. Woo also made a pioneering contribution to the Congress Symposium entitled "Biomechanics in China, Japan, and U.S.A.," the first East-meeting-West Conference held at the beautiful East Lake (Dong Hu), Wuhan, China, in colorful May, 1983.

This writer has held a deep impression on the two papers (and more later) from these symposia by Savio Woo and co-authors on the soft tissues in animals, like tendons and ligaments, as well as their homeostasis with cortical bones. They evidently expounded a horrendous subject involving mechanical, biological, physiological, thermo-physical and countless nonlinear effects pertaining to all the various levels of activities. All these endless variations do exhibit some key features in differing facets. These features are so striking that they retain in mind, like, the first, the nonlinear strain-stress relations for various species of animals, and the different premises in making observations, etc. Another unexpected one reveals that impulsive exertions of these tissues may take hours to all relax.

As pointed out by Dr. Woo, all such underlying mechanisms may reach the molecular level, a penetrating viewpoint. This writer is also wondering what might furthermore arise as unseen phenomena if all the pertinent sorts of energies, including the thermo-physics and dissipation (in generating heat) be also accounted for. If the topic pursued at the Landau Institute in Moscow has any biochemo-physical ground, it may also appear in athletic use of soft tissues, if not only in degrees. That is, when the adenosine triphosphate is dephosphated to ADP, the biochemical energy so generated is found to propagate along DNA molecules in critical nonlinear dispersive waves to run the musculature engine. Looking at the flooding sweat all over athletes in field racing, this writer is further wondering whether similar complex mechanisms underlying soft tissues and cortical bones may be right there too.

Already writing too afar, the foremost wish here is to congratulate Dr. Savio Woo for his 70th birthday and welcome him to the wonderful Kingdom of the Septogenarian Land. There the birds are singing and flowers blossoming. He can have his mind roaming anywhere as he pleases, and pursue whatever he may like, and to cherish much more for his new achievements in serenity and high spirit.

With all kind wishes for many happy returns of creativity with Pattie and your dear family.

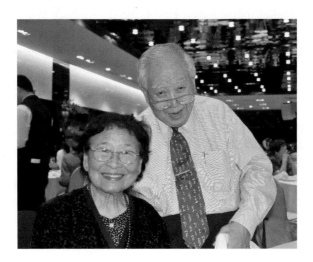

TO MY BIRTHDAY TWIN AND GRANDMASTER OF THE ACL RECONSTRUCTION

Sheldon Weinbaum

The City College of New York, CUNY
New York, New York, 10031, U.S.A.
E-mail: weinbaum@ccny.cuny.edu

It was only at your 70th birthday celebration at the winery at the 2011 Summer Bioengineering Conference in Farmington, Pennsylvania that I first learned that we were both born on July 26, a shared birth date with George Bernard Shaw and Aldous Huxley, Castro's Cuban Independence Day, and if you go back very far, the Battle of Edgecote Moor in the War of the Roses. It always puzzled me why I thought of you as much younger when we were only four years apart. Initially, I thought it was Pattie, who looked so youthful, compared to us, but then I realized that you were really not part of the Sputnik generation like our colleagues Bob Nerem, Don Giddens, Forbes Dewey, and many others dating back to Bert Fung, all aerospace engineers in our first life. You were part of the first of a new generation, a biomechanician from day one out of graduate school. My daughter now teaches English at the University of Washington, your bioengineering roots, and when I go there I do think of you.

Since I carefully avoided working in cartilage, ligaments, and tendons, I tried to recall where we first really bonded. I am sure it was in Wuhan in 1983 at the first U.S., China, Japan Biomechanics Conference at Chou En-Lai's retreat, and here Pattie did play the important role. If I recall there were only two planes a week to Wuhan from the U.S. and the airlines had left both Pattie and my luggage back in the U.S., which arrived five days later. It was obvious to all that we never changed our clothes, which of course was much more critical for Pattie than for me. What I do remember you warmly for, is telling me about Chou En-Lai's barber at the retreat who for $2 gave this luxurious haircut with a fabulous head massage.

You have been one of the shining stars in our biomechanics community over the past four decades, one who has contributed greatly to what we now know about ligaments and tendons. You are also one of the few who has truly lived in the world of orthopedic surgeons and has changed the way these medical practitioners understand joint loading. Since I have an ailing knee with half a meniscus from an old sports injury, it might have been wiser in retrospect to work on soft tissue as opposed to bone, arterial disease, and biotransport, but who is so wise as to know what aches and pains we will have as we grow older.

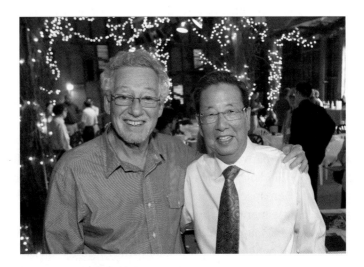

I have greatly appreciated your and Pattie's friendship over the past thirty years. I join you in celebrating life so far and the pleasures and satisfaction that will come from all that the two of you have done.

A FRIEND INDEED!

Ed Chao

Johns Hopkins University
Baltimore, Maryland, 21205, U.S.A.
E-mail: eyschao@yahoo.com

After the divine Venus awarded Paris the most beautiful woman on Earth, Helen, the wife of the King Menelaus of Sparta, Ulysses of Ithaca was drawn into the silly War of Troy. Ulysses spent 10 years away from home to win the Trojan War and another 10 years of going through hair-rising adventures in the Mediterranean Sea before reuniting with his beloved wife, Penelope and their son! Some asked him afterwards, "Why did you do that? It was not your fault in the first place!" Ulysses answered, "Helping a friend in need is a friend indeed!"

Savio, deep down I knew that if it were not you who led the effort and fought for me, I would never have had the chance of being elected to the National Academy of Engineering (NAE). I will forever remember that you came with a bottle of champagne just to celebrate the totally unexpected surprise! I tried to follow your footsteps to win the Olympic Gold Medal; unfortunately, my feet were just too small to fit the big shoes! Thank you very much and Happy Birthday for the 70th time and many more to come! As Confucius would have proclaimed, "Savio may do anything he wants from now on and no one will fault him!" So, when are you moving to Southern California?

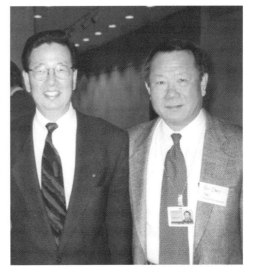

THE BIOENGINEERING FAMILY

Robert M. Nerem

Georgia Institute of Technology
Atlanta, Georgia, 30332-0363, U.S.A.
E-mail: robert.nerem@ibb.gatech.edu

Dear Savio:

We have known each other for almost 40 years, dating back to the Atlanta meeting in the early 1970s. For me it has been a pleasure to have you as a friend and as a professional colleague. Together and working with others, we have helped bioengineering grow from being a research area to being a new academic discipline in engineering, we have worked together to build the bioengineering family. Throughout the years there were several times that we have been together that I would like to highlight.

One of these is the 1983 trip to China for the first China, Japan, U.S. Conference on Biomechanics. This trip started in Beijing, and from there we went on to Wuhan and East Lake where the meeting took place. After the meeting it was down river and on to the Hwang Shan Mountains where we hiked the 4000 steps to the hotel at the top of the mountain. This trip to China was led by our dear friend, Y.C. Fung, and for those of us who were part of this expedition, it was a real "bonding" experience. Although the trip continued to Hangzhou and then Shanghai, the Hwang Shan Mountains were the high point, and the photo below shows our group with Pattie and you almost 30 years ago at the "height of your youth."

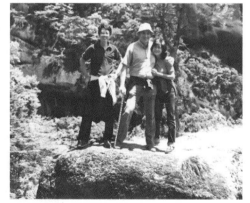

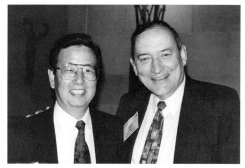

Another highlight for me was our working together on the task force that led to the formation of the American Institute for Medical and Biological Engineering (AIMBE). Not only was this, in my opinion, important for bio-engineering, but over the time of the task force you went from being on the faculty of the University of California, San Diego to being a Professor at the University of Pittsburgh. What a loss for UCSD, but it was a major step for you and the University of Pittsburgh. One of the key meetings in the recruitment process took place in Atlanta at a time when the task force was meeting.

There have been other highlights. This includes many conferences both in the U.S. and abroad as well as site visits such as those of the Whitaker Foundation. Most recently there was the 2011 ASME Summer Bioengineering Conference at the Nemacolin Woodlands Resort in Pennsylvania. At this conference a birthday party was held for you at a local winery. Marilyn and I arrived late, and as we walked in the person at the microphone was extolling your virtues and achievements, which of course are many. He was saying such nice things; however, that I wondered if I had come to a memorial service for you.

Of all that you have achieved, and these achievements are considerable, what I appreciate the most is our friendship and knowing your wonderful partner in life, Pattie, and your two children. As I said at the beginning, we have worked together to build the bioengineering family, and Marilyn and I do feel that all the Woos are family.

Thanks for all that you have contributed to our field and from both Marilyn and me HAPPY BIRTHDAY. We know that the best is yet to come!

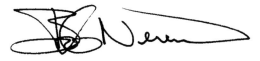

HAVE A WONDERFUL 70TH BIRTHDAY AND MANY HAPPY RETURNS

Albert King

Wayne State University
Detroit, Michigan, 48201, U.S.A.
E-mail: king@rrb.eng.wayne.edu

I have known Savio for some 40 years both professionally and socially. If memory serves me correctly, I reviewed his first proposal to the NSF before I actually met him. Of course, I gave him a good score.

In the mid 1980's, Savio and I were serving on the Executive Committee of the Bioengineering Division (BED) of ASME. The major divisional award at that time was the H. R. Lissner Award (currently the Lissner Medal) which was established in 1977. But it was not a society-wide award which would bring a much higher visibility to the BED. In order to upgrade the award, ASME required a substantial contribution from the BED, well beyond the means of the Division. Savio and I got to work to figure out a scheme to bring this about.

The Award was named after Professor Herbert R. Lissner, a pioneer in injury biomechanics research at Wayne State University. His zeal in research extended beyond the technical aspects of biomechanics. He was a big promoter of training young engineers in this field. When he died in 1965, the BED of ASME named an award in his honor for outstanding research in Bioengineering. I started a memorial fund for him at Wayne State and by the mid 1980's it had accumulated to about 75% of the amount needed for a society-wide award. It took a lot of arm twisting to get Wayne State to agree to transfer the funds to ASME, on condition that we found the rest of the money for the award. Here is where Savio came in. He worked his magic in the Orthopedic Surgery Department of UCSD and through an orthopedic colleague in the department, he managed to come up with the rest of the money. The H. R. Lissner Award became a society wide award in 1987 and the first recipient was Dr. Van Mow. Savio received his award in 1991.

Best wishes from Liz and I on the occasion of your 70th birthday. I am very happy that your friends and colleagues decided to honor you with a commemorative volume of tributes for a lifetime of dedicated research to biomechanics and to the profession. We wish you continued success in your future endeavors and hope to remain in touch. I also want to thank you for serving on the Bioengineering Advisory Board of the BME Department of Wayne State from 2004 to 2010.

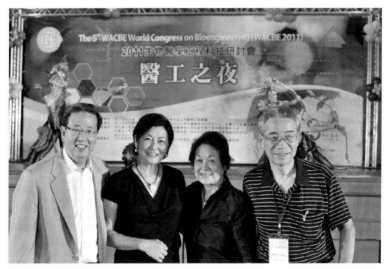

Taiwan (2011)

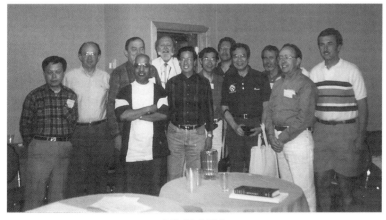

ASME (1986)

SAVIO WOO: WE APPLAUD A PIONEER IN BIOENGINEERING

Geert W. Schmid-Schönbein

University of California San Diego
La Jolla, California, 92093-0412, U.S.A.
E-mail: gwss@ucsd.edu

Dear Savio, congratulations on your 70th Birthday! Enjoy the celebration while looking back on many great achievements with many firsts.

We met the first time in 1972 during one of many lunches with Y.C. Fung in the Basic Science Building listening to your thoughts about cartilage. I soon started to appreciate your pioneering effort in the development of orthopedic biomechanics. The first time I was able to attend one of your seminars was when you spoke about the biomechanics of the eye in glaucoma. It was a fascinating story – showing at the time what was possible in this young field we called Bioengineering. The closeness between your office on the third floor and Bioengineering on the 5th floor made it possible to meet many times, exchange ideas and organize classes and meetings. It was an exciting and trailblazing period in Bioengineering.

Y.C. and I often commented that orthopedic biomechanics at UCSD with you at the helm was in strong hands and spearheading many new directions in bioengineering. Looking today at the Musculoskeletal Research Center of Pittsburgh this observation is short of what you actually achieved.

And then there was a memorable dinner with Pattie, you and Kirstin in a lobster restaurant near Yale University in 1977. Renate and her parents had joined us from New York, and Renate's father fell hopelessly in love with young Kirstin. Later, Pattie sent him Kirstin's picture, and he kept it in his library for several years.

Yes, Pattie, thank YOU for a lifetime of companionship.

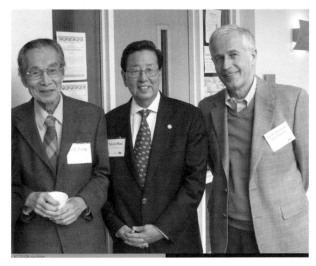

Savio and Geert with our mentor and friend Y.C. Fung at UCSD (2008)

A TRIBUTE TO SAVIO L-Y. WOO

Thomas Budinger

*University of California at Berkeley
Berkeley, California, 94720, U.S.A.
E-mail: tfbudinger@lbl.gov*

Savio was one of the distinguished members of the Whitaker Foundation Scientific Board and that is how we met while he was in San Diego. Perhaps it was the second meeting, when he hosted the scientific board where I began to appreciate his precision of thought, economy of words, firm convictions, and deep respect for others.

We discussed the difficult decision for his move: California vs Pittsburgh and Pittsburgh won Savio and his wife, a prize that made the medical school more famous and in particular, for contributions to the molecular bases of joint disease from the intellect of an engineer.

Our next encounter was at an orthopedic research symposium where he presented new material that gave insights regarding molecular biology of ligament and tendon injuries. I believe he is the first mechanical engineer who had the courage to learn about and apply molecular biology to joint diseases.

Savio L-Y. (there are other Savio Woo's) preceded me as an inductee of the National Academy of Engineering where he played a key role in navigating the academy away from traditional bioengineering to engineering applied to tissue repair.

An admired attribute of Savio L-Y. is his ability to change situations, students, and friends without making a storm of being noticed, thus I have no pictures to share. Congratulations on your seconds of life, your legacy of students and your contributions to healing.

LEADERSHIP, RESEARCH EXCELLENCE, AND GREAT CHINESE FOOD

Steven Goldstein

*University of Michigan
Ann Arbor, Michigan, 48109-0480, U.S.A.
E-mail: stevegld@umich.edu*

It is with absolute pleasure that I have the opportunity to contribute to the tribute to Savio Woo, on the occasion of his 70th birthday!

I have known Savio and Pattie for more than 30 years. As a fellow musculoskeletal biomechanist, we have sat in conferences, served on society committees and study sections, shared the podium, traveled, dined and had fun all over the country and numerous places around the world. Although I have mostly dabbled in bone, my first work in the field was focused on the viscoelastic properties of tendons and tendon sheaths (a little known secret); and much of my work followed the writings, teaching, and discoveries of Savio. His work has led the field, inspired trainees, and advanced treatments for Orthopaedic patients.

Most importantly, he has always been there providing advice, leadership and good cheer! Of course, since we always ate at Chinese restaurants, he also provided descriptions of what we just ordered (items never on the regular menu).

Savio; congratulations on your birthday and thanks for all you have done for our field and for our friendship over these many years!!!!

AN EXTRAORDINARY INVESTIGATOR AND EDUCATOR

John Watson

University of California, San Diego
La Jolla, California, 92093-0412, U.S.A.
E-mail: jtwatson@ucsd.edu

I got to know Savio some two to three decades ago while serving at the National Heart, Lung, and Blood Institute. It was clear that he was an extraordinary investigator and educator. With time, I learned that he is a fine gentleman with great interest in colleagues, students, and family. Over the years, I have always valued our friendship.

Savio, we all have appreciation for your efforts and success in translating your ligament and tendon injury laboratory and clinical research into clinical trials and subsequently, clinical use. Everyday your findings change the clinical rehabilitation paradigms for most orthopedic procedures practiced today both nationally and internationally. Members of my extended family enjoy greater mobility and function as a result of your creative endeavors and desire to improve patient outcomes.

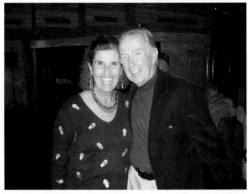

A secret, Savio, is telling one of my favorite stories to my "fitness" friends about one of my bioengineering friends who won the first Olympic gold medal at the Nagano Games in Japan. Who was it, they ask? Dr. Savio Woo! Who! What event did he win? Well he won first place in a special new event, the ACL downhill. Then, of course, I tell them the rest of the story.

So enjoy this well deserved tribute. Diane and I wish you and Pattie the very best, now and in the future.

HAPPY 70TH BIRTHDAY, SAVIO

Kerong Dai

Shanghai Ninth People's Hospital & Shanghai Second Medical University
Shanghai, 200011, China
E-mail: krdai@163.com

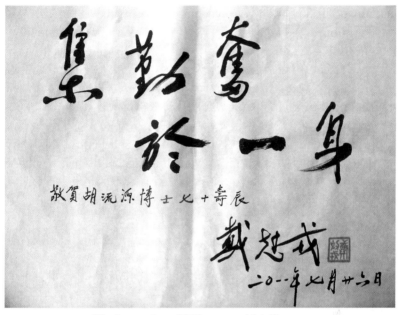

The Incarnation of Diligence and Intelligence
To celebrate Dr. Savio L-Y. Woo's 70th Birthday

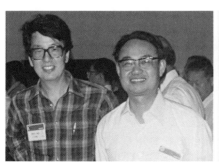
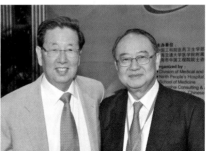

CONGRATULATIONS SAVIO!

Tingye Li

AT&T Bell Labs (Retired)
Boulder, Colorado, 80304-0575, U.S.A.
E-mail: tingyeli77@gmail.com

Congratulations, Savio, on your reaching the venerable age of 70!

As a pioneer in the field, you have contributed uniquely to bioengineering. The discoveries of your research and impact of your work have greatly benefited sports medicine and revolutionized knee injury treatment. I look forward to see your further successes in the field of regenerative medicine. Congratulations to you on your professional achievements!

Edith and I enjoy getting together with you and Patti at the biennial meeting of Academia Sinica in Taiwan and, especially, the annual "Ski Meet" of the OCF group at Vail. We look forward to doing so for many years to come!

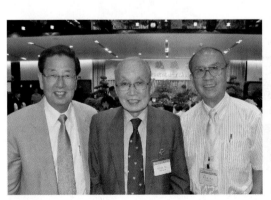
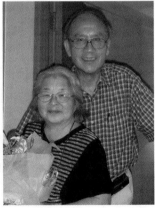

CHICO - IT IS NEXT TO PARADISE

Tim Thomassen

Albuquerque, New Mexico, 87106-2206, U.S.A.
E-mail: tmt402@msn.com

Dear Savio,

Happy 70th birthday! It sounds like you will have a very memorable celebration as greetings, salutations and tributes pour in from family members and friends around the world.

I recall fondly our days together while attending Chico State in the early 1960's. Having you as a roommate was an enriching experience and I am grateful to have had this opportunity. I have enjoyed and valued our friendship ever since.

I remember the times when we would go with others to my parents' home in Paradise on a Saturday and enjoy playing croquet on the back lawn, shooting the basketball or participating in other games. These outings were usually topped off by eating some of "Mama Thomassen's" home-made cooking and desserts. These excursions were welcome breaks from our studies and helped to make my college days more memorable and pleasant.

Over the years, it has been fun to visit with you and your family in Seattle, San Diego, Albuquerque and Pittsburgh. Sandi's parents were sometimes with us and they, too, enjoyed and treasured our times together. We recall the time we went out to eat at a Chinese restaurant and you wrote out the order in Chinese on a blank piece of paper. We had never experienced anything like that before.

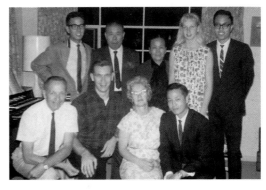

Sandi's mother, Roberta, was very impressed by the tour of your lab in Pittsburgh several years ago. As a retired nurse, she was in awe of and fascinated by the research that you and your associates were conducting. She excitedly related that experience to several of her friends later.

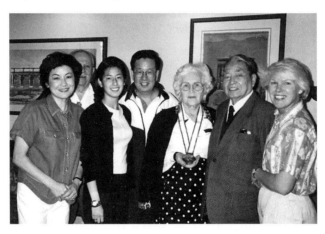

Sandi and I appreciated the respect that you and Pattie extended to Sandi's parents and mine. Both sets of parents felt very close to you and always looked forward to seeing or hearing from you. They spoke of you warmly.

We also admired the dignified manner in which you and Pattie treated Pattie's father. It was a notable example of honoring one's father.

I have been impressed with your many accomplishments over the years. You have certainly been an inspiration and a remarkable success story. I feel privileged and fortunate that our paths have crossed. My life has been enhanced because of our relationship. And I am sure that many others can attest to the impact that you have had on their lives as well.

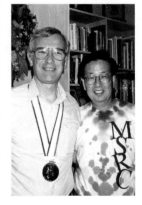

So, it is with esteem that I conclude this message and wish you the best in the days ahead. I am sure that your years will continue to be filled with adventure, excitement and pleasure. Please keep in touch.

MEMORIES FROM COLLEGE LIFE

Jeremy and Barbara Jones
*Scottsdale, Arizona, 85259, U.S.A.
E-mail: libarbian@cox.net*

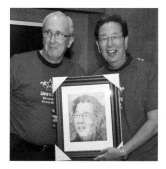

Savio and I had a good time as roommates, but much of what happened during that period has been sworn to secrecy. This was the period when Savio was going to rival Stevie Wonder on harmonica, but just could not get enough time to practice. We barely had time to check out a basketball to shoot hoops somewhere under McMahon Hall. I missed much of what happened due to going to bed by 9 p.m., but we all remember trying to eat the "ice cream" made by another group of engineers across the hall. They used all of the artificial colors in the pack thinking they would get colorful results, but ended up with olive greenish brown. They also reversed the proportions of salt and sugar, so we only ate a cup or two.

Shortly after college, the four of us went for a drive to Whidbey Island and ended up at Deception Pass, a rocky scenic area just right for someone with a Super 8 movie camera to shoot an abstract anti-war movie. This movie is better imagined than seen. Just picture Pattie jumping from rock to rock in the latest fashion and hair down to her waist. Meanwhile, Savio held a pile of weeds on his head for his role as...ummm...now that I think of it, I am not sure what he was supposed to be!

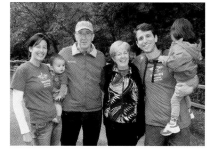

So, my toast to Savio is: May the next seventy years be just as mysterious as the past ones, but may your wisdom provide even better clues about how to enjoy them.

TRIBUTE TO SAVIO WOO

Wayne Akeson

University of California San Diego
La Jolla, California, 92093, U.S.A.
E-mail: orthoake@gmail.com

It gives me great pleasure to give honor to Professor Savio Woo.

I first met Savio Woo when he was completing his PhD requirements at the University of Washington in Seattle, Washington. At that time, I was a faculty member in the Orthopaedic Department at that institution. I had sought out bioengineering collaborators from the faculty of Engineering at the University without much success until Savio's name surfaced. It was with great delight, that I engaged his assistance in a cartilage repair project we had undertaken. It was easy to predict that Savio was a "comer" in the parlance of those days in the late 1960's. He was clearly bright, energetic, and highly innovative with excellent preparation for bioengineering studies.

When I received an invitation to join the new Medical School at the University of California San Diego (UCSD) in 1970, I sought out both Savio and David Amiel to join me there. With our good fortune, Savio and David were lured south to San Diego away from other institutions with competing offers. It was an obvious, though seldom successfully employed concept at that time, that collaboration from basic scientists on clinical relevant basic research was key to improved clinical understanding in the orthopaedic field. Over the following two decades, our collaborative efforts combining clinical insights with biological research and bioengineering met with considerable success. In fact, the basic understanding of the importance of early motion post-operative to facilitate ligament and tendon healing in the recovery from a variety of musculoskeletal injuries was clinically transformative. Over those years, we enjoyed considerable success in achieving critical research support from the Orthopaedic Research & Education Foundation and the National Institutes of Health for which we are eternally grateful.

Savio was naturally highly regarded in the Bioengineering Department at UCSD, headed in those days by the estimable Professor YC Fung, the grandfather of Bioengineering worldwide. Savio naturally garnered national recognition and competitive offers from a variety of institutions as the result of his achievements, and for acquiring premier status in orthopaedic research leadership. In the end, he received an invitation from the University of Pittsburgh that we were unable to match. With regret, but with admiration for his years of productive research on our team, we said goodbye, and with all best wishes.

It is the mixed blessing that when a research team becomes successfully integrated it is difficult to hold together, because other institutions inevitably lavish attractive offers on the team members. Unfortunately, such offers are frequently difficult to meet. But that is the price of success, and while sad, one can only be proud of the achievements of a much beloved comrade from the trenches of collaborative research successes. Savio continued his extraordinary productivity at Pittsburgh as we knew he would. We at UCSD are proud to have shared his achievements in his decades while here and consider him a proud alumnus of extraordinary accomplishment and world renown.

Respectfully submitted,

Wayne H Akeson, MD. Emeritus Professor of Orthopaedics, UCSD

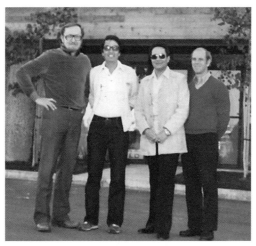

With Savio, David Amiel and Richard Coutts

OUR SPECIAL PARTNERSHIP AND FRIENDSHIP

David Amiel

University of California, San Diego
La Jolla, California, 92093-0863 U.S.A.
E-mail: fshepherd@ucsd.edu

Hi Savio,
Welcome to the world of being 70. It's not too bad; I crossed that bridge a couple years ago.

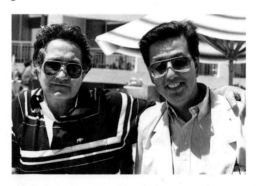

Looking back in time, our long-standing friendship began much before our successful academic achievements. This photo certainly reflects we were part of each other's lives and families, even before Jonathan was born.

Wayne Akeson, you and I came from the University of Washington to southern California to start our academic partnership. A clinician and two scientists, we joined UCSD Orthopaedics with a unique approach; our research was both novel and quite productive. Very seldom was our research not on the cutting edge, and the majority of our NIH grants were well funded.

Besides being close we were also competitive. We spent many weekends on the tennis court, also walking many miles discussing each other's concerns. Besides research topics, we also analyzed & planned our financial future(s).

Our masterpiece during our UCSD partnership was creating the research institute. Our vision created an extended facility, affiliated with the University, for students to perform research and be mentored. It was a sad day in 1990 when, after 20 years, you exited San Diego to establish an orthopaedic research department with the University of Pittsburgh.

In the past two decades we've watched our families grow, have maintained contact, and see each other at meetings. Happy 70th Birthday, I wish you many more.

Your friend, David

P.S. Savio, I thought your birthday was June 3, the same as Nancy. What happened?

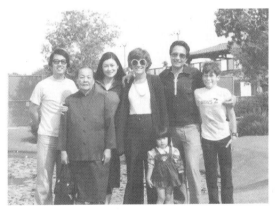

With Savio and his mother, Pattie, Nancy, Kirstin, and Michael (1978)

IT STARTED WITH A BUMP

Peter Chen

University of California, San Diego
La Jolla, California, 92093-0412, U.S.A.
E-mail: pcchen@eng.ucsd.edu

I went to the University of California, San Diego (UCSD) from Hong Kong after finishing high school in 1968 and signed up for a Bioengineering major. There were only 1,700 students at that time and the campus was very quiet. One day in 1970, while rushing across the wooden bridge connecting my dormitory in the Revelle Campus to the Basic Science Building, I bumped into a person walking from the other side. We paused, glanced at each other and in no time started talking in our native dialect, Cantonese. Savio told me he already has a Ph.D. degree and had just started some research programs in orthopedics and bioengineering at UCSD. We worked on different floors in the same building. As we began to part after the brief conversation, Savio turned around and shouted, "By the way, I have a young and beautiful wife." I soon met the lovely and charming Pattie and because of their 'seniority', Savio and Pattie treated me like a little brother, often asking me to go to their place for meals.

After Annie and I got married, we continued hanging out with the Woo's taking advantage of their hospitality. I remember one time Savio invited us and another friend for dinner and a slide show of his recent trip. We were driving back from Los Angeles and hit heavy traffic. There were no cell phones at that time and we were more than 90 minutes late getting to their house. Their immediate reaction was one of relief because they were worried we might have been in an accident. It was then that Pattie started to prepare dinner, they had waited for us. With a growing family they moved to Encinitas and with a big house and a big yard they got a big dog. I was very impressed with how well Savio trained and disciplined 'Ferrous'.

In 1984, Savio organized a symposium honoring Professor Fung's 65th birthday and he asked me to be the treasurer. That was a fun, memorable and successful meeting. We had a picnic and a banquet at that meeting. Attached are two photos of Savio presiding over those events. I bet Savio can still remember the 'truck full of flies' joke he told at the picnic.

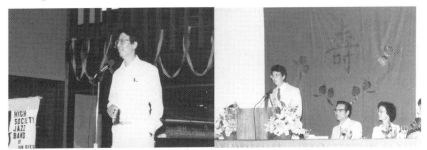

Fig. 1: Delivering a joke   Fig. 2: Honoring Prof. and Mrs. Fung

With careful planning and budgeting we had funds left over after the meeting. Savio came up with the idea of setting up an award to recognize and encourage young scientists working in Bioengineering and through his hard work and inner workings the Y.C. Fung Young Investigator Award was established. I handed the cheque over to Savio.

I missed seeing the Woo's after they moved to Pittsburgh. However, in 1993, I began to collaborate with the Scripps Clinic orthopedics group in San Diego and started bumping into Savio and Pattie again at the annual Orthopaedic Research Society (ORS) meetings. It is nice to be able to check on each other on a yearly basis and I was really thrilled to participate in Savio's 70th birthday celebration and symposium organized by his group during the 2011 American Society of Mechanical Engineers (ASME) Summer Bioengineering Conference in Farmington, Pennsylvania.

Happy Birthday Savio and look forward to the 80th celebration.

THREE CHEERS FOR DR. WOO'S BIRTHDAY

Michael Yen

University of Memphis
Memphis, Tennessee, 38152, U.S.A.
E-mail: myen@memphis.edu

I have known Dr. Savio Woo for nearly 40 years, almost as long as I've known my wife. We first met at the University of California, San Diego, where I was a graduate student and he was a junior faculty member. We spent 10 years working in close proximity in the Basic Science Building, he on the 3rd floor and I on the 5th, often we would get together to discuss our scientific research and we became close friends. Our common mentor was the widely recognized "Father of Biomechanics", Dr. Fung, who we remain in close contact with today. Though Dr. Woo worked on orthopedics and I worked on lung mechanics, we shared a common interest in biomechanics. Eventually, he moved to Pittsburgh, PA and I left for Memphis, TN. Through the years, we have managed to stay in touch through various science review boards, conferences and personal get togethers. Each year we also meet at the annual National Health Research Institute (NHRI) in Taiwan where Dr Woo, Dr Fung and I were the three original bioengineering review committee members.

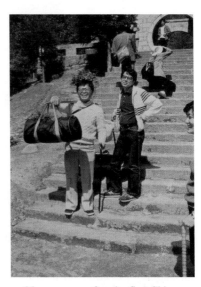

30 years ago, after the first China-USA-Japan World Congress on Biomechanics at Wu Han, Dr. Woo and I took a photo before climbing Huang San.

Savio, as I fondly call him, is a very distinguished scientist with literally shelves of awards. Yet, I think the award he was most coveted and proud of, is the gold medal he received from the Olympic committee for his research contribution for quick recovery from tendon and ligament injuries. His research actually changed the way we think about recovery from this type of injury. It makes me smile to think how he himself benefitted by being invited to the Olympic Games. Yes, as you can easily guess, I was very envious of my good friend's fortune. I watched those Olympic Games on TV while Savio sat in the front row players' box at the stadium.

Though highly distinguished scientist, Savio was always concerned about the future scientists. He believed it was the responsibility of current scientific leaders to pass the baton to future generations by establishing mechanisms that facilitated the superior scientific universe. He founded the World Association for Chinese Biomedical Engineering (WACBE). Today young scientists enjoy an excellent environment to where sharing of ideas and research is common. Thanks to the foresight of men like Dr. Savio Woo

On the family front, his wife, Pattie, and my wife, Min, have been also close friends. Savio, Pattie and I shared a common passion; we love to play tennis. Whenever we meet we always managed to find time and ways to play tennis. Even today, his wife and I are still avid tennis players. Some of my fondest memories of him were playing doubles against other members, like Drs. Ed. Chao and Ben Tsui. Always played in good spirit and friendship, our matches were a true joy irrespective of who won or lost.

Savio and I also share the love of good food. After reviewing proposals, we often enjoyed the sights, sounds and smells of Taiwan visiting local restaurants enjoying many wonderful dinners. It amazes me how Savio had this brilliant knack for finding restaurants that typically were reserved only for locals. One of my most vivid memories was of this restaurant in Hsinchu. The restaurant was a large garden where everything was served in tin buckets. The atmosphere was memorable with city lights in the background and the low chatter of family and friends. We shared a full bucket of the tastiest seasoned prawns on the planet. Often when I think back on these special evenings, enjoying a sprinkle of life's treasures, I am left with a strong sense of gratitude towards Savio for taking me to all those special places, to enjoy good food, conversation and friendship.

I wish Savio a healthy, fun filled and prosperous life. I fervently hope and wish that he will continue to inspire us all. Three cheers!!!

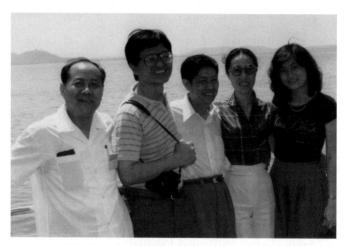

Mrs. Woo (first from right), me (second from left), and other friends on East Lake, Wu Han

PROFESSOR SAVIO WOO
PIONEER AND PROMOTOR OF SOFT TISSUES

Albert J. and Elizabeth Banes

Univ. of North Carolina at Chapel Hill and North Carolina State University
Flexcell International Corporation
Chapel Hill, North Carolina, 27599, U.S.A.
E-mail: albert_banes@med.unc.edu

I have known Dr. Woo and his work since 1976 when I was a post-doctoral fellow at the University of North Carolina working in Dr. Jerry Mechanic's lab on collagen cross-links. Dr. Woo was working in San Diego with The Akeson group, including David Amiel, who would routinely visit Dr. Mechanic to learn about cross-links and how to assay for them. The San Diego projects were based on immobilization and mobilization of rabbit knees to test how motion affected stiffness of joints. This was all ground-breaking work then and Savio was right in the middle of it. About a decade later, a World Congress of Biomechanics was being held in San Diego and Savio was an organizer. I still recall him dressed in Western costume for one of the gala dinners and, of course, meeting Pattie, his dear and glamorous wife on that occasion. They were quite a pair and were always at the center of activity of any meeting in which they participated. Savio and I would meet many times at the Orthopaedic Research Society meetings as we had a common interest in tendons. When I served on the NIH Orthopaedics Study Section in the early and late 1990's, I would sometimes be a reviewer on his grants. I was always honored to read these masterpieces of technology and innovation which scored well. When we served together in the same study section, I noted that the room would quiet down when Savio spoke, belying the high consideration his opinion garnered.

Dr. Woo has an impressive career, not only from the standpoint of his scientific and engineering contributions to our field, but because he has been the pioneer who boldly stepped forward to promote the soft connective tissue fields by establishing the International Society of

Ligaments and Tendons. This was at a time when no other individual had the foresight to step forward to fight for more exposure for our field and hence, more funding from the NIH. As with most leaders, he was attacked behind the scenes for taking some of the tendon and ligament papers from the ORS field and for calling attention to his work. What he really achieved, that probably no one else could have done at the time, was to create a forum for engineers, biologists and medical specialists interested in the under-represented soft tissue fields. This was really a stratagem! Immediately, there was a buzz created for the field and the numbers applying for this intense, one day meeting grew steadily. Naturally, leaders in the fields attended, spoke, interacted with others and promoted young scientists. I think, in the end, Dr. Woo established a brother and sister-hood of investigators in the field who collaborate, interact and continue to promote the field with new investigators from all over the world.

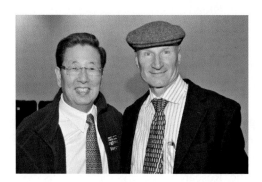

We all have different seasons in our lives, when we are young, we focus on our own careers and do our best to move up the imagined ladder to some goal in the clouds. Whether it is publications, recognition at meetings or funding-these are the early goals. As we mature in our careers, we can help promote others, especially the new investigators - not only in our own departments, but all over the globe. Savio Woo has managed to build his career as an internationally recognized scientist and innovator and create organizations to promote collegiality within our field. This is the tribute to Dr. Woo that belies his passion for science, engineering and medicine, as well as following in the footsteps of his mentor, Dr. Y. C. Fung, who Savio often quotes. Dr. Woo has been a colleague to me in science and both, he and Pattie, have been friends as well to me and my wife, Beth. It is a pleasure to honor him with this humble tribute. In the future, we hope he will share his wisdom with us at scientific meetings as well as the joys and defeats yet to come in our lives as friends. We wish him and Pattie all the best.

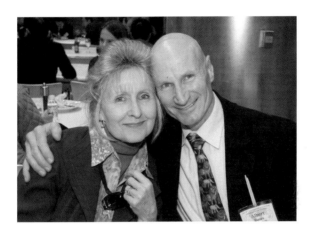

AN EXEMPLARY ROLE MODEL

Eva and Wen-Hwa Lee
University of California, Irvine
Irvine, California 92697, U.S.A.
E-mail: elee@uci.edu & whlee@uci.edu

We have known Savio for almost 30 years and have come to know a remarkable individual, extraordinary professor and incredible scientist. He is a man of strong convictions with passion and compassion for his family, students and friends. For us, he has been an exemplary role model - not only through his accomplishments, but for his beliefs. His bioengineering innovations for the past 4 decades have earned him many deserving accolades and recognition in the translational research of healing and repair of tissues; and his ideas and research continue as he leads today's cutting-edge technology in his field.

When I was a young Assistant Professor at the University of California, San Diego (UCSD), I worked with Professor Woo in the same building and every night before he left work, he would check up on me to ensure that I was still in the lab working diligently. What struck me as an impressionable scientist at UCSD was that Savio Woo organized a large group of faculty members to bring a suit against the University for a miscarriage of justice in the UC policy. I was taken by his strong sense of fairness and impeccable integrity. It was a sad day in 1990 when he left for Pittsburgh and I quickly followed in his footsteps the next year and left for San Antonio.

What I cherish most is our working relationship since 1995 with NHRI on review committees, but what I did not know was Savio Woo could be quite the prankster. Once, to my horror, while extolling the important and innovative biological significance of a proposal, he told me with a straight face that the bioengineering equation of the proposal was wrong. Who knew that Savio had mischief in him to toss some lightheartedness during a serious review? Needless to say, I have never let my guard down again, especially when it comes to reviewing proposals with Savio. What I remember most is the fun I have had during the past 16 years. Eva and I are fortunate to continue enjoying working together with Savio at these meetings.

More recently - during a keynote speech at the 2010 NHRI annual meeting where I was invited to speak on cancer susceptibility to members of NHRI from different and varying fields of expertise - I wrote my speech with only one individual in mind: Savio Woo. I was relieved to learn after the talk that he understood at least 50% of what I was saying.

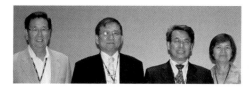

(L-R) Savio Woo, Ken Wu, Wen-Hwa Lee & Eva Lee

Chinese proverb:
前人栽樹後人乘涼;
which translates to *"One generation plants the trees, and another gets the shade"*. Savio L-Y. Woo has planted many, many trees and we would like to thank him for the shade. On this special occasion of his 70th birthday, we would like to wish him well and many more productive and playful years to come.

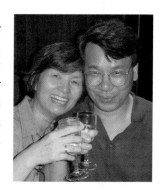

Eva & Wen-Hwa Lee

GOOD HEALTH, GOOD LUCK AND HAPPINESS ALWAYS

Winston and Priscilla Tsang

Nathan International, LTD
Hong Lok Yuen, Taipo, N.T., Hong Kong
E-mail: Winston@nathan.com.hk

We met Dr. Savio Woo at Ames Bio-engineering Department in 1973. He frequently came and visited us while he was at the Orthopedic Department at UCSD Medical School. We also would get together at the Chinese Faculty and Student Association and became good friends. We still keep in touch and see each other occasionally since I returned to Hong Kong in 1975.

Dr. Woo is a very knowledgeable and motivated young Orthopedic researcher! We congratulate Dr. Woo in his accomplishments in the past 30+ years.

Dr. Woo, we wish you Good Health, Good Luck and Happiness Always.

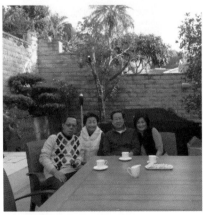
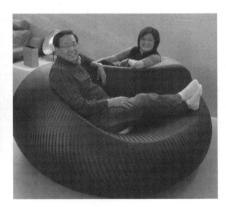

Winston, Priscilla, Savio & Pattie
(2011)

HAPPY 70TH BIRTHDAY TO A DEAR FRIEND

Brad and Loretta Sowers
Tucson, Arizona, 85718-3408, U.S.A.
E-mail: lsowersaz@comcast.net

To Savio,

It has been over 20 years since we have seen you, yet we have heard of your tremendous success. Recognized as a pioneer and leader in Bioengineering and Orthopaedics, you have been inducted into the nation's highest academies, scientific institutes, and professional societies. You have also won an Olympic Gold Medal. To laypeople such as us, that is impressive!

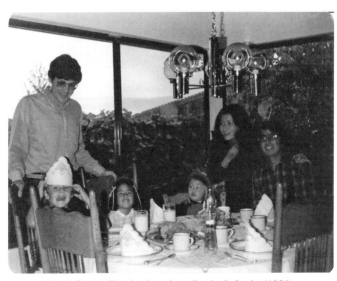

Brad, Ryan, Kirstin, Jonathan, Pattie & Savio (1981)

While we have gone our separate ways, you to the green, green east, us to the southwestern desert, we have not forgotten that you and Pattie were our first San Diego friends: sharing car pools, organizing play dates, celebrating birthdays, and watching our children grow. Most of all, we remember your kind countenance, wise counsel, and sweet smile and wish you continued success, joy and happiness.

Enjoy your 70th Birthday and raise a glass to our continued friendship and love,

Brad and Loretta Sowers

Savio… a wise and kind man who…

Wisely followed his instincts to come to America,
Wisely married smart and beautiful Pattie,
Wisely counseled Kirstin and Jonathan to listen to their Mother,
Wisely chose the University of Pittsburgh to continue his pioneering work.

Kind in his heart,
Kind in his demeanor,
Kind to his team, and
Kind to his friends.

Happy 70th Birthday. We wish you continued success, joy and love.

TO THE CELEBRATION OF SAVIO'S 70TH BIRTHDAY!

Ikuko Seguchi

Kobe University
Kobe, 657, Japan
E-mail: ikukoseguchi@gmail.com

It has passed more than 35 years since the Seguchi Family first met Savio & Pattie! Times Fly! But you always have been a never-failing friendship to us all. I would like to express my appreciation for you in this happy opportunity. May you always be in the best of health, great shape like a youth and warm heart like vintage wine!

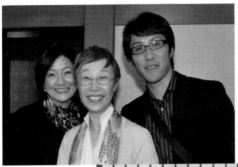

Pattie with Ikuko and Osamu Seguchi (2009)

With Savio, Pattie and Friends in Kobe (1981)

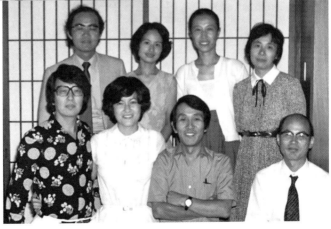

A TRIBUTE TO DR. SAVIO L-Y. WOO FOR HIS DISTINGUISHED CAREER AND HAPPINESS

Tin-Kan Hung and Shunan Cho Hung

University of Pittsburgh
Pittsburgh, Pennsylvania, 15219, U.S.A.
E-mail: tkhung@pitt.edu

胡興醫工新世纪，流暢五洲中外光。
源水長流學術旺，七旬歡慶福壽康。
洪鼎侃　　卓秀南　　賀

The era of biomedical engineering has been significantly contributed and promoted by Dr. Woo. His influence in research and education is "flourished like streams all over the five continents." What a joy to celebrate the blessing, the health, and the longevity of Savio Lau-Yuen Woo on his 70th birthday!

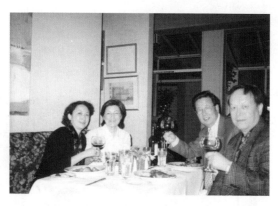

The joy of inviting you to visit the University of Pittsburgh in 1990 has been enriched by witnessing your partnership with our visionary leader, Dr. Thomas Detre, the ceremony of your National Academy of Engineering, other honors and family activities let alone wine tasting and picnics. All the good times with you are matched by our common goals, vision, and dedication to Pitt Bioengineering.

CONGRATULATIONS x 70!

Kai-Nan An

Mayo Clinic
Rochester, Minnesota, 55905, U.S.A.
E-mail: an@mayo.edu

Congratulations on this milestone celebration of your 70th birthday!

It has been my privilege to know you professionally for more than 35 years. You have been my role model since the early stages of my career. I have appreciated the opportunities to learn much from you at conferences, symposia and workshops. Your scientific insights not only set many standards in the field, but also have stimulated and influenced my scientific pursuits. Above all, your encouragement and support have made my professional accomplishments, if any, possible.

In addition, I am grateful for the friendship that has grown between us and our families. We remember fondly the trip to Savannah when the kids were young. Suei-Ching very much enjoyed being with you and Pattie whenever we were together on work trips. Throughout the years, I vividly remember how she constantly reminded me "to be calm and speak slowly and clearly as Savio does." She is now rejoicing from Heaven in celebration of your birthday.

May you enjoy a blessed birthday, and many more, and take extra time to enjoy your grandkids.

God bless you and your family.

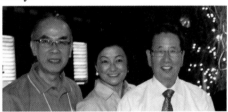

Happy birthday party

CONGRATULATIONS SAVIO: THE FIELD IS A BETTER PLACE BECAUSE OF YOU

Thomas Andriacchi

Stanford University
Stanford, California, 94305, U.S.A.
E-mail: tandriac@stanford.edu

It has been a pleasure to know Savio since 1974. Over the years, we have met at numerous scientific meetings and social events, I visited Savio when he was in San Diego, and also had the opportunity to visit Savio's lab in Pittsburgh. I was always impressed that Savio was able to manage a productive lab while maintaining a pleasant working environment with happy people. Perhaps keeping people happy is one of the secrets of his success. Among the many pleasant times with Savio, Doreen and I had the pleasure of attending the award ceremony for Savio's Olympic Award and hosting Savio and Pattie when Savio gave the Distinguished Lecture here at Stanford. It was also a great experience to have Savio spend a portion of his sabbatical here at Stanford where we were able to have many informal discussions about research, biomedical engineering education and life.

On a personal note, Savio might not remember, but back in 1974 before we met, I sent him a letter seeking his advice about entering the field of orthopedic biomechanics. I had just completed my Ph.D. in mechanical engineering and was considering pursuing this new field of biomechanical engineering. I was uncertain of the wisdom of focusing my career solely on biomechanical research. I had the opportunity to take a position in a medical school or a position in a traditional school of engineering. I was undecided and contacted the small group of scientists working in biomechanical engineering at that time to inquire about the opportunities and future of this new field. Savio's response was memorable. Even though he did not know who I was at that time, Savio responded to my letter promptly with a very warm, thoughtful, and detailed letter on his perspective for the future of the field as well as excellent advice about maintaining the professional status of an engineer working in a clinical department. I still recall his very encouraging response about the potential and need for engineers to address fundamental and applied clinical problems related to musculoskeletal pathology. Obviously, his letter had quite an impact on me as I have remained in the field for more than 40 years and I am very grateful for his encouragement. My experience is only one of many examples where Savio has been very supportive and nurturing to young investigators in this field.

Savio congratulations on your 70th birthday. Thank you for all you have contributed to the field of biomechanics and the many people you have helped along the way. The field is a better place for all you have done and your impact will last long into the future. I wish you continued success and happiness. We all look forward to seeing your continued contributions to the field. Have a great Birthday!!

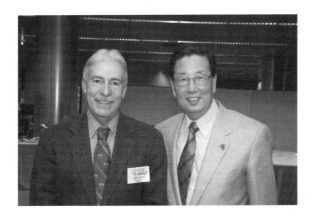

A TRIBUTE TO SAVIO WOO ON HIS 70TH BIRTHDAY

Jody and Kitty Buckwalter
University of Iowa Hospitals & Clinics
Iowa City, Iowa, 52242, U.S.A.
E-mail: joseph-buckwalter@uiowa.edu

Savio and Pattie have been our close friends and colleagues for nearly a quarter of a century. Our families spent a memorable week together in Savannah, Georgia, in June 1987. It was memorable because of the heat, the success of the NIH/AAOS workshop Savio and I had organized and, most important, because our families spent time together. Our children had the opportunity to go deep sea fishing together and caught a large number of small sharks. Savio and I worked hard leading the workshop dedicated to injury and repair of the musculoskeletal soft tissues. Later that week, Savio and I spent long hours editing and organizing manuscripts and became close friends. I do not know of a better example of a workshop that helped advance a series of important research directions and that also led to an important publication. The book that we edited, "Injury and Repair of the Musculoskeletal Soft Tissues," was published in 1988. People continue to seek copies of this book and I still see it cited in publications.

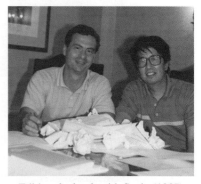

Editing the book with Savio (1987)

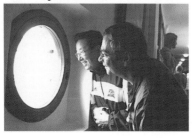

In the years since, our families have enjoyed a number of opportunities to come together at meetings, including an exciting white water rafting trip in Idaho, and renew our friendships.

We wish Savio a very happy birthday and many more.

HAPPY 70TH BIRTHDAY TO MY FRIEND AND MENTOR

Steven P. Arnoczky

Michigan State University
East Lansing, Michigan, 48824-1314, U.S.A.
E-mail: arnoczky@cvm.msu.edu

Congratulations Savio on your 70th birthday. I have had the good fortune to consider you both a friend and mentor for almost 25 years. While it would be very difficult for me to single out your most important contribution to the field of biomechanics over the years, I do know that your most significant contribution to my career was when you invited

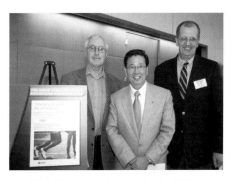

With Per Renström and Savio (2007)

me to be part of the "team" you put together to write your classic textbook *Injury and Repair of the Musculoskeletal Soft Tissues.* Being part of the symposium that generated this epic publication and getting to know the leaders of the field who have since become lifelong colleagues was a pivotal event in my research career. I have not been to a meeting where I learned so much since and I cannot thank you enough for that opportunity. Perhaps it is time for the 25th anniversary edition?

Thank you so much for all the guidance and friendship you have provided over the years. I have become a better scientist and educator because of the lessons I have learned from you.

"Best wishes on this momentous anniversary and I look forward to many more years of your good humor, gentle spirit, and great wisdom."

A TRIBUTE TO MY GOOD FRIEND, SAVIO WOO

David Butler

University of Cincinnati
Cincinnati, Ohio, 45221, U.S.A.
E-mail: david.butler@uc.edu

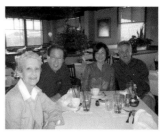

I first met Savio in 1976 when I attended my first ORS meeting in New Orleans. He presented his research using methods that paralleled some of the approaches that we had been taking during my Ph.D. at Michigan State University. After his move to UCSD and my move to the University of Cincinnati, we continued to conduct similar research. Savio visited our group and we visited his laboratory over the next several years and presented our work at similar orthopaedic and bioengineering meetings. Our friendship has grown as the field of tendon, ligament and joint biomechanics has matured and functional tissue engineering has evolved. We have also served on many committees in professional societies.

I have really enjoyed getting to know Savio and Pattie. I had dinner with them in San Diego many years ago and recently Savio and Pattie joined Sara and me for lunch in Cincinnati. They are a great couple and complement each other so very well.

Savio- It has been a privilege to know you and follow your research, including effective experimental designs asking important questions. Even more important has been your leadership qualities. As I mentioned in my talk, you serve as a Connector, Maven, and Salesman! It is all of these qualities that has really accelerated the development of our field.

Thank you!

A TRIBUTE TO DR. SAVIO WOO

Malcolm Pope

University of Aberdeen
Stonehaven, AB39 2BL, Scotland
E-mail: malcolmpope@hotmail.com

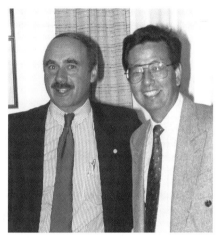

I have known Savio for over 30 years. During my time at the University of Vermont, I worked on the characterization of the ACL, quite complimentary to Savio's seminal work.

I remember we were both honored as a Fellow of the American Society of Mechanical Engineers (ASME) at the same event. It was also my pleasure, while at Aberdeen University, to nominated Savio for the prestigious Carnegie Visiting Professorship. As the Centenary Professor, Savio lectured at Aberdeen University as well as the Royal College of Surgeons in Edinburgh. We had a wonderful time together.

I was also excited to be present and celebrate with Savio in New York when he received the IOC Olympic Gold Medal for his work on sports medicine.

His many honors are testament to his excellent work on soft tissues. Above all a fine gentleman and friend.

VISION, KNOWLEDGE AND WISDOM

Richard Steadman

*The Steadman Clinic and Steadman Philippon Research Institute
Vail, Colorado, 81657, U.S.A.
E-mail: lchase@thesteadmanclinic.com*

Savio,

I am honored to join your many friends and colleagues in this tribute to you on the occasion of your seventieth birthday.

Our friendship began during a time in our lives when we were both considering making great changes in our careers. I remember well the conversations you and I had in Vail as we were contemplating the respective moves that lay before us.

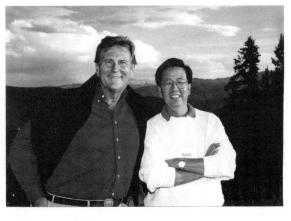

Each of us valued the other's opinion, and we arrived at our decisions to make the major changes in our lives at the same time.

These decisions had significant positive effects on our lives. Both of us expanded our resumes, and consequently, our reputations grew as well. I am thinking today what would have happened if we had taken the easy road and remained in our stable and comfortable positions. Both of our careers would have turned out quite differently!

Since then, your vision, knowledge, and wisdom have enhanced our accomplishments at the Steadman Philippon Research Institute, and we are grateful for your presence on the Scientific Advisory Committee.

I am fortunate to have had the opportunity to meet you, and share in the process of choosing a career path, which turned out as well for me, as yours did for you. Thank you for your friendship and continued valuable contributions to the Institute!

Best wishes on your 70th birthday!

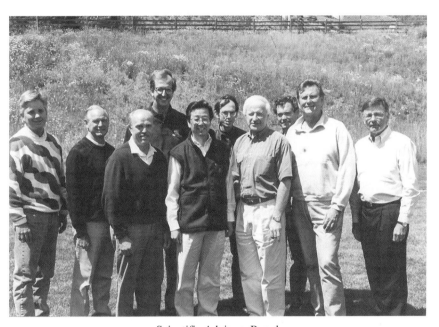

Scientific Advisory Board

UN GRANDE MAESTRO

Giuliano Cerulli

Nicola's Foundation and Let People Move Research Institute
Perugia, Italy
E-mail: g_cerulli@tin.it

Oltre 20 anni fa ho conosciuto il prof. Savio Woo per le sue ricerche innovative ed a volte rivoluzionarie nella bioingegneria e biomeccanica delle strutture dell'apparato locomotore, per il rigore scientifico e le ricadute applicative delle stesse. Con gli anni ho apprezzato il prof. Woo per la sua correttezza intellettuale e comportamentale ed ho incontrato un grande maestro!

In anni di collaborazione con Savio ho ammirato le sue doti umane ed ora godo anche della grandissima amicizia sua, di Pattie e della sua famiglia.

Grazie mio grandissimo amico SAVIO! Ti siamo affettuosamente riconoscenti tutti noi della famiglia Cerulli, della Nicola's Foundation Onlus e Let People Move.

I met Professor Savio Woo more than 20 years ago after reading a number of his innovative and revolutionary research publications. His scientific work in the field of bioengineering and orthopaedic biomechanics has been thorough and contains translational values in the treatment of musculoskeletal injuries. Over the years, I have come to appreciate Professor Woo for his intellect and his high moral standard. I have met a Great Master!

Years of collaboration with Savio have helped me to learn to admire his qualities as a human being. I have particularly enjoyed my great friendship with him, Pattie and all the members of his family.

Thank you my dearest friend, SAVIO! We, the Cerulli family, Nicola's Foundation Onlus and Let People Move, are all deeply grateful to you.

SAVIO L-Y. WOO – A DISTINGUISHED PROFESSOR, TEACHER, SCIENTIST, TENNIS PLAYER AND FRIEND

Per Renström

Karolinska Institutet
Stockholm, Sweden
E-mail: per.renstrom@telia.com

I have had the privilege to know Dr. Savio L-Y. Woo as a colleague and as a friend since the early 1980's. At that time, I started to regularly participate in the meetings of the Orthopedic Research Society (ORS). Savio was, at that time, "the king" of orthopedic biomechanical research not the least because of his great work on ligament biomechanics and healing of ligament and tendon at the cellular, tissue and organ levels published in 1982. I was working at the University of Vermont in 1983-84 and started to get very actively involved in in-vitro strain gauge biomechanical studies. Savio always had an open mind and a great willingness for discussion. When I presented my first paper on strain knee biomechanics at the ORS in 1985, I remember how Savio expressed his support for the work we did. This meant a lot. He has since been an inspiring role model for me.

Together with Ben Kibler and Robert Nirschl, I founded the Society for Tennis Medicine and Science (STMS) in 1991. I remember well how happy we were when Savio early on joined our society, not the least, his and Pattie's participation in the stimulating STMS meeting in Melbourne 1996 and also in our STMS meeting in Stockholm in 2002. We have had some great times together. We will never forget when the Woos, Kiblers and Renströms were at a 3-day tennis training camp at Manitou in Northern Ontario, Canada in 1997. Savio and I were assigned to play tennis with a blond tennis coach of Swedish descent and one day we played for over 5 hours. We could hardly move after this, but some good food, excellent wine, and massage helped. We are very proud over the fact that Savio has been appointed an honorary member of STMS; the only one so far.

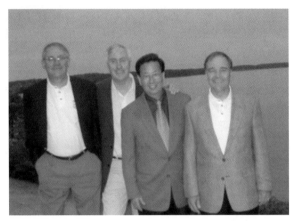
With Savio and tennis friends Peter Jokl and
Ben Kibler outside my home in Sweden

In 1994, The International Olympic Committee (IOC) introduced the Olympic Prize in Sports Science. A jury of eight people was selected by the IOC Medical Commission including two in Psychology, two in Physiology, two in Medicine/Orthopedics and two in Biomechanics. I was selected to be the Orthopedic expert. The jury received nominations on all the most prominent Sports Scientists around the world. A careful process was worked out. The first prize went to Dr. Jeremy N. Morris and Dr. Ralph Paffenbarger in recognition of their pioneering work demonstrating that exercise reduces the risk of heart disease. They received $250,000 US and an Olympic Gold Medal in 1996. During this time, some of us recognized that Savio was a superior candidate in Orthopedics and Biomechanics. Everything he had done was scrutinized. Savio won unanimously the second prize. The Olympic Prize was awarded during a ceremony in New York and then he received an Olympic Gold Medal during the Olympic Games in Nagano 1998.

Savio´s contributions to research and science in Sports Medicine and Biomechanics are outstanding. His lectures are the highlight at most conferences and we all learn from his lectures. We did a consensus work shop on Tendinopathy at the Pre-Olympic Conference in Athens 2003 with most of the best scientists on the topic present. This ended up as an Encyclopedia called Tendinopathy with Savio, Steven Arnoczky and I as editors. I consider this work to be a highlight in my career as it gave me the great privilege to work with these two curious minds and world leading scientists. I am very proud of this experience and honor.

On a more personal note, my wife Lena and I are very happy for our friendship with Savio and Pattie. It is always such a privilege to spend time this them. We have many lasting memories, not the least, due to Pattie´s great expertise with the camera, the results of which she generously shares. Lena and I wish Savio and Pattie many more happy and enjoyable years to come shared with their lovely children, grandchildren and now also grandchildren.

Thank you for a wonderful friendship and for all the good times together. We are honored to be friends of the Woos. A special "skål" to our distinguished friends.

IN FRIENDSHIP FOR SAVIO WOO

Werner Mueller

Riehen, CH 4125, Switzerland
E-mail: w.u.mueller@datacomm.ch

SAVIO is for me the pure gentleman of a scientist.

He is a scientist with by far outstanding knowledge in the field of biomechanical sciences, which has developed from the traditional macro-biomechanics into the field of tissue biomechanics and further into cellular and even molecular biomechanics. This is now really close to the enigmas of life and the adaption of living structures to all type of different natural requirements.

Savio has looked over the clouds of the actual debates far ahead into the future demands of our science, and the clinical requirements have always been in his perspective for the future research.

He has acquired this knowledge by a very well organized brain with a broad and bright philosophical thinking, which helps him to combine all the brick stones even of little findings into a complete construct and explains it so that we can understand it. And all this without any arrogance .....

But beside all these tremendous qualities, he is a wonderful personality and a true friend in life.

I always look forward with great anticipation to meet him and his lovely and friendly wife, Pattie, another time again.

I remember so well a great day with Savio in 1997, when we were visiting together the unbelievably gorgeous Museum of Chinese History, Art and Tradition in Taipei. It was amazing, how we could discuss about the great inventions of the humanity in the Asian culture and often parallel in the European/Western cultures. There were among many others the invention of the wheel, of the measuring of time, wonderful, masterly made art-pieces of porcelain as well as food like the spaghettis, which came also from China. With these inventions, the Chinese have often been far ahead of the rest of the world.

Now, I can give some philosophical saying back to him. Eight years ago, Savio gave me a very special Chinese reminder out of the Book of Etiquette. Now, at this time, I return it to him with our best wishes for Savio and Pattie's future in best health.

At 30 one becomes	independent
At 40 one becomes	self-assured
At 50 one knows	ones destiny
At 60 one is	bothered by nothing
At 70 one can	do whatever ones heart desires

Yours,
Werner and Ursula

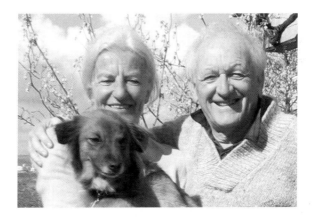

VERY HAPPY BIRTHDAY SAVIO
FROM ALL YOUR FRIENDS IN AUSTRALIA

John Bartlett

University of Melbourne
Melbourne, Australia
E-mail: r.j.bartlett@bigpond.com.au

Happy Birthday to you and may there be many more.

What an honor it is to be able to say "Savio is a friend of mine." I have appreciated your kindness, being welcomed into your home, given a ride in the Porsche, joined you on the tennis court, drank your wine and been part of several of your colorful dinners.

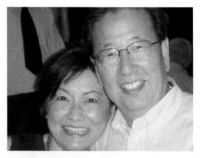

Savio and Pattie, the most generous, loving, & respected people I know

You are so much loved and respected around the world, partly because you are so generous and so willing to share. I recall being asked to deliver the first Master's lecture at the Australian Orthopaedic Association Congress – the title to be "Knee Surgery: Past, Present & Future". You responded to the call for help and I had the "future" by return mail.

Also when I had the opportunity to be a Program Chairman, you were so gracious in agreeing to "open the batting" with the first Keynote Lecture, which was received to great acclaim setting the standard for the meeting.

John Feagin said in Gargonza that "Savio is a national treasure" to which I objected saying "Savio is an international treasure".

For 30 years, I have told my Fellows and Registrars to try to follow your research work and teaching, because therein lie the answers. You have the communication ability to make the complex seem understandable.

Savio we love you so much – my heart goes out to you in admiration and gratitude.

My thanks to Pattie, Kirstin and Jonathan for this opportunity.

Happy Birthday! Enjoy the Day!
John Bartlett

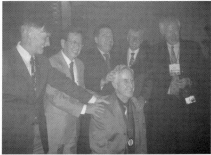
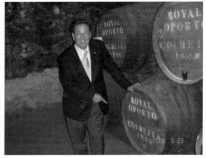
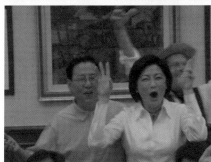

A Little Reminder of your visit to Melbourne for Tennis. Top Left: Roli, Savio, Paolo, JB and Rene anointing Per as next President of ISAKOS. Top Right: ESSKA in Porto and we nearly finished the barrel. Center: To be invited to a party by Pattie and Savio is to be guaranteed a fun time. Bottom Left: Florence and the decorations looked promising. Bottom Right: And the feasting began.

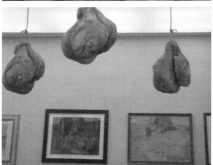
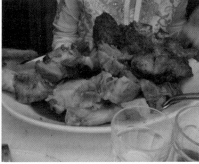

TRIBUTE TO A DEAR FRIEND

Mahmut Nedim Doral

*Hacettepe University,
Turkish Society of Orthop. & Traum./TOTBID
Sihhiye, Ankara, 06100, Turkey
E-mail: ndoral@hacettepe.edu.tr*

Dear Savio & Pattie,
Savio and his precious family have a very special place in Esra, Ceyla, Coşku and I. As everyone agrees, he is a world-class scientist, who is extremely humble, charitable and of course hard-working. He is a teacher!

His contributions to the 3rd Congress of Asia-Pasific Knee Society combined with the 7th Congress of Turkish Society of Sports Traumatology, Arthroscopy and Knee Surgery, which was held in Ankara in 2004 were unforgettable, both scientific and culturally. During this meeting, he accepted Dr. Sinan Karaoğlu for a two year fellowship program and that was the master key for Turkish young Orthopaedic Surgeons for future research. In addition, he has visited Turkey so many times as a teacher.

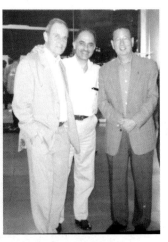

Dr. JC Imbert, France
Perugia (2000)

It is proof of our friendship that he attended my daughter's wedding and we attended his daughter, Kirstin's, wedding from miles away. This was just an example of conventionality to our cultures. We would like to present our kindest regards to his lovely wife Pattie and childrens.

Best from Ceyla, Coşku TURHAN & Esra, M. Nedim DORAL

Tributes from Colleagues and Friends

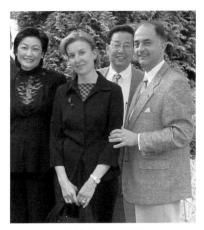

Heidelberg (2008)

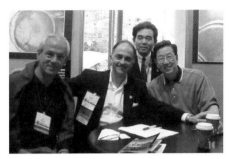

Dr. G Bellier, France and Dr. M. Ochi, Japan
New Zealand (2003)

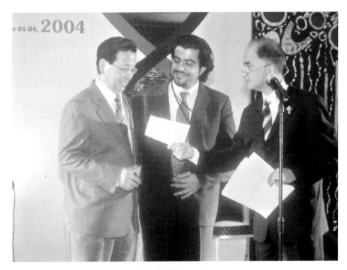

Dr. S. Karaoglu
Ankara (2004)

THANKS FOR WHAT YOU HAVE DONE & ARE STILL DOING

Jose Huylebroek

Parc Leopold Hospital
Brussels, Belgium
E-mail: jose@sportsmedchirec.be

When I first met Professor Woo, maybe 25 years ago, I believe at a meeting of the International Knee Society, today ISAKOS, it was nearly a scientific shock to hear Professor Woo explaining so easily the importance of biomechanics and biochemistry in orthopaedic sports medicine. We, young European surgeons, had the impression that the topic Savio was approaching was something we had never thought of, sometimes never heard of even. We found ourselves so little and unaware of what was going on in the laboratories. Savio made a great impression on us, and particularly, he had such a stimulating effect on our professional life and interference with the engineers he always defended. When we were listening and watching him, he seemed to be the strictest and severe Professor we had ever met! The man, who scared us with his knowledge and his simple way of explaining the most difficult biomechanical findings, later became a close friend who we have even more appreciation as he was not the ex cathedra professor, but a real warm family man, a man with a very open mind, always happy to help or to explain!

One of the nicest "adventures" with Savio and his lovely wife Pattie was the private travel from Ankara to Antalya with another good friend, Mahmut Doral. With an exceptional guide as Mahmut, we discovered quite a bit of Southern Turkey and found a brand new facet in the person of Savio: not only he seemed to be a keen historian, but particularly, a great connoisseur of wine, especially French wines!

Every visit to a restaurant we had the pleasure to accompany with Savio, he proved to be a real oenologue! As European, it is a great pleasure to be with him in a restaurant, wherever in the world. And for every special bottle, he has a story to tell or he remembers the last time he had the occasion to drink that wine. That is another point I would like to bring up: the absolute fantastic memory of Savio. Not only in his field he is a walking dictionary, but of every friend or "connaissance" he has a nice story or joke to tell. He loves jokes, particularly the jokes emphasizing cultural differences as he is probably the best combination himself as a Chinese American or American Chinese. A wonderful person, a magnificent husband for Pattie, a top-scientist: we are grateful to know this person as a good friend!

Thanks Savio, for everything you have done and are still doing for the orthopaedic community and your friends on every continent!

We hope your train keeps going for many more miles.

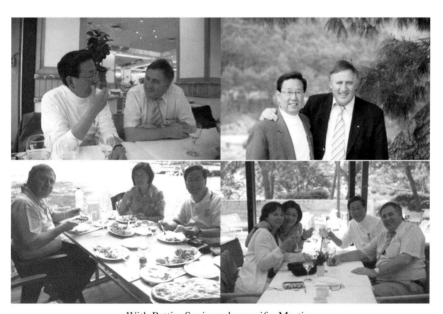

With Pattie, Savio and my wife, Martine

PROFESSOR SAVIO WOO ON HIS 70TH BIRTHDAY

Arnold Caplan

Case Western Reserve University
Cleveland, Ohio, 44106-7080, U.S.A.
E-mail: aic@po.cwru.edu

Savio has always been one of my favorite individuals. He fits the image of the soft-spoken, ageless Chinese scholar. One could imagine him with a long white and wispy flowing beard covering the front of the long flowing silk embroidered robe although it is difficult to "see" the tennis racket he always carries in this out-fit.

I cannot tell you when we met (I'll bet he remembers exactly…), but he has always been at ORS, at his annual tendon meeting, at Gordon conferences, and in his fabulous Pittsburgh basketball seats. What I can say is that Savio has always been there for me, has always had the most positive comments, both personally and professionally and has always supported my activities, ideas and my intrusions of late for Pittsburgh basketball tickets (generously given and hosted).

The very funny story was in March of 2010, Savio gave me three of his tickets for a Pittsburgh basketball game for the last Saturday game. My son and I drove to Pittsburgh at noon from Cleveland on a cold, but beautiful clear and sunny day. When we approached Pittsburgh, we realized that there had been a massive snowstorm which ended about one hour before we arrived. The town was deserted, people walking and taking pictures of the newly fallen snow (streets were unplowed and most side streets impassable with several feet of snow). We parked in a covered lot at the hospital and walked into the stadium to discover that tickets were not being honored (if you could get to the game, they let you in). We saw a great game and weeks later Savio told me that he wanted to join us, but Pattie firmly said "are you crazy…"; a game without Savio ain't the same. Just as he cheers us on professionally, he is an avid University of Pittsburgh basketball fan.

I am lucky to know him. We share many of the same values and, for sure, I highly value my long friendship with him. We Jews and Chinese have many thousands of years of common, family centered, society directed, scholarly progressions and progressive attitudes. The older, wiser, softer spoken Professor Woo has added richness to the lives of all of us he touched. His professional contributions speak for themselves; his personal values are a model for us all.

I am honored to be his friend and cherish our timeless friendship. Happy birthday Savio and many more.

A LONG HISTORY TOGETHER

James C.Y. Chow

Orthopaedic Center of Southern Illinois
Mt. Vernon, Illinois, 62864, U.S.A.
E-mail: ocsi@orthocenter-si.com

I started practicing Orthopaedics in 1972. I heard about Savio Woo for many years and read a lot of his papers. I also had the opportunity to talk to him at several meetings. However, I did not really get a chance to get to know him until we were both invited to Argentina and Greece to meetings within three weeks. Therefore, we spent three weeks traveling together across three continents and sailing the Ionian Sea to Corfu. During that time, we found out that we had a lot of things in common other than I am a few years older than him.

- We both come from the same state in China. Our family's hometown in China is only about 100 miles apart.
- We both grew up in Hong Kong and had to learn Cantonese, which is not our mother tongue. Believe it or not, we even attended the same school.
- We both struggled on the bumpy road as first generation immigrants to America.
- We both have been married once.
- We both have one boy and one girl.
- We both have one child who is a medical doctor.
- We both have kids who lived in California. Until last year when our daughter moved from San Diego to Texas.
- We both live in the Midwest in the United States.
- We are both involved in Orthopaedic research.
- We both have had many national and international fellows over the years.
- Most importantly, we both study and enjoy a bottle of good wine.

We have become good friends over the years. His contributions to Orthopaedics and Sports Medicine are remarkable. To know him and call him "my friend" is a joy and an honor. On your birthday, Savio, as the good old Chinese saying, "long life as the south mountain" and I wish you many happy days to come.

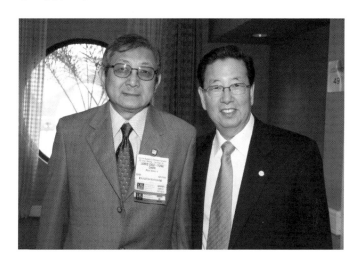

THANK YOU, SAVIO

Peter Katona

Former President, The Whitaker Foundation
George Mason University
Fairfax, Virginia, 22066, U.S.A.
E-mail: pkatona@gmu.edu

Dear Savio, I miss the times when you and I served together on the Scientific Advisory Committee of The Whitaker Foundation in the late 1980s. That was the time when I became acquainted with your talent in science, dedication to education, and skill in expressing carefully considered opinions. Jane and I enjoyed numerous delightful conversations with you and Pattie over walks and meals.

My most memorable conversations with you were in 1990-1991, when The Whitaker Foundation was looking for a biomedical engineer to establish an office in Washington, DC. Being at the right place at the right time, I was asked to consider applying for this position. My initial preference was to go back from a temporary NSF appointment to my permanent faculty position. It was you who set me straight.

Your words were kind, but firm. You emphasized the uniqueness of the opportunity, and argued that the potential impact of the Foundation was much greater than the likely impact a single faculty member could have. You convinced me, and subsequently, I submitted my application. The result was my being fortunate enough to get what would become probably the most attractive biomedical engineering position anywhere.

I was also fortunate to have had the opportunity to visit your institution on several later occasions. It was always a pleasure to see you, learn about your further scientific accomplishments, and to witness your influence on training biomedical engineers of the future.

Although 70 might seem like an advanced age to your students, I want to reassure you that this is considered young by many of us! I sincerely hope that you feel young in body and spirit, and you will continue to advance our chosen profession.

Jane and I congratulate you and Pattie, and wish you a happy and productive combination of work and relaxation. Please say "hi" to us when you are visiting the DC area!

CONGRATULATIONS AND HAPPY 70TH BIRTHDAY

Ron Zernicke

University of Michigan
Ann Arbor, Michigan, 48109-2013, U.S.A.
E-mail: zernicke@umich.edu

Kathy and I extend our sincere congratulations and wish exceptional health and happiness to you and Pattie. We have many memories that we cherish about both of you, and we hope that we will have many more years and experiences to remember as we go forward.

I believe it was around 1975 when we first met. I was a new assistant professor at the University of California, Los Angeles (UCLA), and I came to visit you at the University of California, San Diego (UCSD) to discuss ideas for research; it was a thrill to meet you and to talk with David (Amiel) and Wayne (Akeson). On that visit, I also met a young Cy Frank, who was a fellow at the time in your lab. It is intriguing how lives intertwine, again and again, across the lifespan.

During these many decades, we have continued to interact, on personal and professional bases. We have frequently talked at the Orthopaedic Research Society (ORS), American Society of Biomechanics (ASB), and International Society of Biomechanics (ISB) meetings, and I am very grateful for your recommendation and support of me to become a member of the Scientific Advisory Committee of The Whitaker Foundation. My 12 years with Whitaker were uniquely memorable, personally, and they also generated numerous long-term friendships.

Through the years, you have given me inspiration and served as a role model. Your innovative and pioneering research has integrated multiple fields (engineering, biology, medicine, and physical and life sciences) and has uniquely contributed to the world's knowledge of the biology, mechanics, and adaptive responses of load bearing soft connective tissues. Your superb basic and applied research is widely acclaimed as innovative and significant, and the results of your research have had a pervasive and dramatic impact on our understanding of the mechanisms of injury, treatment, and rehabilitation engineering and medicine.

The impact of your research has been (and continues to be) prodigious. In the past decades, revolutionary changes have occurred in our understanding of soft connective tissue biology, mechanics, and adaptive responses to immobilization and physical activity/loading. Your interdisciplinary, pioneering research was (and is) at the leading edge of this revolution. When you began your seminal work, immobilization was the standard conservative and post-operative treatment for ligament injury. Currently accepted joint injury treatment and rehabilitation protocols—incorporating early mobilization (remobilization)—are built solidly on your basic and applied research. Your research has profoundly influenced current and future generations of connective tissue scientists, bioengineers, orthopaedic surgeons, sport medicine physicians, and physical medicine and rehabilitation specialists, and your published works are the most frequently cited research in this field.

Your scientific and intellectual versatility is legendary. Your inquisitive and intellectually gifted mind has prompted you to use an integrative and hybrid approach to forming hypotheses and solving seemingly intractable problems. Your published work testifies to the excellence in both analytical-quantitative modeling of soft tissue behavior as well as in the experimental manipulation of biological factors that influence tissue adaptation and healing. You are not only comfortable, but also expert at an impressive array of techniques and methods, including continuum mechanics, finite element modeling, multi-body dynamics, robotics, biochemistry, molecular biology, histomorphometry, and gene therapy.

It is abundantly clear that many national and international juries have reviewed your achievements and have selected your work as being preeminent among peers. It is daunting to enumerate your list of honors, including membership in the Institute of Medicine-National Academy of Sciences and the National Academy of Engineering, as well as being the recipient of the *highest* research honors for a host of scholarly organizations (e.g., American Society of Biomechanics, International Society of Biomechanics, American Society of Mechanical Engineers, American College of Sports Medicine, American Orthopaedic Society for Sports Medicine, International Society of Arthroscopy, Knee Surgery & Orthopaedic Sports Medicine, Orthopaedic Research Society, and American Academy of Orthopaedic Surgeons). That brilliant list of awards is mirrored by your Chancellor's Distinguished Research Award from the University of Pittsburgh, the Life Sciences Award from the Carnegie Science Center, and the IOC Olympic Prize for Sports Science.

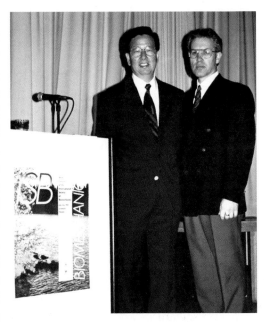

Your continuing influence in science is evident in many, many ways, but the one I highlight, here, is that you, undoubtedly, were a key catalyst in the ascension of orthopaedic bioengineering—nationally and internationally—and at both UCSD and Pittsburgh. You have been and continue to be a masterful mentor and educator; your list of highly qualified trainees is indeed impressive.

... and most importantly, you are a very blessed husband, father, and friend. THANK YOU. Best personal regards and sincere congratulations from both Kathy and me!

TRIBUTE TO A COLLEAGUE, COLLABORATOR & FRIEND: DR. SAVIO L-Y. WOO

Mario Lamontagne

University of Ottawa
Ottawa, Ontario, K1N 6N5, Canada
E-mail: mlamon@uottawa.ca

Relationship, Collaboration and Friendship

Our relationship started in 2001 with a series of famous annual conferences on biomechanics, orthopedics and rehabilitation organized by Dr. Giuliano Cerulli in Perugia/Assisi, Italy. Those conferences reunited the best researchers and clinicians of their respective fields attracting large attendances. These annual events had their regular speakers, which included Savio and I. From the initial relationship through conferences, it evolved to a collaboration to develop the philanthropic vision of Giuliano Cerulli for his Research Institute. From that point, the collaboration has turned to a friendship in the sense of "Amicitia" as described by Ciceron.

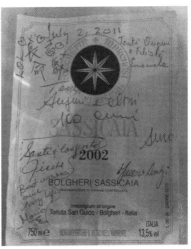

As a tradition Savio & Pattie make you sign a card or in this instance the label of the wine bottle. Sassicaia is produced by Tenuta San Guido in the DOC Bolgheri in Toscana, known as a producer of "Super Tuscan" wine. Its wine is considered one of Italy's leading Bordeaux-style red wines.

Fortunately, his love for Italian food and wine as well as Italian friendships bring him frequently to Perugia and Arezzo. In return, the Research Institute benefits of his invaluable mentorship, experience and wisdom. You may know that Savio is a wine connoisseur. He can tell us the top ranked wines in the Wine Spectator, however, he is the one who drinks the least wine during a dinner. This makes him a wine connoisseur because he can appreciate every drop of wine. To celebrate in advance of his 70th birthday, Dr. Auro Caraffa and his wife (Emanuella) invited us (Savio, Pattie, Mario and Nicole) to the Relais Todini, one of the best restaurant in Umbria. Besides the memorable dinner, we were served two bottles of Sassicaia.

As he turns 70, Savio must be joyful, especially when he looks back at all he has done and realized in his life. You have demonstrated great accomplishments in your career while caring for your very nice family; exceptional wife, son and daughter who has brought to you two granddaughters that are waiting for your love.

Nicole and I wish you a healthy and long life. We hope that we will enjoy many more meetings in Perugia/Arezzo, Italy.

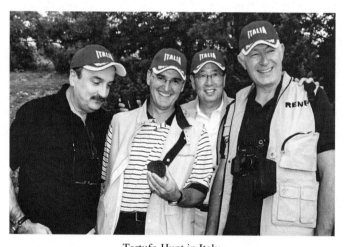

Tartufo Hunt in Italy

THE HIGHLIGHT OF DR WOO'S CONTRIBUTION TO HONG KONG

K.M. Chan

The Chinese University of Hong Kong
Hong Kong Special Administrative Region, China
E-mail: kaimingchan@cuhk.edu.hk

The highlight of Dr Woo's contribution to Hong Kong was probably the 2010 International Symposium on Ligaments & Tendons (ISL&T), held at the Prince of Wales Hospital, The Chinese University of Hong Kong.

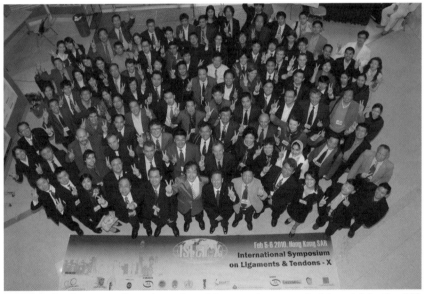

This is the very first time that this meeting was held outside the US after 9 successive and successful meetings. It has really made a difference in this region. The scientific program was superb, the professional exchanges were stimulating and the social event was most enjoyable.

Savio and Pattie are "Hong-Kong...ers" in that they know precisely where to go for the best... their favorite Sheraton Hotel, the famous Shatin pigeon at Lung Wah and the fabulous seafood in Liyumun, etc.

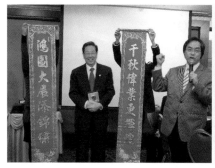 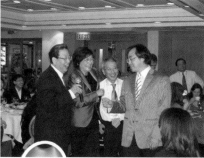

For the past 25 years, we have established a professional and academic link with Savio, not only in Hong Kong and Pittsburgh, but also all over the world, where we showcase the most update research accomplishments on ligaments and tendons.

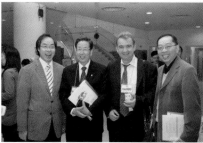 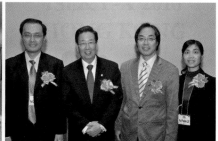

It has been a great honor to work and share some wonderful time with a great scholar, scientist, mentor and above all a friend who cares!!!

AN AGELESS SAGE

Bruce Reider

University of Chicago
Chicago, Illinois, 60637, U.S.A.
E-mail: breider@ajsm.org

I cannot recall for certain when I first met Savio Woo. Like many folks, I had read many of his papers before I met the man himself. I *think* the first time that we actually met personally was when one of his studies was among a group of papers that I was assigned to discuss at a meeting of the AOSSM. I was still fairly young, so you can imagine my trepidation when confronted with the task of discussing the work of such a distinguished and well-known scientist. Nevertheless, I made my best effort to do his work justice. After that, we became friends and often spoke at meetings.

Dr. Woo has made many extremely important contributions to the orthopaedic sports medicine literature. Perhaps because some of my own early clinical research looked into recovery after injury to the medial collateral ligament (MCL) of the knee, I remember particularly vividly his series of investigations about the MCL. I often quote this work to athletes with MCL injuries in order to explain to them how their damaged ligament will heal and the role that active movement will play in the process.

Several years ago, I served as president of the Herodicus Society. One of the most important duties of the presidency is to select a distinguished sports medicine authority to serve as the Godfather of the annual meeting. The Godfather is expected to deliver two interesting lectures and provide the other speakers with frequent sage comments and provocative questions. Although a PhD had never been Godfather before, I could think of no greater sage than Dr. Woo. Needless to say, he did a superb job. My most indelible memory of that meeting, however, was the informal dinner that my wife, Trish, and I, along with a few other officers, enjoyed with Savio and Pattie. Dr. Woo, his lips perhaps lubricated a bit by some good red wine, told us the story of his boyhood, emigration to the United States and subsequent early career. What I learned that evening about Savio only helped me admire his accomplishments even more than before.

Savio, you truly are an ageless sage in the world of sports medicine. Congratulations on achieving yet another milestone in your career. Best of luck to you and Pattie for many more happy and productive years ahead.

Fondly,
Bruce Reider

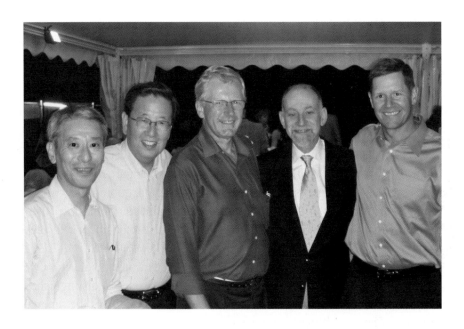

THE BEST IS YET TO COME

John Feagin

Vail Valley Medical Center
Vail, Colorado, 81658, U.S.A.
E-mail: jafduke@aol.com

On behalf of Marty and myself, congratulations on your 70th and all you have accomplished! You and I grew up together in AOSSM, AAOS, the ACL Study Group, and the conundrum of the Knee.

Every step of the way you have been a role model and raised the bar for all. Thank you for the leadership, the integrity and the wisdom you have brought to the profession we have shared. You have made our profession and the world a better place and we are privileged to have shared "the place" with you. You are one special guy and Pattie complements and completes your talents.

As I look backward and think of the role you have played and the effect you have had on our lives, I think of Shakespeare's counsel – "To thine own self be true". That has been one of your many and most salient strengths.

As I look ahead for you and those you lead and inspire, I say "the best is yet to come". The infrastructure

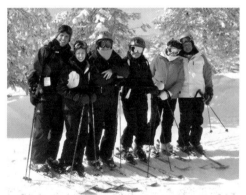

With Adam, Kirstin, Savio, Pattie & my wife, Marty

of "clean thinking and honest dealing" (from the West Point Prayer) will bring you great joy and carry you forward in the marathon of life. You are a winner and we honor your pride of accomplishment on this your 70th Birthday.

With admiration and affection, Marty and John

HAPPY 70TH BIRTHDAY SAVIO

Rene Verdonk

Ghent University Hospital
Ghent, B-9000, Belgium
E-mail: rene.verdonk@UGent.be

We have known each other through the scientific and clinical work we are producing in the locomotor field more specifically on ligaments, tendons, and the menisci. This relationship goes back to at least 1995, if not earlier, when I was touring the US as the godfather of the European Society of Sports Traumatology Knee Surgery and Arthroscopy (ESSKA) travelling fellowship and we were hosted in Pittsburgh. We continued to meet often at U.S. or European international meetings. These encounters were regularly shared by our wives, PATTIE and CHANTAL. The pictures included were taken at a unique Italian location after the ASSISI meeting with PROFESSOR GIULIANO CERULLI on his "private" truffle growing land. We discovered how the truffles were grown and found using trained dogs to do the job. The promenade in the woods up north from ASSISI was a wonderful walk on almost untouched land where nature was dictating the rules and we could enjoy its fruits. Memories we will share forever!!!!!!!!!!!!!

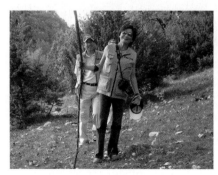
A famous U.S. couple walking the truffle woods in the Assisi Mountains

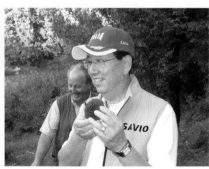
A truffle found to enjoy or …what science brings to life!!

SMART, APPROACHABLE, KIND

David B. Root

D.B. Root & Company
Pittsburgh, Pennsylvania, 15219, U.S.A.
E-mail: dbrootjr@dbroot.com

Savio and I have known each other for many years and I have enjoyed learning about his career and personal endeavors. He is as smart as he is kind, and I always admired his enthusiastic ability to share his knowledge and experiences. I remember the time Savio stopped by my office and found out that I recently had back surgery. It was not long before he was on the ground contorting himself to demonstrate palliative back exercises and stretches! It was classic Savio and indicative of his well being for others.

His career accomplishments are humbling to great men, although he manages to be approachable and kind. I am grateful to have met Savio and even more so to have become friends with him. He is a loyal companion to any Pittsburgh sporting event and I look forward to sitting next to him on the road to another Stanley Cup. I am also especially appreciative of his and Pattie's professional confidence for over twenty years.

Cheers, Savio!

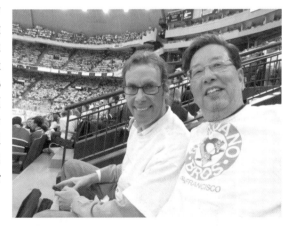

THE SCIENTIFIC OLYMPIAN

Benno Nigg

*University of Calgary
Calgary, Alberta, T2N 1N4, Canada
E-mail: nigg@ucalgary.ca*

There are only a very few people who have shaped the scientific field of Biomechanics in the last 100 years. One of the most important people in this respect is Dr. Savio Woo. He has shaped the thinking of biomechanics all over the world and is one of the main reasons that biomechanics and biomedical engineering is now a leading field of science.

One special recognition for Dr. Woo's professional work was being awarded the IOC Olympic Prize for Sports Sciences! Dr. Woo received the first gold medal of the 1998 Olympics in Nagano, Japan - for his research contributions to the field of sports medicine.

It is an honor and a privilege to celebrate with Dr. Woo, from a distance, on his 70th birthday.

With my best wishes for many more fruitful years, from Calgary.

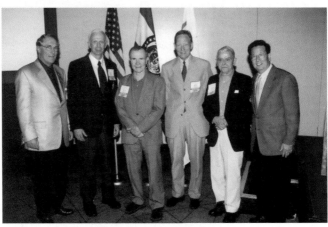

With IOC Olympic Prize Winners
Professors John Holloszy, Ralph Paffenbarger, Bengt Saltin,
Jeremy Morris and Savio Woo

SHARING GOOD TIMES

Ben and Betty Kibler

Lexington Clinic
Lexington, Kentucky, 40504, U.S.A.
E-mail: wkibler@aol.com

Betty and I have known Savio and Pattie since 1993. We have shared many times together, ranging from the Kentucky Derby (do not ask Savio to pick any horses to bet on - he lost every bet he placed), eating Chinese food from Melbourne, Australia to Vancouver, Canada (he always picks out the food), watching Pittsburgh Pirates baseball, and playing a lot of tennis (Stockholm, Sweden, Miami, San Diego, Pittsburgh, Hawaii, and 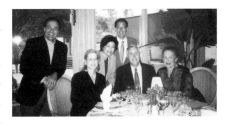 places in between). We have enjoyed their company at many dinners, and always have felt their warmth and honesty in conversations.

Congratulations, Savio, on your accomplishments - the sports medicine world is much better for your accomplishments, in science, in mentoring and encouraging many other scientists, and in being a good friend to many in all fields of sports medicine.

This picture is from one of our most memorable and enjoyable tennis trips, to the Inn at Manitou in Canada, in 1997, the Woos, the Kiblers, and the Renstroms. The food was great, the tennis was competitive, and the companionship was the best. It is these types of activities that remind us what is most important in life - good friends, taking time to enjoy each other, and building memories.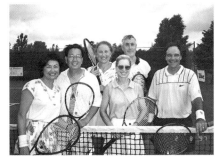

HAPPY 70TH BIRTHDAY TO MY GOOD FRIEND, SAVIO

Robert J. Johnson

University of Vermont
Burlington, Vermont, 05405, U.S.A.
E-mail: Robert.J.Johnson@uvm.edu

What a pleasure it is for me to have the opportunity to write a letter of congratulations at the time of your 70th birthday. I cannot remember when we first met. I am sure it was at least 30 years ago, but I cannot remember the details (you will be as forgetful as me when you reach my age). I have had the pleasure of being on many faculties with you throughout the years at many interesting places around the world. I have learned a great deal from you not only from your presentations at meetings as mentioned above, but also in your written work. Clearly you have contributed a tremendous addition to the knowledge that all orthopaedist need to practice good orthopaedic surgery.

I remember one of the first times that I got to know you quite well was at a Gordon Conference in New Hampshire during the summer Olympics. It may have been the Korean Olympics. It was most impressive when you and the rest of the "Chinese Mafia" loudly cheered for the Chinese teams as we watched the Olympic events late into the evening. I also recall another time that Shirley, Pattie, you and I were hosted by Tassos on a wonderful yacht trip through the Greek Islands. What a good time to get to know each other better in a beautiful environment.

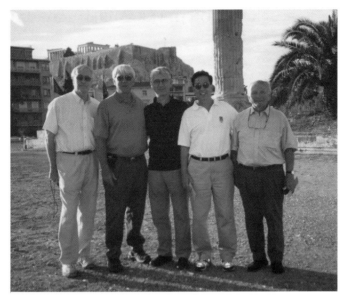

Good friends in Greece.
With Per Renström, Anastasios Georgoulis,
Savio, and Ejnar Eriksson.

I certainly wish to congratulate you for all you have done for the field of biomechanics as it applies to orthopaedic surgeons. I greatly appreciate all you have taught me through the years and I certainly wish you a very happy 70th birthday. I look forward to the continuation of our long friendship.

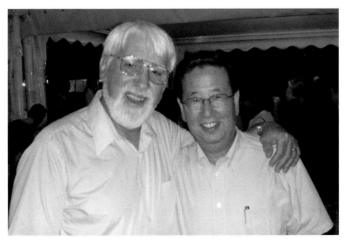

A NATIONAL TREASURE

Scott F. Dye

University of California, San Francisco
San Francisco, California, 94114, U.S.A.
E-mail: sfdyemd@aol.com

I have known Savio for over 20 years, having been a visiting speaker at the University of Pittsburgh on several occasions. I have always been impressed by his thoughtful and meticulous approach to his research. He has been called by many a "National Treasure". This is an obviously accurate description. In 2007, Savio was awarded the "Lifetime Achievement Award" given annually by the Bay Area Knee Society. This award is considered by many as a kind of "Nobel Prize of the Knee". The legacy of his work and leadership within biomechanical engineering and orthopaedic surgery is secure. I feel fortunate to be one of his many friends. Congratulations Savio, on your 70th birthday. May you be blessed with many more.

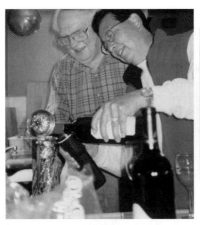

Pop and Savio

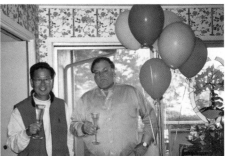

Happy Birthday to Savio in my home

SABIO

Ramon Cugat

Hospital Quiron
Barcelona, 08023, Spain
E-mail: ramon.cugat@sportrauma.com

Thanks a lot for the enormous honor of being able to collaborate in the collective creation of your special present. My family and I are honored to know you and be part of your friends.

Writing about you is very easy for Spanish speakers. In Spanish, there is a word spelled SABIO, but pronounced similarly to SAVIO.

Sabio translates to English as **Savant:** A person in possession of wisdom making his conduct prudent in life and business. Also with a deep knowledge of Physics, Exact and Natural Science, along with their opposites: Humanistic Science and The Arts.

With all due respect Savio, you are a Sabio. Your name defines you.

Family Cugat. Ramon, Montse, Debora, Coco and Pepe
CONGRATULATIONS!!

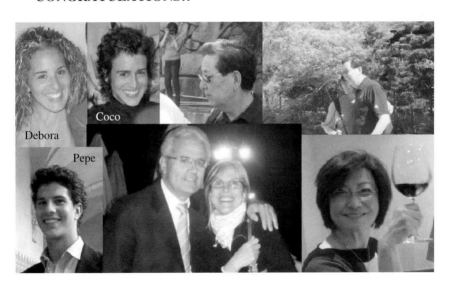

TO MY "OLD" FRIEND SAVIO WOO

Giancarlo Puddu

Clinica "Valle Giulia"
Roma, 00197, Italy
E-mail: giapu@tin.it

Dear Savio,

From all of us, happy birthday to a very special friend! We have known each other for many years and it is always with renewed pleasure when we get together all over the world. If there is one regret, it is that we would like to see you and Pattie more often!!

Now between you and me, I will always remember when standing in Union Square in San Francisco I asked you "why should there exist competition between a butcher and a fisherman? One is selling and teaching how to prepare a roast beef and the other how to prepare a dover sole." It was the only time when you answered a difficult question: "I don't know!"

Dear Savio enjoy until the year 9999. A big hug on your 70th birthday from Giancarlo, Agneta, Isabella and Cristina.

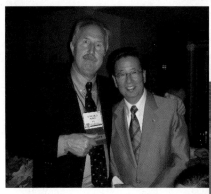
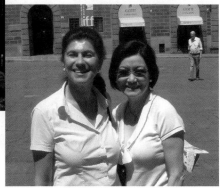

TRIBUTE TO SAVIO WOO

Peter and Linda Jokl

Yale University
New Haven, Connecticut, 06510, U.S.A
E-mail: peter.jokl@yale.edu

Linda and I want to send you our heartfelt best wishes on the celebration of your 70th birthday!

We have enjoyed so many good times with you and Pattie watching some great tennis competitions and playing tennis with you.

Your contributions to clinically relevant biomechanics and making them applicable, in your always clear and concise scientific articles or in your lectures, have contributed greatly to the Orthopaedic knowledge base. Your seminal studies have been widely applied in our clinical practices to the great benefit of our Orthopaedic patients.

We look forward to many more productive and happy years for you and Pattie.

A YOUTHFUL DR. WOO

Zong-Ming Li 李宗明

Cleveland Clinic
Cleveland, Ohio, 44195, U.S.A.
E-mail: liz4@ccf.org

I first met Dr. Savio Woo during the Fourth China-Japan-USA-Singapore Conference on Biomechanics in 1995, when I was an orthopaedic researcher at the Shanghai Institute of Orthopaedics and Traumatology, Rui Jin Hospital. During the meeting, I was attracted by Dr. Woo's lecture showing knee biomechanics with a robot. At the banquet, I managed to take a photo with Dr. Woo.

After finishing my PhD studies at Penn State in 1998, I took a faculty position at Walsh University. While there, I decided to write to Dr. Woo for advice. To my delight, he wrote back complimenting my work, pointing me in a research direction, and most importantly, inviting me to visit him. Later, I went to Pittsburgh to see Dr. Woo (of course, taking along the 1995 photo). The visit went well; at the end of our meeting, Dr. Woo told me that he might have a position open in the near future. Sometime later in 2001, a faculty position became available; I applied and accepted Dr. Woo's offer.

During my MSRC years, I was glad to have an office next to Dr. Woo's. Our interactions were instant and frequent – in offices,

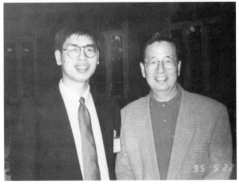

Dr. Woo and I first met in China (1995)

meetings, labs and restaurants. When Dr. Woo was in town, we always went to lunch at the Fifth Avenue Golden Palace, where the chef entertained us with special "Woo Dishes." We also drove to Mount Washington for lunch – good view, good food, and, of course, good chat.

It was common that our lunch conversations lasted for 2-3 hours. This intensive mentoring might as well be seen as brainwashing!

My experiences working closely with Dr. Woo for MSRC business, symposia, societies, and grant reviews have been invaluable. One cannot help admiring his finesse and dedication to professional leadership and service. Most recently, he founded the World Association for Chinese Biomedical Engineers, for which I was the secretary. I look forward to keeping up his high standards when I serve as President of the association in 2013.

Dr. Woo and I (and families) have traveled together to many places, such as Chengdu, Beijing, Shanghai, Hong Kong, Bangkok, Taiwan and Munich – for work and for leisure. Life is truly enjoyable being around Dr. Woo.

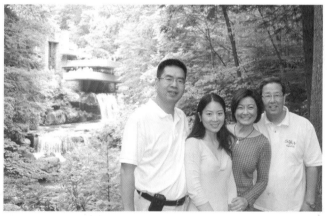

Woo and Li families at Fallingwater,
the famous Frank Lloyd Wright house in Pennsylvania

Now at the age of 70, Dr. Woo continues to be full of energy doing research, teaching students, lecturing to colleagues, and serving our profession. It is, as a Chinese saying goes, "three thousand fruits still counting, seventy years of age just as young."

桃李三千犹未满
人生七十正年轻

MAZEL TOV AND L'CHAIM

Harvey Borovetz

University of Pittsburgh
Pittsburgh, Pennsylvania, 15219, U.S.A.
E-mail: borovetzhs@upmc.edu

It is with the utmost pleasure that I send this note on behalf of Savio's 70th birthday. Savio and I have known each other professionally for more than 20 years now. Savio's recruitment to Pitt by our dear friend and mentor, Dr. Tom Detre, was an occasion of true joy for me. I say this because I knew that if Savio Woo would join the University of Pittsburgh, then the potential for excellence in bioengineering was a real possibility at Pitt. And, thanks in so many ways to Savio's exceptional contributions, we can claim with considerable pride that we have achieved excellence in bioengineering at Pitt!

I can also say with pride that throughout our 20+ year association, Savio and I have never had a disagreement. For this, I would like to take the lion's share of credit. By that I mean that almost from the day I first met Savio, he would brag about his family. In good times and not so good times, Savio always would break into a big smile if I would ask about the "Woo children." So, whenever Savio and I would meet about a challenging topic (e.g., budget), I would always make sure to begin our meeting asking about his children. And, talk about a doting grandpa, it must be true that this phrase was coined to describe how Savio dotes on and loves his grandchildren. Savio is the consummate grandpa who is always happy to show me a picture and talk about his next planned visit to California. Savio is so happy now, and his joy rubs off on me and everyone around him. The end result is that whatever academic assignment I ask Savio to undertake, be it serving for three years on the Promotions Committee or teaching a core undergraduate bioengineering class in the dead of winter in Pittsburgh, Savio agrees to do so. I simply could not ask for anything more.

So on this wonderful occasion of Professor Savio Woo's 70th birthday, I am so delighted to inform the readers of this tribute page how happy Savio is, how wonderful a colleague he is, and how fortunate we have been and continue to be for all that Savio does on behalf of our students, fellows and young faculty. Among all of Savio's many remarkable accomplishments and awards, I would rank as #1 the impact Savio has had on the young people he has educated and trained, for they are his legacy to our profession now and for years to come.

MAZEL TOV! and L'Chaim (To Life!), Savio. Fran and I wish you, Pattie, your children and grandchildren the best of everything, always.

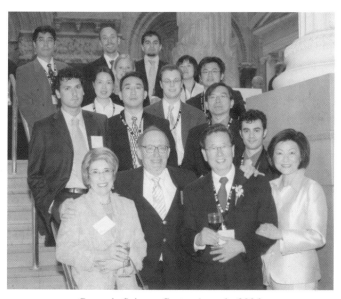

Carnegie Science Center Award - 2006

PROFESSIONAL DEBT OF GRATITUDE

Sanjeev Shroff

University of Pittsburgh
Pittsburgh, Pennsylvania, 15219, U.S.A.
E-mail: sshroff@pitt.edu

Greetings Savio and Pattie. Thank you for the opportunity to say a few words at this joyous occasion; I am pleased and honored to do so. I am not going to say anything about Savio's academic and professional contributions and accomplishments – you all know this very well and more importantly, if I did talk about his professional life, then I would simply be stating the obvious. So, allow me to say something about Savio as a person instead, a person who is faced with the same professional and personal challenges that all of us face and who, like all of us, does not always know the "right" or "perfect" answer. Although I knew of Savio for a long time, it is only over the past 5 years or so that I have had significant interactions with him. In spite of this relatively short interaction time, I have learned something very valuable from Savio – the idea of "professional debt of gratitude." Clearly, our professional lives are in a very competitive arena, wherein an inward-looking focus is of prime importance – my goals, my needs, my accomplishments, etc. I have learned from Savio to also look outwards – for he strongly believes that each one of us is standing on the shoulders of those who have come before us and it is just a matter of honest introspection to identify the professional debt of gratitude one owes to these individuals. Of course, this idea of professional debt of gratitude is not limited to those who have come before us; it extends to our contemporaries and those who will follow us, i.e., our students. Although this type of thinking is not a magic bullet, it has helped me in my decision-making process, particularly those that involve human interactions and I have Savio to thank for this wonderful lesson.

I am not the only one who has noted Savio's remarkable humanistic qualities. Allow me to share quotes from two very accomplished individuals – I am sorry I cannot divulge their identity, nor can I divulge the context in which these quotes were made. Most of you are in the academic arena – so you should be able to figure out the context for yourselves.

"Finally, Professor Woo is a person of impeccable character, unimpeachable ethics, and high moral values. He has always represented himself, his profession, and his institution in the highest standards." (Quote-1)

"In addition to the academic achievements, which are so abundantly evident in his publication record and the number of successful researchers he has trained and groomed, what makes Professor Savio Woo a remarkable leader in academia is his deep sense of humanity and a desire to influence others, often by his own example." (Quote-2).

Savio – Surya and I want to wish you a happy 70th birthday and many more. Thank you for your friendship, advice, and inspiration.

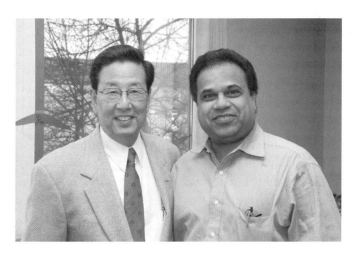

A TRIBUTE TO DR. WOO: FROM RECRUITMENT TO PITTSBURGH TO A VALUED MENTOR AND FRIEND

David Vorp

University of Pittsburgh
Pittsburgh, Pennsylvania, 15219, U.S.A.
E-mail: VorpDA@upmc.edu

While a PhD student in the late 1980s at the University of Pittsburgh, Department of Mechanical Engineering, performing my dissertation in the area of (cardiovascular) biomechanics, I, of course, was familiar with Dr. Woo's work. This period of time was an exciting era of growth at the University of Pittsburgh and the University of Pittsburgh Medical Center (UPMC). Giants – such as Dr. Albert Ferguson, the pioneering Chair of Orthopedic Surgery, Dr. Henry Bahnson, the legendary Chair of Surgery, Dr. Peter Safar, who pioneered CPR, and Dr. Thomas Detre, who was the architect behind the formation of UPMC – were still walking the hallways. With Dr. Detre's recruitment of Dr. Thomas Starzl, Pittsburgh became the World's foremost center for organ transplantation science and clinical medicine. Analogous to this for the field of biomechanics was the news that the University was attempting to recruit Dr. Woo. There was an air of excitement surrounding the recruitment efforts, and all of us in the bioengineering community in Pittsburgh were excited. Being one of the few graduate students at the University of Pittsburgh at the time working in the area of biomechanics, and being a native Pittsburgher, I was asked to do my part by helping to "sell" the University, and Pittsburgh in general, to Dr. Woo's graduate students who were then with him at UCSD. I was told to take the students to a "nice restaurant", but being a poor graduate student, I had no idea what that was! After seeking the input from some friends, I ended up driving all of the students 12 miles into the northern suburbs to a restaurant that I would not place in the area's top 50 today.

When I was recruited by the Department of Surgery to initiate a focused research program on vascular biomechanics, I requested help from Dr. Woo, who graciously allowed me to use some of his equipment for the generation of critical preliminary data, which eventually led to my first grant funding. I am forever grateful for his kindness and generosity in those early days of my faculty appointment. Since then, I have continued to learn from and be the recipient of Dr. Woo's graciousness. My wife, Allison, and son, Justin, have also come to love Dr. Woo and his beautiful wife Pattie. We will forever cherish the wonderful dinners that we often have together, where we occasionally get to see Dr. Woo's culinary skills (Fig. 1). And who will ever forget the amazing Sunday brunch at Lautrec at the Nemacolin Woodlands Resort (Fig. 2) after the 2011 Summer Bioengineering Conference, where I was fortunate to be honored with the ASME Van C. Mow Medal the same year that ASME recognized Dr. Woo on the occasion of his 70th birthday.

Congratulations, Dr. Woo, on your milestone birthday and on all of your tremendous accomplishments! Paraphrasing from Allison's great-grandmother on the occasion of her 100th birthday: Remember, the first 70 years are the hardest! Enjoy your next, easier 70 years!

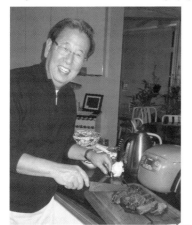

Fig. 1: Dr. Woo cutting filet for one of the dinners with the Vorps and Shroffs at his home

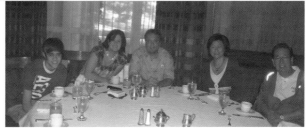

Fig. 2 (right): Brunch at Lautrec (2011). From left: Justin, Allison and David Vorp; Pattie and Dr. Woo.

A PARTNER IN TRIUMPH – BIOENGINEERING AT THE UNIVERSITY OF PITTSBURGH

Jerome S. Schultz

University of California, Riverside
Riverside, California, 92521, U.S.A.
E-mail: jerome.schultz@ucr.edu

I joined the University of Pittsburgh, School of Engineering in 1987 to lead the development of the Center for Biotechnology and Bioengineering. Initially this was tough going as there was a general perception of faculty in the School of Engineering that starting a new initiative would take away limited resources from other programs in the School. Also there was some hesitancy in developing joint programs with the "800 pound gorilla" School of Medicine.

In order to facilitate joint programs with the School of Medicine, we decided to formulate a joint academic graduate program leading to a Ph.D. in Bioengineering. Another function of this new program was to enhance joint research projects between the School of Engineering and the School of Medicine. A national search for the Directorship of this new School of Engineering program was undertaken, and Savio Woo was the unanimous choice of the selection committee. Dr. James Herndon, Chair of Orthopaedic Surgery was on the selection committee and saw a broader role for Savio at Pittsburgh, and made a counter offer to Savio as the Director of a new Musculoskeletal Research Center within the School of Medicine.

Savio wisely chose this great opportunity and we benefited by his decision to join the University of Pittsburgh. The subsequent significant impact of Savio on the explosive growth of Bioengineering at Pittsburgh was manifested in many ways, but most importantly, he was a major factor in our ability to obtain support from the Whitaker Foundation. These grants were the key factors for the start of a new independent Bioengineering Department within the School of Engineering.

With Savio's support, we were able to attract an energetic and talented group of faculty that have been the essential ingredients of this successful enterprise.

One testament to the national recognition of our bioengineering program was the induction of both Savio and me to the National Academy of Engineering in 1994.

Pitt Bioengineering also had a major role in the establishment and operation of the American Institute for Medical and Biological Engineering (AIMBE). The picture below shows a group of us celebrating the 1992 Inaugural Event of AIMBE at the National Academy of Engineering in Washington, D.C. I organized this event with the assistance of Savio and other Bioengineering faculty.

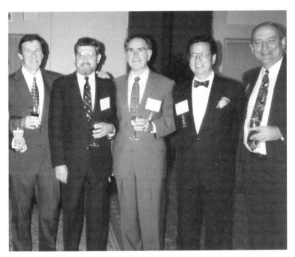

With (l-r) Cliff Brubaker, Sidney Wolfson, Savio and Robert Nerem

A SIGNIFICANT SUCCESS STORY

James Herndon

*Massachusetts General Hospital
Boston, Massachusetts, 02114, U.S.A.
E-mail: jherndon@partners.org*

Congratulations, Savio! I hope you, your family and friends have a special and wonderful celebration of your 70th birthday.

It was a real honor for the University of Pittsburgh - Department of Orthopaedic Surgery and the School of Engineering - when you agreed to join the faculty and re-establish your laboratory at the Medical School. Your major contributions continued and you brought our Department and our Sports Medicine Division to new levels of scientific excellence.

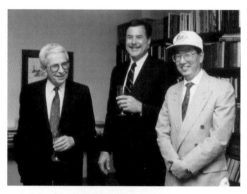

With Drs. Thomas Detre, & Woo (1990)

I continue to have fond memories of our friendship and our families' friendship as well as your many successes in bringing orthopaedic bioengineering research to Pitt: NIH research funding, an unbelievable number of distinguished research fellows, scientific presentations and publications, a terrific teaching program for our residents and students, and even a new division of bioengineering in Pitt's School of Engineering.

Yours has been a significant success story. Congratulations again! Gerry and I wish you and Pattie many more continued years of happiness together.

A TRIBUTE TO DR. WOO

Mark S. Redfern

University of Pittsburgh
Pittsburgh, Pennsylvania, 15261, U.S.A.
E-mail: mredfern@pitt.edu

It is an honor to be able to write this note to Dr. Woo, acknowledging his contributions to biomechanics, bioengineering, and clinical treatment of musculoskeletal disorders. I knew Dr. Woo by reputation for decades. Being in the biomechanics field, I followed his research discoveries with great interest and admiration. When he decided to come to the University of Pittsburgh, I was thrilled and excited that such a prominent and distinguished research scientist was going to be a colleague. I felt that Dr. Woo's stature and knowledge of biomechanics would be a catalyst here at Pitt to grow a world-class biomechanics research effort across the campus. I must say, Dr. Woo did not disappoint. When he arrived, he built the Musculoskeletal Research Center (MSRC) into one of the leading orthopaedic biomechanics research facilities in the world. His personal research efforts in ligament structure-function and other work in biomaterials have been outstanding. In addition, he built a Center that includes other top researchers with the same ultimate goal of improving the treatment of musculoskeletal disorders. He also has mentored many students and junior faculty along the way, who have since gone on to also do great work in biomechanics. Now, he provides leadership to the Department of Bioengineering and continues biomechanics research towards his goal of improving patient care that he established at the start of his amazing career.

Congratulations on an outstanding career. Your leadership and research efforts have led to new discoveries that have impacted the care of patients. I look forward to your continued contributions to the field of biomechanics and your help leading Pitt Bioengineering to even greater heights.

LONG MAY YOU RUN

Patrick Loughlin

University of Pittsburgh
Pittsburgh, Pennsylvania, 15261, U.S.A.
E-mail: loughlin@pitt.edu

Dear Savio,

It is my great honor and privilege to be included among the many family, friends and distinguished colleagues that have been invited to mark the happy occasion of your 70th birthday by offering a few words of congratulations and reflection. Although I have known you for but a relatively brief period of your very distinguished career, it has indeed been a pleasure to get to know and learn from you.

You are a man of great compassion, humility, intellect and thoughtfulness. When I formally switched my primary appointment from electrical engineering to bioengineering just a few years ago, you were the very first faculty member to respond to Dr. Borovetz' email announcement and warmly welcomed me into the department – a most kind, thoughtful and very genuine gesture on your part. Your kind words and gentle counsel over the years have been equally welcomed and inspiring. While you are rightfully renowned and respected for your many scientific accomplishments, I believe your actions and words have likewise made a very positive, indelible impression on a host of students, colleagues, friends and family.

I wish you all the best on your 70th birthday. As the song goes, "long may you run," and may you, Pattie and your dear family and friends have trunks of memories to come!

"ENGINEERING NOBILITY"

Alan Russell

Carnegie Mellon University
Pittsburgh, Pennsylvania, 15213, U.S.A.
E-mail: alanrussell@cmu.edu

Dear Savio,

On this important birthday, it is my great pleasure to congratulate you on a remarkable career that has been filled with glittering highlights. As a young faculty member, I remember well hearing about "Dr. Woo's" recruitment. I went to the internet (which was in its earliest form) to learn more. As I read of your accomplishments, I was struck by two thoughts. First, I thought it a real statement that the University of Pittsburgh would be able to attract such "engineering nobility". Second, as I looked over the resume, I was struck by a desire to one day come close to your stature and accomplishments.

Although I never achieved your stature and accomplishments, I am proud to say that something much more important happened. You became a close friend and advisor. As careers move forward, professional relationships are important, but real friendships transcend and outweigh everything else. It is humbling to know you as a friend and I look forward to many more years of hearing your calm advice and wise counsel.

Happy Birthday, Savio!

YOU ARE THE BEST

Jag Sankar

North Carolina Agricultural & Technical State University
Greensboro, North Carolina, 27411, U.S.A.
E-mail: sankar@ncat.edu

I came to know Dr. Woo in 2007, when we were discussing ideas to apply for the NSF Engineering Research Center (ERC) grant with the University of Pittsburgh. Since then, I have to come to know him very well.

He exemplifies character that everyone wants to emulate. His smooth, soft spoken, vision driven style has taught the entire ERC family well. One thing I always noticed is the aura of wisdom that he brings with him when he walks into any gathering without saying a single word….. truly remarkable. I sincerely feel this is because of all the wonderful things he has done to so many in his life.

Dear Dr. Woo, have a great 70th birthday and many, many more. I know, by hanging with you some of your greatness may rub on all of us.

With warmest regards and many, many happy years to come.

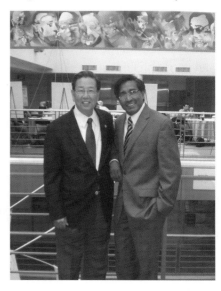

A TEACHER AND MENTOR

William T. Green, Jr.

University of Pittsburgh
Pittsburgh, Pennsylvania, 15243-2039, U.S.A.
E-mail: wtg@pitt.edu

Savio, as a fellow septuagenarian, I welcome you to the age of personal evaluation. "We stand on the shoulders of giants." As teacher and mentor, you have played this role for many.

My father and teacher – I did much of my surgical training under my father and understand his devotion to orthopaedic surgery – emphasized the importance of basic science in clinical medicine. He felt that a basic scientist ought to be part of the leadership of a healthy department of orthopaedic surgery. I believe you would agree with him.

I want to thank you for inviting me to attend your afternoon conferences in the School of Medicine during which you moderated presentations and discussed current research projects under your direction. It gave me the opportunity to learn and by my discussion, to connect the projects with clinical orthopaedic surgery. I was disappointed that more of my clinical colleagues did not take this opportunity and attend. Perhaps it was the increased business pressure on the faculty to bring more income into the academic health center, a pressure that I consciously resisted.

Leaders of academic medicine should find a pathway towards this goal for the future. MDs must respect and work with their PhD colleagues. Even in the business world, success comes with an appropriate investment in research and development.

Dorothy and I wish you, Pattie, and your family health, happiness and prosperity in the future.

A REMARKABLE SCIENTIST AND PERSON

Marc J. Philippon

The Steadman Philippon Research Institute & The Steadman Clinic
Vail, Colorado, 81657, U.S.A.
E-mail: drphilippon@steadmanclinic.net

It is with great pleasure that I take part in this celebration of Dr. Woo's 70th birthday. I first met Dr. Woo in 2001 when I became a new faculty of the Department of Orthopaedic Surgery at the University of Pittsburgh Medical Center (PMC). I came into the department as the Director of Sports Medicine Hip Disorders and Dr. Woo was considered the best in biomechanics in the world. Dr. Woo's research of the knee had influenced the way knee injuries were being treated.

I remember meeting him in his office. I was extremely excited to have the opportunity to discuss research ideas. Dr. Woo was very supportive and gave me a very important pearl that has helped me throughout my career. He shared with me the importance of formulating a precise research question – If I had too many hypotheses, I would never get projects finished. Since our first meeting, our relationship has progressed. I moved to Vail, where Dr. Woo is a member of the Steadman Philippon Research Institute Scientific Advisory Board. He visits several times a year providing insight into our research.

Everyone who comes in contact with him not only learns from the experience, but enjoys spending time with him. Dr. Woo is a remarkable scientist and person. I will always remember what he taught me about clarity and how to approach a research question. Research is Dr. Woo's career, but he is also an excellent person and I enjoy spending time with him. He always has a smile on his face and I wish the best to him in all his future adventures. Best wishes on your 70th birthday!

HAPPY 70TH BIRTHDAY SAVIO!

Larry J. Shuman

University of Pittsburgh
Pittsburgh, Pennsylvania, 15261, U.S.A.
E-mail: shuman@pitt.edu

Congratulations Savio! What a wonderful 20 years it has been! I fondly recall the first time we met – T.K. and I picked you up at the airport and showed you the city. We told you our dreams for Bioengineering at Pitt; dreams that you shared. Amazingly, those dreams have been realized and then some! Certainly you deserve a large share of the credit for helping to provide a solid foundation from which to build such an outstanding program. One of my most enjoyable moments as interim dean was the reception we held in honor of you and Jerry Schultz being inducted into the National Academy of Engineers together – an event that occurred soon after you joined us. It was an important national recognition; it further indicated that our Bioengineering Program and our new Department were on their way to national and now international prominence.

Every time I visit La Jolla, I marvel as to how we were able to twist your arm to leave sunny California for Pittsburgh! I am sure that there were many winter days when you must have asked yourself the same question. We are delighted you made that decision – as I recall your request to come to Pittsburgh included 50 yard line and center court seats among a few other things!

Barbara and I send our best wishes to you and Pattie on your 70th birthday. Enjoy your grandchildren as we are doing the same.

Best,
Larry and Barbara Shuman

A MENTOR, A COLLEAGUE AND A FRIEND

Harry E. Rubash

Massachusetts General Hospital and Harvard Medical School
Boston, Massachusetts, 02114, U.S.A.
E-mail: hrubash@partners.org

I met Dr. Woo early in my career at the University of Pittsburgh. Dr. Woo was an important mentor for me as I began to formulate my initial research interests in the field of total joint arthroplasty. His invaluable guidance in the areas of musculoskeletal research and bioengineering eventually helped me to bridge the disciplines of clinical medicine and basic science to better understand the biomechanics and failure mechanisms of total joint arthroplasty (TJA) in the hip and knee.

Congratulations Dr. Woo on this very special birthday. I wish you all the best and thank you for the tremendous impact you have made on my career!

Jon JP Warner

Harvard Medical School/Massachusetts General Hospital
Boston, Massachusetts, 02115, U.S.A.
E-mail: JWarner@partners.org

Savio played a very important part in my early academic career. His guidance in matters of research helped me ultimately win the Kappa Delta Award for original research in shoulder biomechanics. It is doubtful I would have achieved such recognition if not for his input, teaching and support. On a personal note, he and Pattie were always very kind to my wife, Geraldine, and myself, and we shared many experiences of our children as they grew and developed. There is no question that I am a better Surgeon Scientist for having known Dr. Woo and I am pleased to have the opportunity to say so.

All my best wishes.

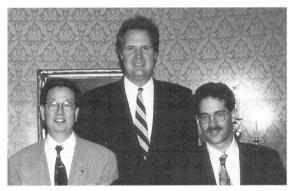

Drs. Woo, Rubash and Warner

James Kang
*University of Pittsburgh
Pittsburgh, Pennsylvania, 15213, U.S.A.
E-mail: kangjd@upmc.edu*

I wish you a very Happy 70th Birthday and congratulate you on your great accomplishments. I wanted to personally thank you for your early mentorship and the support that you provided me (and our budding spine research team) as I started my clinician scientist career. I wish you continued good health and many more momentous birthday celebrations.

回憶科學耕耘二十年

Cheng-Wen (Ken) Wu **吳成文**

National Health Research Institutes
Zhunan, Miaoli County, 350, Taiwan
E-mail: ken@nhri.org.tw

台灣經過將近三十年的耕耘，生命科學研究逐次與世界先進國家接軌，除了學術界力爭上游之外，背後尚有一股龐大的奧援：有一群華裔的學者，秉持著回饋民族的心情，二十多年來，每年如同候鳥一樣，飛到台灣，以其專精的學術經歷，提供諮詢，參與研究計畫的審查並導引方向。這一群學人對台灣生命科學的發展，有著實質的意義，功不可沒。胡流源院士就是一位這每年返鄉的候鳥，我與胡院士的結緣，也因此疊綿了二十多年。

胡院士來自香港，於美國華盛頓大學獲得博士學位，之後在美任教與從事學術研究，學術成績斐然，獲得國際大獎無數，並在1996當選中研院數理組院士，是一位謙恭溫和，任事認真的科學家。

我與胡院士在90年代初結識。那時我方回台灣不久，為家鄉生命科學學術研究拓墾撒種，我發現當時台灣的研究計畫其研究經費不足，研究時程侷促，同時因為國內研究人員有限，研究評審制度未建立，難以揀選出優異的計畫，非常不利於需要長期深研的科學發展，因此我排除萬難，先在中研院生醫所設立了整合性醫藥衛生研究計畫，希望以較高的研究經費、多年期的研究時程，以及嚴謹的評審制度，鼓勵與篩選出卓越的研究計畫。

這其中評審制度的建立最為重要，一定要藉助國際上同領域、研究有成的科學家，參與國內研究計畫的審查，來濟補台灣學術人才不足的難處，這即是我國引進國外學術評審制度同儕審查(peer review)的初端。

而華裔在國外學術有成的科學家們，成為整合性醫藥衛生研究計畫的最佳後盾。胡院士從最初整合性計畫開始，每年均風塵僕僕地回台，就其專精的醫學工程學術領域，參與計畫審查，並主持計畫的決選。爾後國家衛生研究院成立，整合性計畫移至國衛院，胡院士始終如一，還是年年如候鳥一樣往訪台、美兩地，為台灣這一塊初萌芽的科學領地，貢獻學術智慧與時間，二十餘年如一日，默默地付出奉獻。

除了整合性研究計畫的審查，國衛院成立醫學工程研究組之刻，胡院士為該組組主任遴選委員會委員以及學術諮詢委員會委員，從費心為國衛院尋找優秀的組主任，到參與審查學術進度、提供醫工組最佳的發展意見，無不用心至極，這一份對台灣科學土地的關愛，非常值得一書。

因為生醫所以及國衛院之緣，我有幸與胡院士成為好友，我也曾造訪他在匹茲堡大學的實驗室，以及他任教的系所，一睹其學術奧堂，內心非常敬佩。有時，藉著國內或是國外會議，以及學術審查之便，與胡院士及夫人一起相聚用餐，兩人話題總是環繞如何提振台灣的學術競爭力，與如何激勵卓越的計畫上。同是學人心腸，兩份學術交誼，轉眼已經二十餘年。

今日大家都是七十耄耋，這時候，還是企盼胡院士一秉初衷，繼續為台灣的生命科學博智效力，有生之日，讓加總起來已經超過三甲子年歲的我們，還能清悠閒話科學家常，一路說說候鳥過往——這一長串耕耘的回憶。

也祝胡院士永遠健康、永遠快樂。

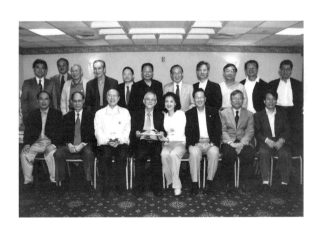

A GREAT TEACHER

Monto Ho

University of Pittsburgh and National Health Research Institutes, Taiwan
Pittsburgh, Pennsylvania, 15241, U.S.A.
E-mail: monto@nhri.org.tw

It is my pleasure and honor to participate in the celebration of your seventieth birthday. You look and act so much younger that it is hard to believe that you have attained those years. Really though, medicine has advanced so much that one can no longer say that "Life begins at Forty", rather we should go back to our ancient Chinese philosopher, Confucius, who said that "At age Seventy, One follows what the heart desires, without fear of transgression." You are a true model of that ideal.

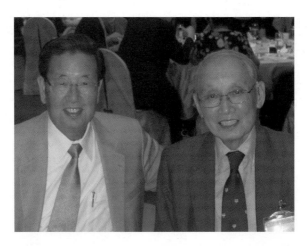

One is overawed if one looks over your accomplishments. Besides having attained the renown of an internationally recognized researcher in your field, you have become a great teacher. That was already the case in 1996, when you were elected to Academia Sinica of Taiwan and we first got to know each other. Your activities there attest to your greatness as a teacher. Since the establishment of the extramural research program of the Academy you have been the director of its bioengineering program.

That program is the most important teaching instrument of us academicians who have become instructors in the program. It is strictly voluntary and giving. There has been an enjoyable camaraderie among leaders of this group, shared by our wives.

I read an account of you in the Internet that the Musculoskeletal Research Center (MSRC) had in 1991-2007 over one hundred fellows who spent two years with you. This is further testimony of your fame and ability.

Carol and I wish you a Happy Seventieth Birthday, and Many Happy Returns.

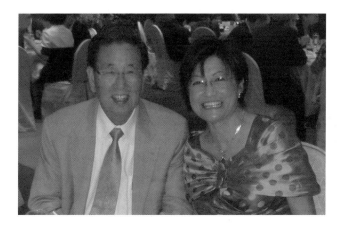

A TRIBUTE TO SAVIO WOO

Chien Ho

Carnegie Mellon University
Pittsburgh, Pennsylvania, 15213, U.S.A.
E-mail: chienho@andrew.cmu.edu

Happy 70th Birthday to you! You have reached a respectable age!

We have been friends for over 25 years. I have always valued our friendship as well as your advice and am an admirer of your scientific accomplishments.

Since 2000, it has been a great pleasure to work with you as the Chair of the Biomedical Engineering Review Committee of the National Heath Research Institutes (NHRI). Through your leadership, your Scientific Review Committee has done an outstanding job in promoting biomedical engineering research in Taiwan and the quality of the research projects has improved greatly. You should be proud of your accomplishments!

I am enclosing two photos that were taken during past meetings of the NHRI Scientific Study Review Committees and Scientific Council. Even though one of the pictures was taken 7 years ago, you look the same as today. This is no doubt because Pattie has taken good care of you!

Nancy joins me in sending our very best wishes to you and Pattie on your 70th birthday.

Tributes from Colleagues and Friends 315

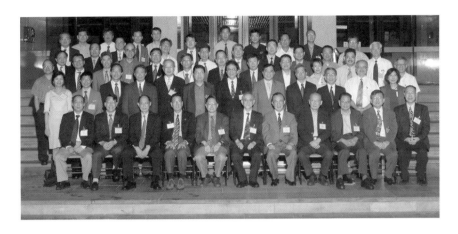

九十三年度國家衛生研究院院外研究計畫學術審查會 8/24-26, 2004
2004 NHRI Scientific Review Meeting

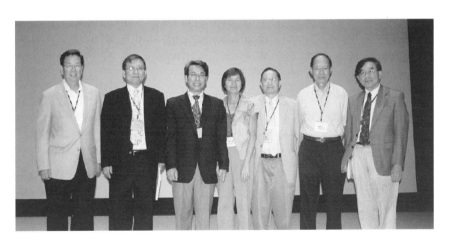

2010 NHRI Biomedical Research Symposium

A LIFETIME MENTOR

Daisy Tsai

Academia Sinica
Taipei, 115, Taiwan
E-mail: daisy306@gate.sinica.edu.tw

In January of 1993, The National Health Research Institutes (NHRI) had its first study session meeting in New York for granting life science projects throughout Taiwan. Dr. Woo was one of the reviewers in the Medical Biology (MB) study section for which I served as executive secretary. That was the first time I met Dr. Woo. In 1995, the NHRI study session meeting moved back to Taiwan and in the meantime, the Medical Engineering (ME) study section was branched from MB, and Dr. Woo has served as the chair of ME ever since. So we started to have more opportunities to work together and discuss with each other.

In those sessions, Dr. Woo generously shared his insights and wisdom, not only as a scientific mentor, but also as a trusted friend. His advice more than helped and guided the operation of the review process, it has also shed light during intersections in my life. His support has been an important driving force in every milestone during my career. When Dr. Woo and I first met, I was just a junior staff. He has accompanied me on each step of the way since then. The Extramural Research Affairs Department was officially established along with the NHRI in January 1996. All through my promotion to program manager, senior program manager to deputy director, Savio is always the source of constructive advice, heartfelt encouragements, and unreserved recommendation.

In his gentle way, Savio taught me how to be a professional woman by treating me as his equal. During a meeting in 1993, he saw me trying to serve tea to the reviewers. He then whispered "Daisy, don't do that, you are a professional person, don't make yourself the water girl. This is America, men can serve themselves." In return for his support, I want to make every meeting with Savio a special occasion. One time, I found he loved pickled bird pear, which is only available in Taiwan. Since then, it has now become our little secret that we will have such pickled pear as our coffee time desert in every meeting I organized.

Savio always speaks softly and slowly, but with dignity and nobility. Before Savio, I never met anyone who could say my very mundane Chinese name "Shu-Fang" with such elegance. In that deep and resonating voice, I found the friendship with the greats can be enjoyed even in such small matters as hearing my own name called. A portrayal of Savio is not complete without Mrs. Woo. Whenever Pattie came to a meeting with Savio, she always packed her own schedule and had lots of fun while Savio was on duty. Yet, she still managed to draw the spotlight in the banquet or social events. She makes me believe that there is always an independent woman behind every successful husband.

I appreciate that my dear friend always challenges me to move forward and achieve more and to always be true to myself. In 2003, I was fearless to take the more challenging post in Academia Sinica. I would not be who I am without Savio's guidance and encouragement. I wish that everything that is 70 years old is as awesome as Savio. Happy Birthday, to a timeless classic, who will never go out of style.

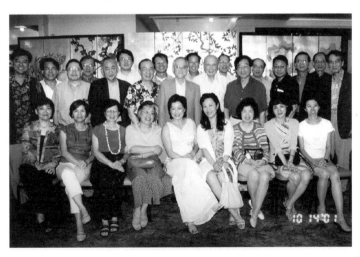

NHRI Scientific Council Meeting
Hawaii (2001)

THANK YOU FOR YOUR INSPIRATION

Zhi-Pei Liang

University of Illinois at Urbana-Champaign
Urbana, Illinois, 61801, U.S.A.
E-mail: z-liang@illinois.edu

As you all know, Savio is a legend in the field of biomedical engineering. His name was known to me as soon as I entered graduate school to study biomedical engineering at Case Western Reserve University in 1983. However, the opportunity to get to know Savio *personally* came 17 years later, mostly by luck: In 2000, Savio was looking for a reviewer with MRI expertise for his National Health Research Institutes (NHRI) Study Section. I believe that my name came up when he asked his National Academy of Engineering colleague, University of California at Berkeley Professor Tom Budinger for recommendations. I was delighted to receive his invitation to serve and accepted it without any hesitation, despite earlier visa difficulties associated with my travel to Taiwan. For the past 11 years, I have always looked forward to the annual NHRI Study Section meeting!

Savio is truly an amazing person. There is no need for me to elaborate on the fact that he is a great researcher and technical leader whose work has impacted the field profoundly; there is no need for me to say, either, that he is a fantastic mentor who cares deeply about his students and colleagues. But let me share an observation of how inspiring a teacher he is.

The flagship annual international conference of IEEE Engineering in Medicine and Biology Society (EMBS) was held from September 1-5 in San Francisco (http://www.fresno.ucsf.edu/embs2004/). As the Program Chair, I had the privilege and honor of inviting Savio to give one of the four plenary lectures. Savio's lecture was on *biomechanics*, which was not a sexy, popular topic for EMBS members. I have to admit that I was a bit "worried" that his Plenary might not be well attended, which would make him and our Society look bad. However, my "worry" turned out to be not justified at all as Savio's reputation attracted a large crowd to his lecture. In addition, Savio gave such an inspiring lecture that the conference committee invited him back to give another Keynote lecture in the subsequent IEEE-EMBS annual meeting held in Shanghai, September 1-5, 2005. It is interesting to note that although EMBS has had many luminaries (such as Nobel Laureates Paul Lauterbur, Steve Chu, Andrew Fire) as plenary/keynote speakers for its flagship annual meeting, Savio is the only person so far who has been invited to give a plenary/keynote lecture in two consecutive annual meetings. What can I say? Savio just has a unique talent to teach and inspire!

There is a Chinese saying, "人到七十古来稀 (one is blessed to live to age 70)." So, July 26 is truly a special day for Savio and for his family and friends, a day for celebration! Without further ado, let me extend my warmest congratulations to Savio, a role model and inspiration. I would also like to use this opportunity to express my sincerest appreciation for having had the opportunity to work with and learn from him; I shall value the experience for the rest of my life. I wish Savio a very happy 70th birthday and many happy and healthy years to come!

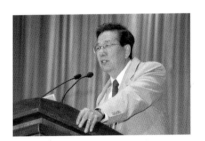

Savio delivering an inspiring plenary lecture for the 26th Annual Int'l Conference of IEEE-EMBS, Sept. 3, 2004, San Francisco.

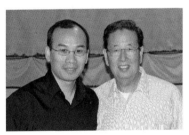

Drs. Woo and Liang
2011 NHRI Study Section Scientific Review Committee on Medical Engineering in Taiwan

A PRIVILEGE TO KNOW YOU

Kam W. Leong

Duke University
Durham, North Carolina, 27708, U.S.A.
E-mail: kam.leong@duke.edu

It is with the greatest pleasure, and honor, that I write as a colleague, mentee, and "student" to pay tribute to a giant in biomechanics and biomedical engineering.

When I received your invitation to serve in National Health Research Institute (NHRI) in the late 1990s, my hair was black, my waistline thinner than a sumo wrestler, and my professional view confined to struggles in my small lab. Since then I have grayed, ballooned, and expanded my thinking on what should I do as a researcher and an educator. The last two developments are attributed to you--actually the first one too, with all those pressures to finish the reviews on time. Your introduction of good food directly or indirectly during all these NHRI visits has corrupted my simple culinary requirement; for that I will hold you responsible forever. At the same time, your inspiration on how to approach science and education with innovation, integrity, humility, and generosity has left me with a deep impression; for that I will be grateful forever.

You may not remember my visit to your Musculoskeletal Research Center in January 2005, but it was one of my most enjoyable seminar trips to any university: the dinner in the club house, the basketball game (Pitt vs. Georgetown), the discussion of science. I shall always treasure this "non-biodegradable" memory.

It has been a privilege to know you. I have learned much from you: your strife for excellence, scholarship, integrity, and most of all, humanity. You inspiration will stay with me. I shall always remember your kindness and generosity, and repay you by passing on your legacy in my humble way to my students and the next generation of scientists.

I wish you the best as you devote more time to your family, and look forward to seeing great things you and Pattie are achieving with your philanthropic effort to help deserving international students and orthopedic scientists.

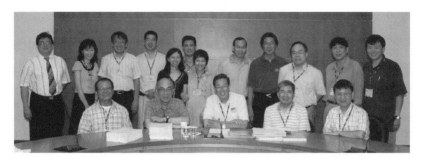

NHRI Panel chaired by Dr. Woo (2010)

THE SAVIO I KNOW – MENTOR, CONNOISSEUR, SCHOLAR

Abraham "Abe" Lee

University of California at Irvine
Irvine, California, 92697-2715, U.S.A.
E-mail: aplee@uci.edu, aplee@cal.berkeley.edu

I first met Savio during one of the last Whitaker Foundation grant review panel meetings in Washington, D.C. in April 2003. I was a rookie serving this monumental organization (Whitaker Foundation is arguably the most instrumental in establishing Bioengineering/BME as a discipline in the US) for the first time, though most others in the meeting were regulars and heavyweights in the field. Furthermore, it was only my second year as a faculty member at UC Irvine. I must have done okay reviewing the proposals as Savio approached me during one of the breaks and asked more about what I did. He subsequently invited me to serve on the National Health Research Institute (NHRI) Scientific Review Committee that was to meet in August that year. My first impression of Savio was someone eager to meet and promote young faculty/researchers despite his high esteem and glowing achievements. He was gentle and encouraging, and made those around him feel a sense of affirmation and willingness to work with/for him. Savio is a leader to those around him and I consider him one of my first mentors as a Biomedical Engineering academician.

In subsequent years, I would meet Savio every summer at the NHRI Scientific Review Meetings in Taiwan, first at Academic Sinica and more recently at NHRI campus in Zhunan. I invited him to give a talk at UC Irvine and even attempted to recruit him to our campus.

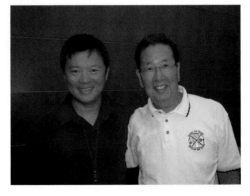

I would also see him at various conferences (e.g. BMES and EMBS annual meetings) and got to know more about the seminal work he had accomplished over his illustrious career. I also was made aware of the charitable work he founded (ASIAM Institute) including the scholarship for young biomechanics researchers and was involved with his efforts to start the World Association for Chinese Biomedical Engineers (WACBE). I witnessed a special person up-close with vision, with passion, and with the delicate skills to lead a team of highly accomplished individuals from all around the world to collectively help the younger generation make it in the ever-competitive research environment.

Aside from Savio's academic and leadership prowess', I have seen his attention to details and zeal for excellent work spill out to the lighter side of life. I have found Savio to be a connoisseur's connoisseur of food, always seeking out delicacy in the most adventurous locations. We would sneak out of different review meetings to taste the best food in town – be it greasy-fried dough for breakfast or super fresh fish we got to pick out from a large tank at the entrance of the eatery. These restaurants were not fancy some even without air conditioning in the sizzling Taiwan summers, yet the tasty food and the memorable "group outings" have left an indelible, if not mischievous, smile on our faces every time we meet. Life is that much more enjoyable when one is around Savio!

Savio, it is hard to imagine that you are celebrating your 70th birthday! You are young at heart, vibrant in life, and willingly hang out with young lads (not so much any more) like us. In fact, I think you make all of us younger each year and willing to do more to contribute to the field to the betterment of human health and life quality. I wish you a most deserving and joyful birthday. May you and Pattie continue to amaze us with the fountain of youth that you seem to never run out of!

A LEADER WITH FORESIGHT AND CONVICTION

K. Kirk Shung

University of Southern California
Los Angeles, California, 90089, U.S.A.
E-mail: kkshung@usc.edu

I have known Savio for more than 15 years, both as a professional colleague and as a friend. I got to know him well after I joined a review group in Taiwan in the 90's. Savio has served as the chair of a panel in reviewing grant applications related to biomedical engineering. The review panel actually was given a heavy responsibility of fostering biomedical research in Taiwan by the government. The quality of biomedical research including biomedical engineering in Taiwan now compared to that in the early days is simply day and night. This impressive achievement can be attributed to the effort of Savio and a few others. Professor Woo is particularly interested in helping young scientists. He always reminds the review panel that special attention should be given to budding young investigators because they are the future and must be properly nurtured.

Savio's knack for good Chinese food also becomes apparent during these meetings. He is particularly fond of Chinese breakfast, fried cruller (You Tiao) and soy milk (Dou Jiang). He would inquire our local colleagues about places well-known for Chinese breakfast and have someone drive a few of us there early in the morning to tame our wild Chinese stomachs, because most of us have lived in the U.S. for many years and rarely have opportunities to enjoy such delicacies. After the meeting, he would invite us to join him again usually for an exquisite meal in a restaurant that he has researched for good food and service. It is always a joyful evening, after 3 long days of hard work, for us to share a laughter or two.

More recently, Savio has paid much of his attention to international cooperation of Chinese biomedical engineers and under his leadership the World Association of Chinese Biomedical Engineers (WACBE) was formed. Savio became the founding president. The first meeting of the society was held in Taiwan in 2001. Since then, three more meetings have been held in China, Thailand and Hong Kong, respectively. In 2011, the meeting was held in Taiwan again. The attendance has grown from a couple of hundred to more 500. I am the current president of WACBE and will follow the model that Savio has established in faithfully carrying the torch forward. For the meeting in 2011, Savio and Mrs. Pattie Woo generously endowed several travel fellowships to support outstanding students to attend the meeting. I am thankful that we have a leader with such a foresight and conviction in nurturing young scientists. Professor Savio Woo is a role model for many of us to emulate.

Savio, I wish you the happiest 70th birthday and many happy years to come.

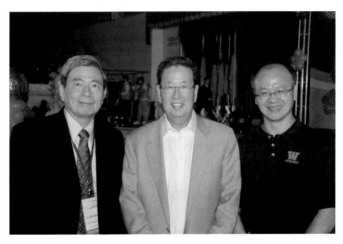

A happy gathering of three UW alumni (L-R: Kirk Shung, Dr. Woo, Patrick Hsieh)

A ROLE MODEL AND FRIEND

Richard Cheng-Kung Cheng

National Yang Ming University
Taipei, 112, Taiwan
E-mail: ckcheng@ym.edu.tw, ckcheng2009@gmail.com

Dear Savio:

Thank you for your guidance and kind help in the past years, especially for your kind contribution to Taiwan's National Health Research Institutes (NHRI) and the Biomedical Engineering Society. You are really my role model. Congratulations for your 70's birthday. As a Chinese, I thought I should write down congratulatory words in Chinese as below.

恭祝 胡院士七秩華誕：
胡公七秩，鱟江仙鶴臥雲松；　典型樹範，桃李成蹊盡化龍。
七十不稀，正是千山極目時；　澄潭影現，仰觀皓月鎮中天。

晚 誠功 敬賀

Happy Birthday!

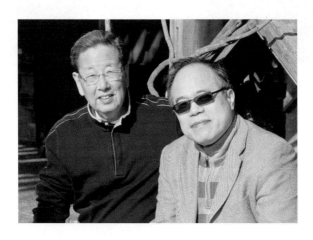

YOUR LEGACY CONTINUES

Jeremy Mao

Columbia University
New York, New York, 10032, U.S.A.
E-mail: jmao@columbia.edu

Savio is a giant in the fields of orthopedics and bioengineering. As extraordinarily accomplished as he is, Savio is extraordinarily generous. He has shown remarkable generosity to spend time with junior scientists, myself included when I first started my career, despite his impossibly busy schedule at all times. Savio offers help to junior scientists in a way that he expects no return, except a gentle reminder here and there that you need to do the very best science that you possibly can. I recall the story of 'picking horses'.

Savio cares deeply about the fields of orthopedics and bioengineering to an extent that is matched by few. His understanding of the past is luminary for the present and even aspects of the future. Savio thinks broadly, and yet has tireless rigor to focus on the scientific problems that he attempts to solve. As complex and multifaceted as the fields of orthopedics and bioengineering are, Savio is among the masters who, for decades, have applied knowledge has gained in fundamental sciences towards the solving of clinical problems.

As extraordinarily accomplished as Savio is, he is laid back and easygoing. He speaks slowly so others have a chance to reflect and respond, and at times, is eloquently blunt to get his points across with precision and purpose. Savio respects his colleagues and listens carefully even when others disagree. He is a great colleague to have, and one, along with Patti, that is great fun to have dinner with.

Happy birthday, Savio, on the occasion of you being 70 years young! Your legacy continues.

SAVIO - A GIANT IN HIS OWN RIGHT

Wei-Shou Hu

University of Minnesota
Minneapolis, Minnesota, 55455, U.S.A.
E-mail: wshu@umn.edu

Ever gracious, ever joyful,
Ever gentle, ever kind,
His words soothing,
His smile healing,
Quarrels melt in his hands,
Storms calm upon his wave,
Steel strength in invisible stealth,
Fountain of wisdom in unpretentious disguise
Forever wise,
Forever grace,
Savio incarnates morality,
Savio embodies greatness.

On his 70th birthday, Savio Woo, forever my role model.

DR. SAVIO WOO'S SINGAPORE CONNECTION

James Goh

National University of Singapore
Singapore
E-mail: biegohj@nus.edu.sg

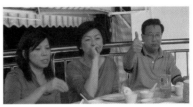

Mrs. Monica Goh, Mrs. Pattie Woo and Dr. Woo enjoying a plate of Singapore's world famous Chilli Crab

Upon my return to Singapore in 1982, I joined the Department of Orthopedic Surgery at the National University of Singapore. I was the first Bioengineer that the School of Medicine had hired to pioneer the field of Orthopedic Biomechanics research. It was a daunting task and I felt rather isolated. I had to turn to a number of renowned experts in the field to help me along. One of them is my good friend and mentor, Dr. Savio Woo. I had followed his excellent work on soft tissue mechanics for many years and had sought his advice on various issues. I managed to persuade Dr. Woo to visit Singapore for the first time in 1988. He gave an inspiring Plenary Lecturer at the 3rd Singapore Biomedical Engineering Symposium. Indeed, Dr. Woo has been an inspiration to me in my career. Since then I had the privilege of meeting Dr. Woo in numerous occasions, i.e. the World Congress of Biomechanics, Orthopaedic Research Society meetings and the International Symposium on Ligaments and Tendons meetings. In 2002, Dr. Woo visited Singapore again, this time accompanied by his charming wife, Mrs. Pattie Woo. He spoke on "Contribution of Biomechanics to Clinical Practice in Orthopaedics". I like the idea of demonstrating the relevance of biomechanics in clinical practice.

Dr. Woo's passion and enthusiasm for research on ligaments and tendons is contagious. The International Symposium on Ligaments and Tendons annual meetings that he established has grown steadily, pushing the boundaries of basic and applied science in this field.

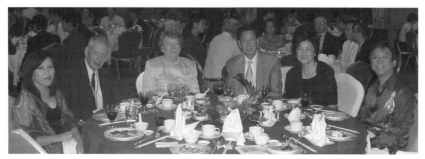

(L-R): Mrs. Monica Goh, Dr. John Paul, Mrs. Betty Paul, Dr. Savio Woo, Mrs. Pattie Woo, Dr. James Goh (2002)

A visionary leader that he is, Dr. Woo recognized the growing pool of Chinese Biomedical Engineers and the need to harness their strength to advance the field of Biomedical Engineering. He, therefore, founded the World Association of Chinese Biomedical Engineers (WACBE) and the WACBE World Congress on Bioengineering series. I have the privilege of being associated with the founding of WACBE and organizing the 3rd WACBE World Congress on Bioengineering in Bangkok in 2007. Dr Woo gave a wonderful Congress Lecture. The highlight was a rare opportunity for Dr. and Mrs. Woo, Dr. Arthur Mak and I to have an audience with Her Royal Highness Princess Maha Chakri Sirindhorn at the Sra Pathum Palace. Her Royal Highness has a special interest in bioengineering, in particular, its application in improving healthcare. The congress was a memorable event for all, particularly for me and my friendship with Dr. Woo.

I would like to take this opportunity to wish Dr. Woo a happy 70th birthday and with many more to come.

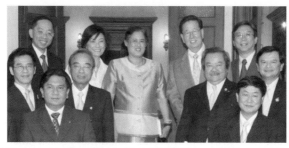

Her Royal Highness Princess Maha Chakri Sirindhorn with Dr. and Mrs. Woo and delegates of 3rd WACBE World Congress on Bioengineering

PROFESSOR SAVIO L-Y. WOO – OUR HONORARY DOCTORATE

Arthur Mak

The Chinese University of Hong Kong
Shatin, New Territories, Hong Kong
E-mail: arthurmak@cuhk.edu.hk

Previously at The Hong Kong Polytechnic University
Hung Hom, Kowloon, Hong Kong
E-mail: arthur.mak@polyu.edu.hk

There are many things I can write as a tribute to celebrate Professor Savio Woo's 70th Birthday. I choose to write about Professor Woo as the recipient of an Honorary Doctor of Engineering from The Hong Kong Polytechnic University (PolyU). This is the highest honor PolyU can bestow upon an individual with outstanding achievements. I choose to write about this because among all the honors and decorations Professor Woo receives, this recognition probably is closest to his home and nearest to our heart.

Probably not too well-known - Savio was once a student at the Hong Kong Technical College, which evolved later to become the present PolyU. Before Savio completed his study at PolyU, he decided to further his study in the United States. So Savio did not graduate from PolyU. That was in the early 60's.

I recall in the conferment ceremony in 2008, Professor Woo was cited as a world-renowned scholar, not only with outstanding academic achievements that won him the memberships of three distinguished national academies, but also bringing much translational values from his laboratories to the clinics, benefitting the health and well-being of millions. This fits in very well with the PolyU motto – "to learn and apply for the benefit of mankind".

So, forty some years later, Savio finally received his degree from PolyU. That was in 2008.

We count Professor Savio L-Y. Woo very much our own and his being a PolyU graduate our honor.

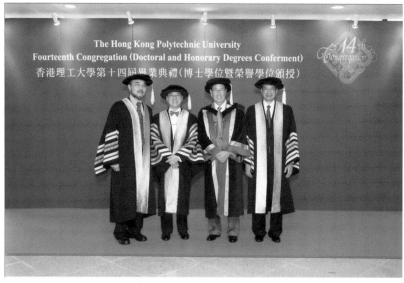

Chair of the University Council, the Honorable Victor Lo,
The Chief Executive of Hong Kong, the Honorable Donald Tsang,
Dr. Woo, and University President,
Dr. Chung-Kwong Poon

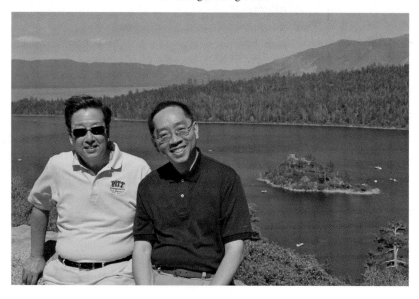

MY MENTOR AND FRIEND

Shiyi Chen

Fudan University Sports Medicine Center, Huashan Hospital
Shanghai, 200040, PR China
E-mail: cshiyi@163.com

I met Dr. Savio Woo at a scientific conference in Hong Kong in 1990 where he invited me to visit Pittsburgh. In 2000, I received the 47th American College of Sports Medicine International Scholar Award to support my scholarship to visit the USA. I spent most of my time at the University of Wisconsin-Madison and had planned to visit the famous UPMC Sports Medicine Center and the MSRC. I contacted Dr. Woo to ask if he could host me for a short visit. He was so generous to provide me with the return flight tickets to visit his MSRC.

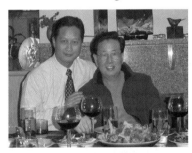 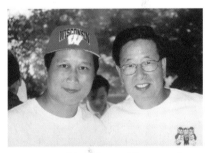

During my visit, he treated me like an old friend teaching me how to manage a biomechanics lab, how to organize seminars and develop research plans. He also showed me how to play unique American sports, such as baseball. Dr. Woo and his wife also hosted a dinner in their home. I had a memorable stay at the MSRC in UPMC, which made us into long-term friends. After my return to Shanghai, I asked Dr. Woo to visit Shanghai several times. He contributed a lot through his presentations and helped Chinese doctors to do ligament research in ACL biomechanical research. Dr. Woo was invited as an Honorary Professor in Huashan Hospital, Fudan University in 2002 and gave a presentation in Shanghai 2nd Medical University. We maintain a long time friendship.

As his student and friend, I congratulate Dr. and Mrs. Woo on very good health and vibrant research forever. We look forward to celebrating his 80th birthday.

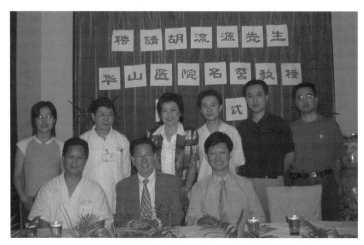

Dr. Woo installed as an honorary professor in Huashan Hospital, Fudan University, Shanghai, China (2002)

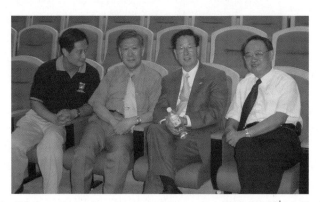

Dr. Woo was invited to give a special speech at Shanghai 2nd Medical University in Shanghai, China on ACL Reconstruction in Biomechanics and Biology (2002). Pictured with (l-r) Dr. Chen Shiyi, Prof. Gu Yudong, Prof. Savio Woo, Prof. Dai Kerong

A GREAT LEADER IN BIOENGINEERING

Fong-Chin Su

Taiwanese Society of Biomedical Engineering
National Cheng Kung University
Tainan, 701, Taiwan
E-mail: fcsu@mail.ncku.edu.tw

On behalf of the Taiwanese Society of Biomedical Engineering, I would like to extend our appreciation for Professor Woo's great leadership and contributions to bioengineering research in Taiwan. Dr. Woo is one of my most respected scholars, mentors, and educators.

In the 1st World Congress of Biomechanics in 1990, my first international conference after completion of a Ph.D. degree, I heard Dr. Woo's name in San Diego. Since then, his image has been deeply impressed and has stayed on my mind. My first close talk with Dr. Woo occurred at the International Society of Biomechanics (ISB) 1995 Congress XV, Jyvaskyla, Finland, where Dr. Woo received the Muybridge Award, the most prestigious award of the Society for career achievements in biomechanics. Except being inspired by Dr. Woo's most amazing lecture, I look up to him as my role model.

Dr. Woo is a super bioengineer and has always presented beautiful talks in a simple standard format with a sense of humor. His initiative, wisdom, creativity and persistence inspired me to start my career in biomechanics.

Dr. Woo coordinates the extramural research grants in bioengineering, at the National Health Research Institutes of Taiwan and provides a lot of help and support for young investigators. Often, I have met Dr. Woo in Taiwan and enjoyed his truly beautiful lectures because he is enthusiastic to share his initiatives, knowledge, and experiences with young bioengineers.

In 2007, I served as the scientific program chair for the ISB 2007 Congress and invited Dr. Woo to present the opening lecture in, Taipei. Dr. Woo also accepted President Michael MC Lai's invitation to visit

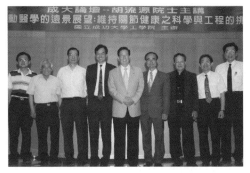

National Cheng Kung University (NCKU) to deliver the President Distinguished Lecture in Tainan, Taiwan. All lecture attendees were inspired to create their own wonderful research career. I was surprised that Dr. Woo shared his secret related to NCKU with us at this special event.

The 1st World Congress for Chinese Biomedical Engineers was held in Taipei, 2002. Professor Woo is the founding president of the World Association for Chinese Biomedical Engineers (WACBE). I was most excited to organize the 5th WACBE Congress integrated with the 2011 Annual Meeting of the Taiwanese Society of Biomedical Engineering in Tainan, August 2011. A special symposium was organized to celebrate Dr. Woo's 70th birthday. It was really special that Dr. Woo visited NCKU again.

Confucius Say "At seventy, I could do what I would without going beyond what is right." The next decade will probably be the most fascinating years of Dr. Woo's career. You are a really unique and special person who deserves respect and honor. I wish you the best of health and enjoy a happy life.

Happy 70th Birthday!

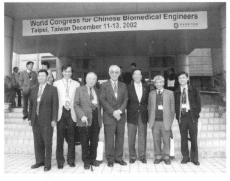

1st WACBE Congress in Taipei (2002)
(l-r) YL Chou, FC Su, YT Wu, VC Mow, SL-Y Woo, GL Chang, SW Yang

松柏長春 福如東海

AN EXTRAORDINARY CAREER AND LEGACY

Lori Setton and Farshid Guilak

Duke University
Durham, North Carolina, 27708, U.S.A.
E-mail: setton@duke.edu, guilak@duke.edu

We are delighted to give Professor Woo our heartfelt congratulations on his 70th birthday. We have known Professor and Mrs. Woo for over 25 years as friends and colleagues in the field of bioengineering. We met Professor Woo during our early years of graduate school while we were working with Dr. Van C. Mow. After hearing many of Dr. Mow's anecdotes and stories of Professor Woo's work in tendon and ligament biomechanics, Farsh had the opportunity to meet him for the first time at the meeting of the American Society of Mechanical Engineers. At Lori's first meeting with Dr. Woo (at the 1990 First World Congress of Biomechanics in La Jolla – see photo below), Dr. Woo immediately exchanged nametags with Lori for the duration of the meeting. That was quite a shock to a young graduate student and gave many of us a chuckle! Professor Woo treated us like his own students, always taking time out to talk to us at meetings and providing encouraging words on our research, as few senior professors would do.

Since our time as graduate students, we have had many opportunities to travel together around the world to many exotic places and stimulating scientific conferences. One of our most memorable trips was to the US-China-Japan-Singapore meeting in Taiyuan, China in 1995. The memories we have of our several days of exciting science, meals, and travel brought us even closer together.

We would like to take this opportunity to congratulate Professor Woo on an extraordinary career and legacy of science and trainees that he has accomplished so far. We are looking forward to seeing many more years of his outstanding work.

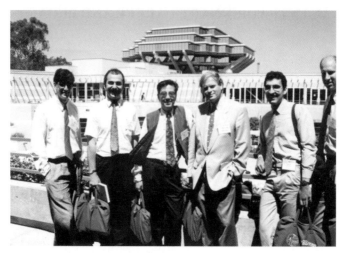

Gerard Ateshian, Kyriacos Athanasiou, Savio L-Y. Woo, Rik Huiskes, Farshid Guilak and Lou Soslowsky at the First World Congress for Biomechanics in La Jolla (1990)

KNOWLEDGE, HUMILITY, LEADERSHIP & FRIENDLINESS

Javier Maquirriain

*High Performance National Sports Center
Argentine Tennis Association
Buenos Aires, Argentina
E-mail: jmaquirriain@yahoo.com*

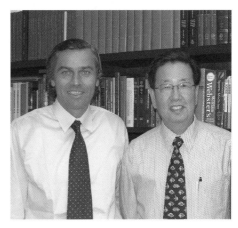

I was really impressed after meeting Dr. Woo for the first time. I was invited to the Board meeting of the *Society for Tennis Medicine and Science* in Rome at the end of 1999, and several topics were being discussed by the committee. Dr. Woo, the man who has published uncountable articles and books, was listening and taking notes silently. Finally, when he was asked about a difficult decision, he pointed out the best solution.

Since then, I have met Savio at many conferences of the Society worldwide. I particularly remember the Barcelona Congress in 2001 where we played tennis with Savio and Pattie at the Real Club de Tennis. We enjoy playing and I was excited to share a sunny afternoon with such nice people.

A couple of years later, he invited me to his fantastic Center in Pittsburgh. I could feel the respect and admiration of all his colleagues, students, and employees. But, I will never forget what happened when I arrived to Pittsburgh late in the night: Yes, Professor Savio L-Y. Woo was waiting for me at the airport!

Savio represents many values: knowledge, humility, leadership, and friendliness, among others.

I really appreciate to be part of your international friends and I hope to welcome you in Buenos Aires in February of 2013.

Happy Birthday!

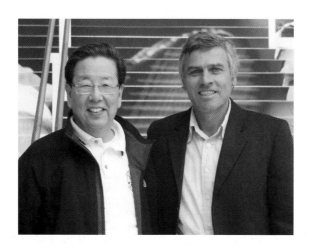

CELEBRATING DR. WOO, RESEARCH PIONEER AND INSPIRATIONAL MENTOR

Helen H. Lu

Columbia University
New York, New York, 10027, U.S.A.
E-mail: hhlu@columbia.edu

Happy Birthday Dr. Woo!!! It is an honor to be able to offer a few words of thanks on this auspicious occasion. Dr. Woo has been an inspirational mentor for me and my students, and through the years, we have benefitted much from his kindness, exemplary scholarship and leadership in the field of ligament and tendon research.

I first met Dr. Woo in 2001 at the ASME Summer Biomedical Engineering Conference, as a freshly-minted Assistant Professor. In fact, it was July 1st and my official start date at Columbia. Dr. Woo's contributions to ligament biomechanics are, of course, well recognized and his seminal studies on the mechanical properties of the anterior cruciate ligament (ACL) were fundamental in our efforts to design a tissue engineered ACL graft during my post-doctoral work. While I am familiar with the extensive body of work from Dr. Woo's group, I had never had the opportunity to meet with him in-person. When we were first introduced, he said with a smile, "oh I hear you are going to be at Columbia…" With a warm handshake and a few words, he readily put me at ease and then listened patiently while I went on and on about the soft tissue-to-bone interfaces, a topic that he already knows much about!

The rest, as they say, is history. Dr. Woo became my mentor, and I was simply lucky to have been able to draw on his wisdom from the very beginning of my career, whether while attending the annual ISL&T conference, which always guaranteed the best Chinese Food in the city, or from having the privilege of working with fellows and students whom Dr. Woo had trained and personally inspired. Whenever our path crossed and throughout our interactions, he was always generous with his time and advices. Dr Woo's messages, peppered with historical anecdotes,

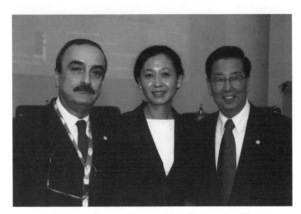

With Professor Woo and Professor Cerulli,
Perugia (2005)

were always delivered in a way that accentuated the positive while delineated the challenges at hand and the likely best course. He often left one with the sense that you are on the right track, while challenging us to think broader and delve deeper into the problem at hand. I shall always be grateful for Dr. Woo's guidance and inspiration through the years.

Over time, I also had the good fortune to get to know Dr. Woo and Mrs. Woo personally. They shared many of their life stories, from juggling the work-life balancing act to where to find the best extra virgin olive oil in Perugia, or the newest culinary delight in New York City. Sharing genuine warmth and a great sense of humor, they are simply a joy and pleasure to be with.

At this year's ASME summer bioengineering meeting, I was honored to be able to speak about our interface work at a special Woo Symposium organized by Dr. Albert Banes. For me, it almost feels as if everything has come full circle. As the day went on, with each talk I heard in the session and later in the many warm personal tributes and stories shared at Dr. Woo's birthday celebration, it became clear what a tremendous mentor Dr. Woo is and has been for many generations of researchers in the ligament and tendon field.

In closing, *Happy Birthday and Many Happy Returns*, Dr. Woo!! Thank you again and wishing you and Mrs. Woo all the best in the years to come!

TRIBUTE TO A PIONEER AND MENTOR: DR. SAVIO L-Y. WOO

Catherine K. Kuo

Tufts University
Boston, Massachusetts, 02155, U.S.A.
E-mail: CatherineK.Kuo@tufts.edu

My first International Symposium on Ligaments & Tendons (ISL&T) meeting was in 2005, where I first met Dr. Savio Woo. Before meeting Dr. Woo in person, I already knew he was a world- renowned researcher in the fields of orthopaedics and biomechanics by the astounding volume and quality of his publications. When I started research in the tendon and ligament area during my first year as a post-doctoral fellow, it seemed that every other paper and book chapter I read was authored by Dr. Woo. A true pioneer in the field of bioengineering, he had published hundreds of original research papers, book chapters and review papers, delivered nearly a thousand lectures, and edited numerous books. A member of the U.S. National Academy of Engineering and Institute of Medicine, and recipient of countless prestigious awards, Dr. Woo's name and reputation preceded him.

At that same ISL&T meeting, I also learned firsthand that in addition to these impressive accomplishments, Dr. Woo has spent much of his career devoted to promoting and advancing the field of ligament and tendon research. Dr. Woo's efforts in this arena are in part reflected by the success of the ISL&T meetings. Dr. Woo founded the annual ISL&T meeting to convene the world's premier ligament and tendon research scientists, clinicians and engineers to exchange ideas, strengthen networks, and forge new research directions.

Even more impressive to me was how Dr. Woo described his wish for ISL&T meetings to be a mechanism through which the field would develop longevity. He specifically highlighted the need to nurture junior investigators and encourage their retention in the ligament and tendon field. It became clear to me by the end of the day, Dr. Woo had successfully made his wish a reality, which was evident by the significant number of student and fellow attendees, presentations at the ISL&T meeting given by these junior scientists, and the competitions designed to recognize these trainees for excellence in research, supported by Dr. Woo and his esteemed colleagues.

Since first attending that ISL&T meeting as a fellow in 2005, I have yet to miss an ISL&T meeting, in the States or overseas. During my post-doctoral fellowship, I was fortunate to benefit from the unique opportunities ISL&T provides, ranging from feedback on scientific data to advice on career decisions to collaborative opportunities. Now, as an assistant professor, I have started bringing my own students to the ISL&T meeting and have had the pleasure of seeing them present, and also to be among the first recipients of the Savio L-Y. Woo Young Researcher Award, established in honor of Dr. Woo by Dr. and Mrs. Albert Banes, to recognize graduate students and post-doctoral fellows who are performing highly significant research in the field. Dr. Woo himself presented the award to my student, and later spent time chatting about his own experiences as a researcher with my student, as he did many times with me over the years.

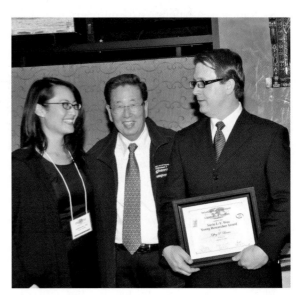

With my student, Jeffrey Brown, ISL&T Savio L-Y. Woo Young Researcher Award Winner (2011)

Congratulations, Dr. Woo. It is with the deepest gratitude that I thank you. Words cannot convey the incredible impact your efforts have had on my career. Serving on the International Advisory Committee and several Program Committees for the ISL&T, it is a pleasure to have had the opportunity to work with you, and to be continuing along your path of giving back to the community and providing opportunities to future generations of ligament and tendon researchers. I am grateful for the support and encouragement you have extended over the years, ranging from personal congratulations to stories about your successes and challenges. I hope that your achievements and unwavering support of this critically important field of musculoskeletal research are recognized by this well-deserved tribute to you and Mrs. Woo and your families, biological and academic.

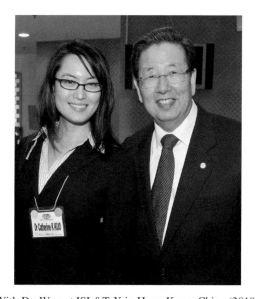

With Dr. Woo at ISL&T-X in Hong Kong, China (2010)

HAPPY BIRTHDAY SAVIO!

Mitsuo Ochi

Hiroshima University
Hiroshima, 734-8551, Japan
E-mail: ochim@hiroshima-u.ac.jp

Happy Birthday to you!

It is unbelievable that you are celebrating your 70th birthday. Whenever I meet you in Japan, the USA or Europe, you are so active, not only in the academic sense, but also regarding your sporting activities and the fact that you look so young.

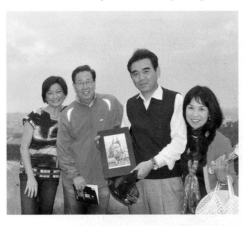

Our numerous meetings, including your wonderful lectures, have always inspired my motivation for basic and clinical research. In 1983, I decided to send Dr. Deie to Pittsburgh, in order to study the spirit of basic research under your direction. Thanks to your wonderful instruction, he is now a Professor at Hiroshima University and continues his research on osteoarthritis knee mechanics.

As you know, in Japan, maybe just like in China, we revere and celebrate certain special ages to show our respect to the elderly. Specifically, these ages are 60, 70, 77, 80, 88, 90 and 99. I have heard that your family, students and friends are planning to hold a special party for you. I wish I could be there to see you and Pattie.

I am sure that this will be one of many wonderful parties yet to come: your 88th, 90th, and 99th birthday parties are awaiting you!

Take good care of yourself, and enjoy yourself at the party. I will be thinking of you, and I will raise my glass in your honor.

Tributes from Colleagues and Friends

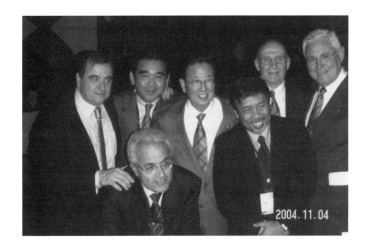

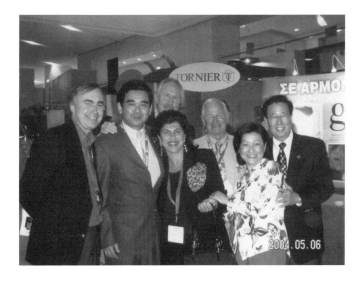

A TRIBUTE TO SAVIO WOO

Robert Hsu

Chang Gung University
Kweishan, Taoyuan, Taiwan
E-mail: wwh@adm.cgmh.org.tw

It must be traced back around 20 years ago, when we moved back from Mayo Clinic (Rochester, Minnesota) after I had completed fellowship training in the orthopedic department. J.J. (Wu) introduced Savio and Pattie to Rita and me in many academic and social activities hosted by Taiwan Orthopedic Sports Medicine Society conducted by J.J. Wu and Professor Y.S. Hang. Between 1988 and 2000, I was actively involved in the care of sports injuries of Taiwan National Olympic athletes. Thereafter, we met on many meeting occasions inside the island and out of the country. Those occasions included ORS, AAOS, ASA, APOSSM, ...and so on. We even had a chance to visit Savio and Pattie at the University of Pittsburgh. I am deeply inspired by Savio at many formal and informal talks about the philosophy of restrict, honest, and persistent properties in the science research. Beside the academic activities, Savio is also involved in the affairs of Taiwan National Health Research Institutes (NHRI). Thus, Savio and Pattie came to Taiwan more frequently. Some times we got together to celebrate the big October birthday parties (J.J., Pattie and Rita), and enjoyed lots of fun. Those were quite interesting memories. Here, we congratulated Savio on his 70th birthday, and we know, Savio and Pattie will certainly plan an interesting life in the future. God bless Savio and Pattie and all of us.

Tributes from Colleagues and Friends   349

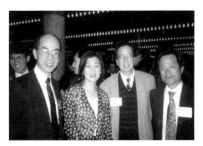

An, Rita, Savio, and me
AAOS/ORS meeting (1993)

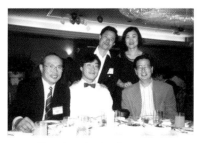

HA, KM, Savio (front row)
me and Rita (back row)
KOSM/APOSSM meeting, Sydney
(2000)

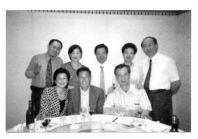

Savio, Pattie and good friends of
Taiwan, had wine-tasting dinner party,
in Taipei, Taiwan (1996)

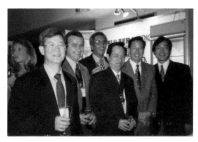

Savio with Board members
KOSM/APOSSM meeting, Sydney
(2000)

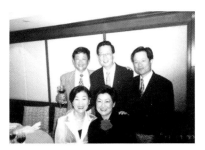

Pattie, Rita (front row) and
J.J., Savio and me (back row)
celebrated the Big October birthday
in Taipei, Taiwan (1997)

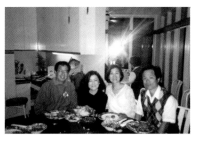

Savio, Pattie, Rita and me
at Savio's beautiful home (2005)

A MENTOR FOR US ALL

Braden C. Fleming

Warren Alpert Medical School of Brown University
Providence, Rhode Island, 02903, U.S.A.
E-mail: Braden_Fleming@brown.edu

As a master's student at the University of Vermont, I attended my first meeting of the Orthopaedic Research Society in 1987. It is there that I first observed Dr. Woo in action and was thoroughly impressed by the discussions he initiated following most papers in the ACL and ligament biomechanics sessions at the meeting. At that time, I was glad that I was not a presenter, but I quickly realized that Dr. Woo was a leader in the field and a pioneer in establishing important links between soft tissue mechanics and the biology of healing.

Over the years, I have had the good fortune to get to know Dr. Woo personally. I continue to follow his work with great interest and routinely utilize many of the testing protocols he developed many years ago. Each year, I look forward to the International Symposium on Ligaments & Tendons, the premier ligament and tendon research meeting of the world, which he successfully initiated to foster international communication and collaboration in 2000. It was an honor to serve as a Program Committee Chair for the meeting in 2008 (Fig. 1). Another career highlight was my visit to the Musculoskeletal Research Center at the University of Pittsburgh in 2008. Dr. Woo was an amazing host. The visit was educational and fun. It was truly impressive to see his laboratory in action.

Although I am not a student who studied directly under Dr. Woo, I consider him one of my primary mentors. Over the years, he has taught me much about the science of biomechanics. I am very grateful for all of his contributions to the development of my career and the field of orthopaedic biomechanics in general. I wish him the happiest of birthdays and I am looking forward to the many more to come. Thank you Dr. Woo! Congratulations!!

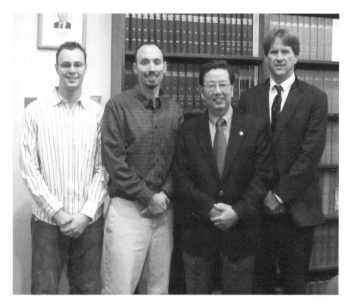

Fig. 1: The ISL&T-VIII (2008) Planning Committee (l-r);
Matthew Fisher, Steven Abramowitch, Savio Woo,
Braden Fleming

HARD WORK, DEDICATION AND COMMITMENT

Lou Soslowsky

University of Pennsylvania
Philadelphia, Pennsylvania, 19104, U.S.A.
E-mail: soslowsk@upenn.edu

As a Ph.D. student of Van C. Mow in the mid to late 1980's at Columbia University, I got to know of the famous Dr. Savio L-Y. Woo almost 25 years ago. In fact, I was Van's first student to develop ligament testing protocols at Columbia (most of Van's work prior had been in cartilage) and essentially all of my work at that time was based on the pioneering work represented in Dr. Woo's publications. We were the first to determine the mechanical properties of the inferior glenohumeral ligament (IGHL) of the shoulder, a topic still being investigated today. From the Video Dimensional Analyzer (VDA), to the use of Dr. Fung's Quasilinear Viscoelastic Theory (QLV) that was popularized for ligaments by Dr. Woo, to the use of laser-based cross-sectional area measurement techniques, and many others, I followed the work of Dr. Woo very closely as his work was, and continues to be, the gold standard. For me, this was the classic "standing on the shoulders of giants" for my own work (and although I am 6 foot 4 inches tall, it is clearly Dr. Woo who is the giant!). In addition to his rigorous and impactful research, one of the early traits that I recall clearly about Dr. Woo was his sincere interest and desire to foster young researchers to investigate ligaments and tendons. In fact, on many occasions, I heard him

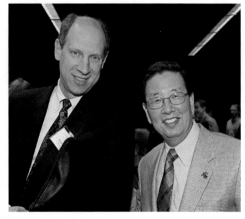

With Savio at a recent ISL&T

implore young researchers to join our field! Indeed, more than 10 years ago, he founded the International Symposium on Ligaments and Tendons (ISL&T), a truly revolutionary and landmark event in our field where young and more seasoned (not old!) researchers could get together in a focused environment and discuss the latest tendon and ligament research. This meeting continues to grow and has quickly become the premier event for our field, clearly due to the hard work, dedication, and commitment of Savio Woo. Our field owes him immense gratitude for this.

On this occasion of your 70th Birthday, I wish you many happy returns and your continued leadership for our field!! With best personal regards....

福如东海长流水，寿比南山不老松．

Nigel Zheng

University of North Carolina, Charlotte
Charlotte, North Carolina, 28223, U.S.A.
E-mail: nzheng@uncc.edu

I first heard about Professor Woo in the early 1980's from my advisor, Professor B. F. Kou, M.D. (过邦辅教授) at Shanghai Jiaotong University, Shanghai, China, and later in 1990's from James R. Andrews, M.D. and William G. Clancy Jr. M.D. at American Sports Medicine Institute, Birmingham, Alabama. In 1999, I visited Dr. Woo and his research center at the University of Pittsburgh. Since then, he has been my respectful mentor and a true friend. Although I have not had an opportunity to study or work in the research center led by Dr. Woo, I have been treated as an alumnus on many occasions. I am really honored to have such a privilege and appreciate his advice and help over the years. Thank you, Dr. Woo.

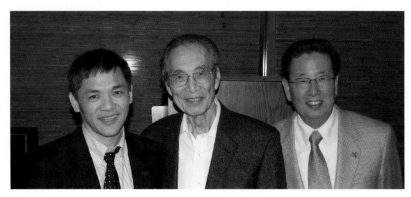

With Professor Woo and Professor Fung (2007)

Dr. Woo, I am very proud of the residents from Ningbo, China (海外宁波帮). They have donated 7.2 billion yuan in the past 25 years, 80% of which went toward education in China. There are about 100 academicians who listed Ningbo as their birthplace or hometown. You are one of them who has made significant contributions to education and science and are honored by the people there. As one of the young generation from Ningbo, China, I would like to tell you that people in our hometown are very proud of you and your achievements. Happy 70th Birthday!

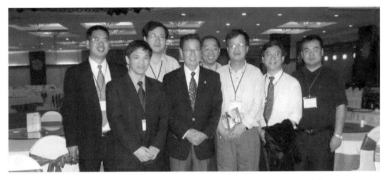

Professor Woo and his WACBE crews in Beijing (2004)

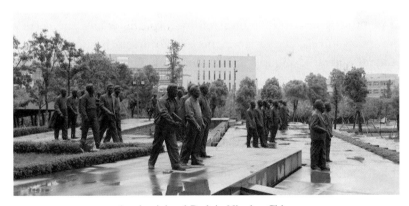

Academicians' Park in Ningbo, China

MENTORSHIP AND INSPIRATION
BUON COMPLEANNO!

Michael Torry

Illinois State University
Normal, Illinois, 61790-5120, U.S.A.
E-mail: mrtorry@gmail.com

Happy 70th Birthday Dr. Woo!

I have chosen to eulogize this joyful occasion with a Chinese proverb which (I think) appropriately and concisely celebrates your life and achievements thus far.

"One generation plants the trees, and another gets the shade"

I believe the proverb exemplifies your commitment to your family. I cannot think of Dr. Woo without thinking of Mrs. Woo; and now with your children and grandchildren, the tree has grown and the "shade" gets larger and larger for the entire Woo family and for those of us lucky enough to be a part of that family.

As one looks at your contributions to science, the proverb emphasizes your commitment to your profession by inspiring young engineers and scientists to solve complex problems and to dream big to achieve new heights of scientific inquiry and exploration. The "shade" provided by your mentorship and inspiration has sparked remarkable achievements across diverse fields of science. Yet, your advice is always rooted in traditional scientific theory and discipline which keeps all of us firmly grounded in the fundamental principles and ethics that guide our decisions.

Lastly and as to underscore the fact that I chose an original Chinese proverb as you achieve your own chronological milestone, I am always impressed with the education you have provided me with regard to your Chinese heritage. I, being of Italian decent, was shocked to hear that the spaghetti noodle was in fact a Chinese invention. My own research has concluded you were right – we stole that recipe. While this somewhat challenged my psychological well being, I find solace in that "We" invented those items most people remember after a spaghetti meal – the vino and gelato!

You have provided "shade" for many people Dr. Woo, so enjoy yourself being in the "sunlight" on this special day!

Buon Compleanno! And many more.

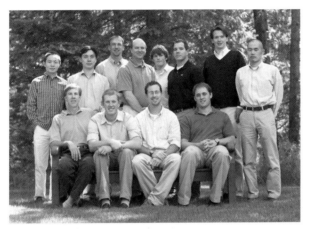

Dr. Torry's group at
Steadman Philippon Research Institute

AN EXTRAORDINARY TEACHER, A KIND MAN

João Espregueira-Mendes

Hospital de Sao Segastiao
Santa Maria da Feira, 4520, Portugal
E-mail: joaoespregueira@netcabo.pt

It is an honor for me to have had the chance of getting acquainted with Professor Savio L-Y. Woo at the beginning of my professional career. It is a greater honor to have him as my friend.

Savio Woo is a true and amazing human being and an excellent Professor. He has renowned the Musculoskeletal Research Center as one of the most important worldwide.

My path has been built around excellent teachers, as Savio Woo, to whom I will be always thankful for providing me knowledge and vision to become a better man and doctor.

Our acquaintance brought together the shared bonds we have. Due to Pattie, Woo's wonderful wife, who comes from Macau, the Portuguese culture is among their life, Portuguese traditions are familiar to him. So, we share the same love towards FADO and PORTO wine with 100 years old.

As a man and colleague, he has been able to grasp life's meaning and become an extraordinary teacher and above all, a kind man.

Happy 70th Birthday!

Your friend,
João Espregueira-Mendes

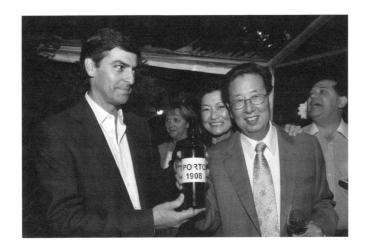

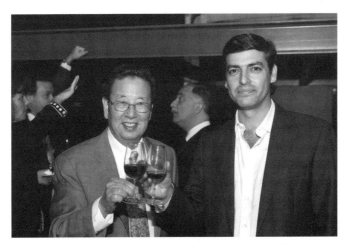

Offering Dr. Woo a taste of 100 year old port (2008)

A SPECIAL FRIEND

Gian Luigi Canata

Koelliker Hospital and University of Torino
Torino, 10129, Italy
E-mail: canata@ortosport.it

I am happy for the opportunity to express in these few lines my esteem and affection for a special friend.

I met Dr. Savio Woo many times in the past during congresses around the world. I was impressed by the knowledge and capability with which he expressed and made clear complex and innovative biomechanical concepts.

I had the joy to know Pattie, his lifelong companion with whom he shares an extraordinary artistic talent. Among many episodes, I remember when they sang in Hollywood, FL, traditional Italian songs that involved all colleagues enthusiastically. It was an unforgettable evening.

I was proud to have him among the faculty members in Torino when I organized a congress for Universiade 2007. On that occasion, he gave me his latest book with an affectionate dedication I still remember.

He invited my wife, Donatella, and I to his ASIAM Institute dinners where we could appreciate his links with the native land and the warmness of his friendship even more.

He is a great man able to connect in the best way - work, science, family and friendship.

Dear Savio, thank you!

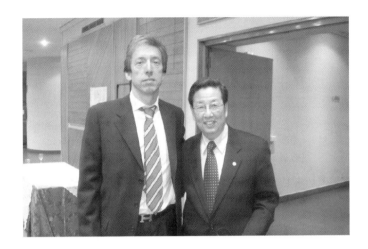

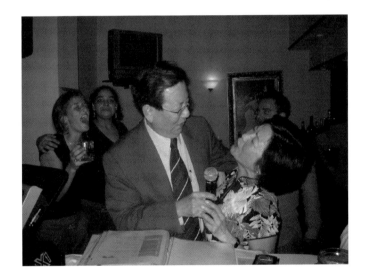

MY SPECIAL MENTOR

Norimasa Nakamura

Osaka Health Science University
Osaka City, Osaka, 530-0043, Japan
E-mail: norimasa.nakamura@ohsu.ac.jp

It was when I started my sports medicine fellowship that the name of Savio became special to me. My mentor in Osaka, Shuji (Dr. Horibe, currently the Director of Orthopaedic Sports Medicine, Osaka Rosai Hospital), used to be a fellow of Savio's at the University of California, San Diego. Shuji educated me in many aspects from basic research to clinical practice and his research background had been developed through his fellowship under the supervision by Savio. In this regard, I was trained indirectly, but with much influence by Savio. In addition, I completed a research fellowship in Calgary under the supervision of Cy (Professor Frank, University of Calgary). He was also a fellow of Savio's and the famous American Journal of Sports Medicine paper published in 1983. This paper on the study of ligament healing particularly inspired me to embark on basic research of joint tissues. Without the encounter with this paper, my career might have developed in other ways. Now it is clear. Although, with no chance to be directly supervised, Savio is one of my special mentors and he has deeply influenced my career development.

It was ten years ago that I had the chance to share time together with Savio. It was thanks to all my friends from all over the world. Above all, the chance to work together in the International Society of Arthroscopy, Knee Surgery and Orthopaedic Sports Medicine (ISAKOS) scientific committee was a special experience, where we worked to spread the significance of basic research throughout the committee and the whole society. Personally, it was a special memory for me that we, with your wonderful wife, Pattie, enjoyed chatting and discussions over wonderful cuisine and wines with many of our good friends.

Savio, I am so happy to be able to celebrate your 70th birthday and the wonderful history of your family with Pattie. Congratulations!!

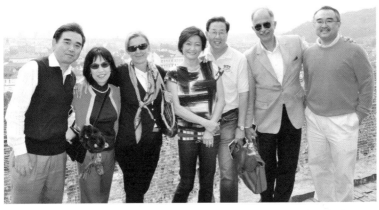

Dr. and Mrs. Ochi, Mrs. Doral, Mrs. and Dr. Woo, Dr. Doral and Dr. Nakamura

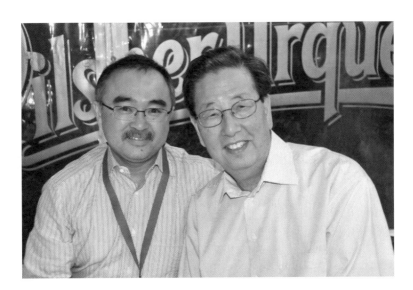

THE HIGHEST LEVELS OF SCIENCE

Nicola Maffulli

Queen Mary University of London and Mile End Hospital
London, E1 4DG, England
E-mail: n.maffulli@qmul.ac.uk

At one stage, I did have hair (or at least more hair than I have now), and a lot less kilos to carry. I had just finished my training in Trauma and Orthopaedics in Aberdeen, Scotland, and I was on my year out. The place was Hong Kong, the town that I still regard as my second home. I was working as a Lecturer at the Chinese University of Hong Kong, with Kai-Ming Chan, having great fun in establishing the laboratory and adapting to a life in such a different culture. No doubt: I was struggling to come to grips to different ways of seeing the world, of interpreting science, of relating to patients, and of developing my personal relationships with my colleagues. Hard work, but a great opportunity and a unique experience. Life was starting to flow, when, preparing for a seminar, the academic staff were told that a great scientist from Pittsburgh would come to listen to what we were doing. Who did not know Savio? A legend was coming to visit, and I would have been able to share ideas with him!

I have always been respectful of authority. My parents instilled in me the awe of seniority and of intellectual superiority in the intrinsically conservative education of a doctor's family in the South of Italy, started in the 1960's, but that I still retain, fully engrained in my genes, and which I hope to be transmitting to my own son. No first name basis allowed, always the proper adoption of the academic title, and, in European fashion, the liberal

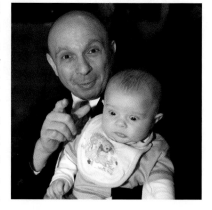

use of the Professorial appellative. I was really stuck, not just tongue stuck. I knew how to deal with orthopods, but this was on another intellectual level. Professor Woo was coming to listen to us, and to actually talk to me!

Salivation was zero and the concentration to listen to the lecture on the biomechanics of anterior cruciate ligament total. Then, a formal introduction, me the only gwei lo of the department, and the possibility to exchange a few words with Professor Woo. Above all, the pleasure to stand in a corner and to actually be listened to. The realization that Professor Woo was not just having polite conversation, but was actually interested in what we were doing (at the time, a simple model of tendon healing *in vitro*). At the end, a smile. For a second, a glint of mischievousness in those lively eyes when asking a question that he knew I was going to answer, and "Do not call me Professor Woo, Savio will be fine".

I remember to this day the pleasure to realize that I was being treated as a peer, and the certainty that I would see Savio again. This has happened at least twice a year since that day in 1995, and I have been part of Savio's extended family ever since, able to share with him and his wife, Pattie, great moments of joy: graduation of their children, the birth of their first grandchild, and my own appointment as a chair in orthopaedics. A humane face to the highest levels of science. Thank you, Savio!

A TRUE INNOVATOR IN OUR FIELD

Scott Rodeo

The Hospital for Special Surgery
New York, New York, 10021, U.S.A.
E-mail: rodeos@hss.edu

It is a real pleasure to offer congratulations to Dr. Savio Woo on the occasion of his 70th birthday.

As a clinician-scientist with an interest in tendon and ligament biology, Savio has taught me as much about the basic aspects of these topics as anybody. His contributions to the literature are legion. There are very few individuals who have had such a profound impact on their field. Savio's work has truly "moved the needle" and has advanced the fields of connective tissue biomechanics and biology. He is a true innovator in our field.

I have always admired Savio for his clear thinking and critical analytic ability. He has contributed to orthopaedic meetings with his insightful comments and questions. His willingness to share his knowledge with others and provide constructive feedback is another way in which he has contributed significantly to our field. When Savio Woo stands up at a meeting to make comments, everyone listens. He has universal respect in our field.

On a personal note, it has been great to see Savio so excited about his grandchildren. He always speaks about them with such pride! They are going to fuel him with energy for years to come, and an invigorated Savio Woo is a great thing for orthopaedic science.

Congratulations, Savio!

SAVIO WOO AT 70

Michael Turner (UK)
Babette Pluim (NED)

The Lawn Tennis Association
London, SW15 5JQ, England
E-mail: Michael.Turner@LTA.org.uk

Babette and I have so many wonderful memories of being with Savio and Pattie over the last 17 years.

The Society for Tennis Medicine and Science (STMS) conferences in the 1990s, Wimbledon in 2000 when they sat in the front row of the International Box with Ben Kibler and Cy Frank, playing doubles tennis in Barcelona ('Woo and Woo') and more recently at the House of Lord's Reception prior to the Arthritis Research UK Conference – 'Tackling Osteoarthritis in Sport'.

Savio and Professor Lars Engebretsen are watching the presentation of the Duke of Edinburgh Prize to Per Renstrom and Lars Peterson – Pattie is talking to the Countess of Ulster, Dr. Halina Fitzclarence (and taking photos!)

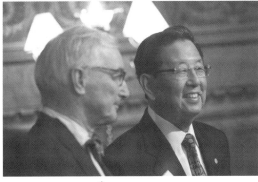

Wishing Savio all the very best for his 70th birthday and a special hug to Pattie for keeping him so fit!

Michael and Babette

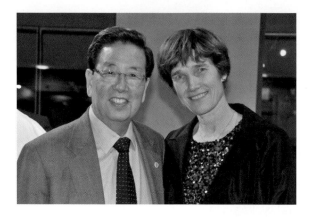

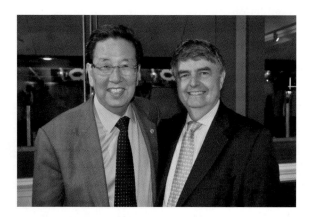

HEALTHY, ENERGETIC AND CORDIALLY FRIENDLY

Milan Handl

University Hospital Motol, Charles University
Prague 5, Czech Republic
E-mail: milanhandl@seznam.cz

Dear Savio,

It is a great pleasure for me to become a member of a great family of your friends from all over the world. First, I want to express my deep wish for you to continue to be healthy, energetic, cordially friendly to everyone, and optimistic as I have shared with you whenever I have had the chance to meet with you. Keep yourself as fantastic as everyone in the world knows you to be!

Looking back, I am not sure about the time we met for the first occasion. Probably in Assissi, Italy, I can estimate it for 2003, during one of the great conferences organized by Giuliano Cerulli with the coordination of Ejnar Eriksson. Of course, I have known you from the orthopaedic literature a couple of years before this first meeting of ours.

It is difficult to tell any exact story we have enjoyed together. I just want to remind and to thank you so much for having accepted my invitation to you and Pattie to come to Prague, Czech Republic during 2009. About 50 very close friends with their spouses from all over the world were able to attend and enjoy The Prague Arthroscopy Symposium on Cartilage Surgery in the heart of my hometown, the capital city of my country. As I could have recognized, all of you felt very satisfied here, which makes me really happy.

Dear Savio, I wish you happy 70th birthday! Keep smiling, you are still on the run and your track is really long! And many long healthy years for you and your Pattie!

Cordially yours
Milan Handl

Prague, August 15, 2011

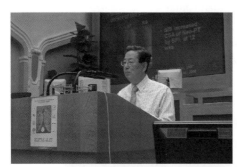
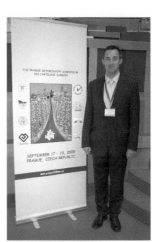
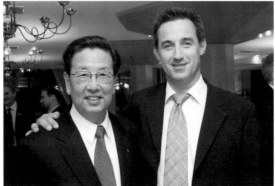
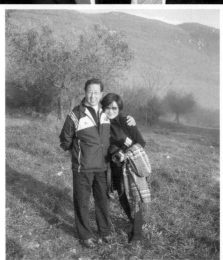

A TRIBUTE TO DR. WOO
SAVIO THE SAVIOR

King H. Yang

Wayne State University
Detroit, Michigan, 48201, U.S.A.
E-mail: aa0007@wayne.edu

We have all heard of the political giants in China: Mao, Zhao, and Hu. In my early days as a bioengineer, my colleagues and I had our giants as well in the field of biomechanics: Van Mow, Ed Chao, and Savio Woo. We always hoped to spot one of them during professional conferences and have a chat. When attending the annual Orthopedic Research Society meetings, I found that Savio seldom asked questions about a presentation despite the fact that he had done the same study years before. On the rare occasion that he skillfully pointed out possible shortcomings of a study, he did so in a crystal-clear, non-confrontational way, unlike many other "mean-spirited" questioners. Savio demonstrates the importance of being humble despite how high a status one may possess in the field. I have learned a great deal from the way he constructs his questions and hope that someday I can act like him.

An event that brought me closer to Savio involved one of his papers published in the Journal of Biomechanical Engineering. Limited by the number of pages allowed, one of the formulas listed did not show its derivation. When I tried to derive it myself, I found that my solution was slightly different from what was published. I wrote him a letter and he quickly responded that the journal misprinted a minus sign in the middle. As a result, my derivation did not match the one that was published. What impressed me the most was that Savio informed the editor right away and published an erratum in the next issue. Since then, I have continued to bother Dr. Woo for suggestions on new research directions, recommendation letters in acquiring jobs and promotions, and soliciting his service on my Center's advisory board. Despite his busy schedule, he always finds time to help me out. Savio is a true savior to me.

On this coming 70th celebration of his birthday, I wish him great happiness for another 50 more years to come. I believe that he will continue his inspirational role in teaching young bioengineers how to make this world a better place.

TO A PIONEERING BIOENGINEER AND LEADER
HAPPY BIRTHDAY, DR. WOO

X. Edward Guo

Columbia University
New York, New York, 10027, U.S.A.
E-mail: ed.guo@columbia.edu

I first read Dr. Woo's name (Savio L-Y. Woo) in the famous translated book of Professor Y. C. Fung "Biomechanics of Living Tissues". I was intrigued by Dr. Woo's work in soft tissue biomechanics and his Chinese name "胡流源". I was also surprised to read Dr. Woo's early work on the effects of exercise on bone properties using pigs running on a treadmill, which is still a classical work in the Bone Bioengineering field. I had the fortune to meet Dr. Woo in person in 1993 when I interviewed for a faculty position in the Department of Mechanical Engineering at the University of Pittsburgh. It gave me a chance to finally meet a giant in the field of Bioengineering. I am among a lot of fortunate Bioengineers who benefited greatly from Dr. Woo's mentorship and guidance in the field. I still remember Dr. Woo's advice on mentorship, "A great adviser will find the unique strengths in all students and shape them to their greatest potential".

Later on, I was fortunate to be involved in the World Association of Chinese Biomedical Engineers (WACBE) and served on its founding Council. I learned a great deal from Dr. Woo's tireless efforts in promoting and educating Bioengineers with Chinese heritage. As a Bioengineer born during the Culture Revolution in the Mainland of China, I was lucky to receive my mentorship and guidance from a world-class leader and pioneer in Bioengineering, Dr. Woo. I would not have been able to make it without Dr. Woo's advice and support! I am so proud and pleased to be your extended academic family, Dr. Woo! Happy Birthday, Dr. Woo!!!

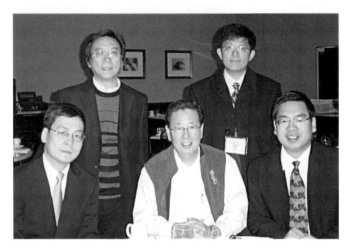

With Dr. James Goh, Dr. Woo, Dr. Jaw-Lin Wang, and Dr. Zong-Ming Li
WACBE Council breakfast

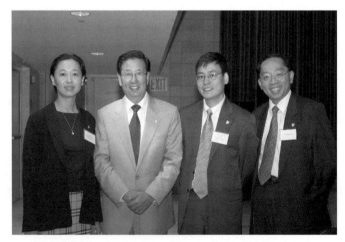

With Dr. Helen Lu, Dr. Woo, and Dr. Arthur Mak
Columbia 250 Biomedical Engineering Symposium

A LEADER AND GIANT

James Tibone
University of Southern California
Los Angeles, California, 90033, U.S.A.
E-mail: tibone@usc.edu

I have always been interested in research and I started my career doing kinematics and EMG analysis in athletes. Then having read Dr. Woo's biomechanics clinical papers on the knee, this influenced me to try to do similar biomechanical research on the shoulder. I became connected with one of your students, Dr. Thay Lee and have been working in his lab for the last 20 years. I still remember presenting my first basic science paper on some aspect of biomechanics of the shoulder at an ASES meeting with you being my discusser. At that time, I knew very little about biomechanics. You nicely complemented my paper, but criticized the use of the terms stress strain when I was analyzing the data when it should have been really load elongation. At that time, I did not know the difference between the material and structural properties of tissues. With your brief critique, I have never forgotten the difference. Since then my knowledge on biomechanics has increased tremendously, with your help, Dr. Thay Lee, and with your formation of the International Symposium on Ligaments and Tendons (ISL&T), which is always my favorite meeting.

Thank you for your help and inspiration as I have always looked up to you as a leader and giant in the field of orthopaedic biomechanics. Best wishes on your future as I am sure you have many more contributions to make to this exciting field. Thank you again for all your leadership and dedication.

A GREAT HEART IN SAVIO WOO

Rogerio Teixeira da Silva

NEO Orthopedic Sports Medicine Research Center
Brazilian Orthopedic Sports Medicine Society
São Paulo, Brazil
E-mail: rogerio@neo.org.br, rgtsilva@uol.com.br

Dear Professor Woo,

To be there in Pittsburgh for a while was a great pleasure, because I had the opportunity to meet a very nice person, not only because of the knowledge of his field, but also the great heart of a man that loves his work and family.

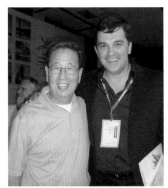

I also had the pleasure to be there as a "tennis science friend", sharing concepts on biomechanics and about life.

Those moments together with Savio and Pattie made me believe that human beings are made for peace and love.

Congratulations for the 70's, and I hope to be there for the 80's.

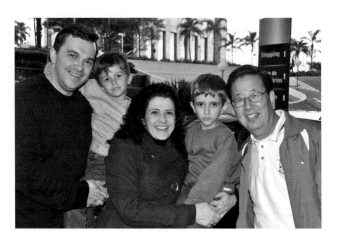

HAPPY 70TH BIRTHDAY AND WARM WISHES

Noshir A. Langrana

Rutgers the State University of New Jersey
Piscataway, New Jersey, 08854, U.S.A.
E-mail: langrana@rutgers.edu

Dr. Savio Woo is one of the handful of researchers who are responsible for the great advancement of Biomechanics. I met Savio when I became the Program Chair of the American Society of Mechanical Engineers (ASME) Winter Annual Meeting in 1985. Since then, through the ASME Bioengineering Division, I have always valued Savio's opinion and comments. This became important to me when I was on the Bioengineering Executive Board 1995-2000. I admire his courage and enthusiasm to promote and support upcoming young investigators.

Savio is an exceptional researcher, a great teacher, a wonderful mentor of Master and PhD students, and has been clearly an outstanding recipient of the many awards including an Olympic Gold Medal. In my opinion, at this time, Savio is the only one who has made significant contributions in the clinical problems related to soft tissue. Savio is truly a leader in the field of soft tissue biomechanics whose work has been of tremendous importance to our patient population. I would rank him at the very top amongst internationally known and recognized researchers in bioengineering. I wish him lots of good health and happiness. Looking forward to his 80th Birthday bash.

YOU ARE A LEADER

Moises Cohen

UNIFESP (University of the State of São Paulo)
São Paulo-SP, Brazil
E-mail: m.cohen@uol.com.br

When I first met Dr. Woo, twenty years ago, I was impressed with his interest in the kinematics of joints and how organized the Musculoskeletal Research Center was. The use of robotic technology to study the function of the knee and shoulder was something totally new for me. His pleasure in teaching us helped us to better understand joints and their surgeries. Once you visit him, you will change your view of biomechanics.

His name is attached to many outstanding research and original papers in biomechanics. Moreover, Dr. Woo is a dedicated man who is focused on the success and development of musculoskeletal research. He contributes everyday to make the study of the joints easier and desirable. Undoubtedly, an example for the Brazilian and worldwide orthopaedic surgeons, You are a leader! Thank you very much for helping me and my fellows with your kind way of making everyone feel at home in Pittsburgh.

It is a pleasure to congratulate Dr. Woo on his 70th birthday and his family, with this tribute. It was wonderful traveling with Dr. Woo and Pattie and to receive you at our beach house in Brazil. The photo book that Pattie created from the Beijing Olympic Games is wonderful and has exquisitely detailed that exclusive trip that was a pleasure for me, Estelita and my daughters to share with you all.

We wish you all the great things in life, hope this day will bring you an extra share of all that makes you happiest and your year filled with the same joy you bring to others. Hoping your wishes come true year after year.

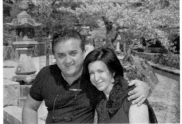

A GREAT LEADER IN ORTHOAPEDIC BIOMECHANICS

Toru Fukubayashi

University of Waseda
Saitama, 359-1192, Japan
E-mail: fukuba@tky.3web.ne.jp

Dear Savio,

Congratulations on your seventieth year birthday (古希). We have been good friends for more than thirty years, though we have not been able to work together. The attached picture was taken in your laboratory at the University of California, San Diego. I am on the right side. You were so young, and you still look young now, though I lost my hair. I hope you would remain a great leader of orthopaedic biomechanics, now and in the future!!

Sincerely,
Toru Fukubayashi, MD

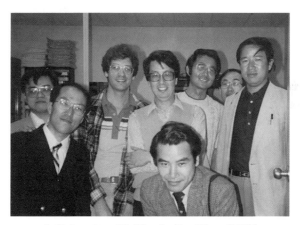

At University of California, San Diego (1983)

TRIBUTE TO MY FRIEND, SAVIO WOO

Ken Kuo

*National Health Research Institutes
Zhunan, Miaoli County, 350, Taiwan
E-mail: kennank@nhri.org.tw*

Welcome to the Seventy club, I am sure that you will enjoy it.

I have known you for almost 30 years since you were in San Diego. We have done many things together including the Chinese Speaking Orthopaedic Society, for that, I will always appreciate your input.

Savio, you are a real scholar, teacher, researcher and organizer. In addition, you are really a good friend. I always remember when we dine together; we talk about good food, wine and enjoy the good time. I hope with your retirement, we will have more time together to reactivate the good old days.

I do not think you will be definitely "retired". You will revitalize and continue to do your best for the orthopaedic research and promote it.

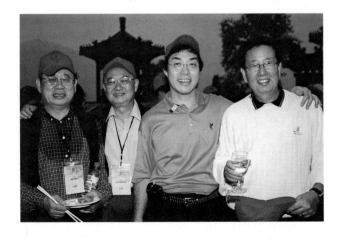

"THE AGE OF RARITY"

Michael Lai

Columbia University
New York, New York, 10027, U.S.A.
E-mail: wml1@columbia.edu

It has been a great privilege for me to be among Savio's professional and personal friends, to have co-authored a paper with him on soft tissue biomechanics, and to be an admirer for his immense contributions to the field of soft tissue biomechanics. On this occasion of his reaching what is known by Chinese as "the age of rarity," Linda and I would like to wish him a very happy birthday and many, many more. Almost ten years ago, when I reached seventy, Savio offered me the advice that "being seventy means that I should be able to do whatever I want with the rest of my life." I have indeed followed his advice to the best I can. Now that he will have reached seventy soon, I am reminding him of what he told me and wishing him well in whatever he will be doing, old stuff or new adventure.

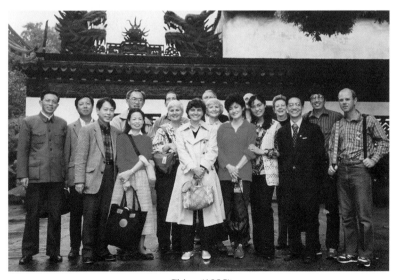

China (1985)

THANK YOU PROFESSOR SAVIO WOO

Ching-Jen Wang

Kaohsiung Chang Gung Memorial Hospital
Kaohsiung, Taiwan
E-mail: w281211@adm.cgmh.org.tw

We are extending our congratulation thousand miles away from Taiwan on Professor Savio Woo's 70th birthday.

Professor Woo is the most renowned scholar and the most respected scientist of the decade. In addition to his academic achievements, he has devoted his time and effort in teaching young scientists, and providing community service to societies around the world. His professionalism has set a role model of our society today. I am privileged and honored to have a professional affiliation with him.

Professor Woo will stay on top of his professionalism and provide assistance to the peers and colleagues even after his 70th birthday. We like to take this opportunity to say thank you to Professor Savio Woo and wish him a wonderful birthday with his family.

PC Leung

The Chinese University of Hong Kong
Shatin, Hong Kong
E-mail: pingcleung@cuhk.edu.hk

I wish to congratulate Savio on his 70th Birthday. In that we are brothers! Savio has enlightened orthopaedic surgeons so much. Savio has taught me not only bone biomechanics but also tissue healing. After Savio's enlightenment, it becomes so clear to us that healing processes require the combined biological, mechanical and chemical forces that converge on multiple targets of activity. Thank you Savio.

A GENTLEMAN AND A SCHOLAR

Steve Burkhart

The San Antonio Orthopaedic Group
San Antonio, Texas, 78258, U.S.A.
E-mail: ssburkhart@msn.com

It was a great honor and privilege to visit Savio Woo's lab in Pittsburgh in 1995, just after I had given Grand Rounds. He had me sign his guest book. As I looked at all of the famous scientists and surgeons that had visited him, I felt very insignificant, yet Savio was so gracious and kind to show me the vast array of research that was under his direction. He knew that I was a surgeon with an engineering background, and he encouraged me a couple of times during my career with personal notes when I really needed encouragement.

Congratulations, Savio, on your 70th birthday. You truly are a gentleman and a scholar.

Gideon Mann

Meir University Hospital
Kfar Saba, Israel
E-mail: gmann@sportsmedicine.co.il

I have been thinking of this project for the last two weeks. I love and admire Professor Woo and the Woo's as a couple. Even so, I could not find something to write which would truly emphasize his open and generous personality or his scientific greatness.

A SPECIAL MENTOR AND FRIEND

Evan Flatow

Mount Sinai School of Medicine
New York, New York, 10029, U.S.A.
E-mail: Evan.Flatow@mountsinai.org

I do not recall the first time I met Savio, but I first got to know him when I was a junior attending working in Van Mow's lab. Van got me involved in the first edition of the AAOS's book "Orthopaedic Basic Science" and Savio was the senior author of the ligament section. I recall Van pointing out, as we reviewed some figures, that every year Savio moved the age dividing line up a year so that Van's ligaments were "old" and Savio's were still young! Those were magical years, and I could not believe my luck to be able to talk to, let alone work with, the giants of the field. Ever since, Savio has been a special mentor and friend, encouraging me to keep toiling in the fields of soft-tissue research.

Best wishes and congratulations Savio!
Evan Flatow

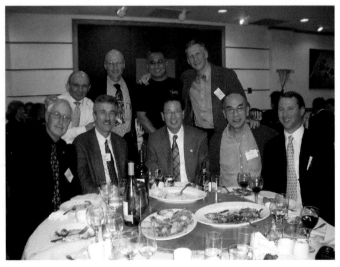

ISL&T-VI

Chapter 6

The Story of One Blessed Academic

THE STORY OF ONE BLESSED ACADEMIC

Savio Lau-Yuen Woo
胡流源

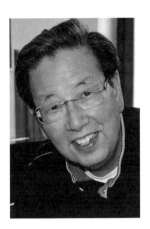

1. A Note of Appreciation

I am astonished that I have reached 70 years of age! I certainly do not feel this age, and it helps that many people tell me I do not look it. Apart from a little morning stiffness, a few more grey hairs, and the difficulties of recalling names and more recent happenings (like what I just had for lunch), I basically feel and function like I always have for as long as I can remember.

Much of this good fortune can be attributed to my surroundings. As much as I believe that everything is genetic (I must, since my younger brother is a leading expert in this field), I also firmly subscribe to the tenet that we are products of our environment. To that end, I am extremely thankful that I was raised by loving parents and grew up with wonderful siblings. I have been educated by great teachers, surrounded by caring friends and colleagues, helped by many able assistants, and so on. I married the best bride on earth, then was blessed with two wonderful children, followed by two (the best yet) granddaughters. All of this has truly made my life complete! With everyone's support, I have been able to concentrate on my work without being distracted by too many unpleasant events.

Another important factor is that I have had the distinct pleasure of interacting with a large number of students and research fellows over the last 42-plus years. The fact that new students, residents and fellows of similar ages arrive each year to study has made me, consciously or unconsciously, think that I, too, remain the same age. Further, my philosophy in life (which I often will unto them) and my passion for learning and teaching have also remained close to constant through time. So, I have very little to remind me that years have indeed gone by and they have gone by so quickly.

The overwhelming number of tributes written for this beautiful book is truly heartwarming. I have read and re-read all of them. Thank you all so very much! I can humbly say that I am not remotely as good as these accolades that have been affectionately showered upon me. But, I am encouraged by the flattering words and plan to work diligently for the rest of my being to live up to some of what has been said.

For my allotted pages, I wish to first share with you my experience in the "extreme" celebration of my 70th birthday. Then, I would like to tell you the humble beginnings of my family and the very blessed journey of my life. With your indulgence, I will then recall some lessons that I wish to share. I sincerely hope that you will enjoy reading (all, or part of) my story as much as I have enjoyed writing it.

2. The "Extreme" Birthday Celebration

At the onset, it may be helpful to clarify which date is my real birthday. I was born on leap June 3rd of the lunar calendar (there were two months of June for that particular year). So, when I recorded my date of birth for official documentation in the 1950s, I wrote June 3rd, 1942. It was not until many years later that my father-in-law, Mr. Antonio Cheong In-Cheong (张賢长), helped us calculate that according to the western calendar, my birth date is July 26, 1941. For a number of years afterward, I celebrated both dates as my birthday, hoping that I would receive double the greetings, birthday cakes, presents, and so on.

But, my scheme also brought confusion to many people. Subsequently, some (who shall remain nameless) used this as an excuse when they forgot one or both of my birthdays. They would say, "Oh! I thought you celebrated your birthday on the other date!" Realizing that my greed did not accomplish anything, I grew wiser. Beginning on my 60th birthday, I chose July 26 as the sole date for my birthday.

As my 70th birthday approached, Pattie and a number of close friends and family asked me what kind of birthday celebration I wished for. I immediately remembered the special celebration for my 60th birthday. My family, mentors, friends and students surrounded me for a full day's scientific program, which included 16 memorable lectures. This was followed by a beautiful banquet of over 300 people, complete with many sweet toasts and humorous roasts. I told everyone that I wanted to keep all these fond memories intact, since this event could not (and should not) be topped. Instead, I suggested a few smaller and more intimate gatherings with friends throughout our planned travels for 2011.

Well, as it turned out, we were pleasantly surprised that there were quite a number of "not-so-small" celebratory events that began in June and lasted for several months! I have treasured these memorable moments and wish to express my deep gratitude to those who took the time, effort and energy to organize and execute them.

2.1. *Let the Celebration Begin*

Thanks to Drs. David Vorp and Jennifer Wayne, a special symposium celebrating my lifetime achievements in bioengineering took place from June 22 - 23, 2011 at the ASME Summer Bioengineering Conference held at Nemacolin Woodlands Resorts in Farmington, PA. My students and friends organized four, 2-hour sessions covering the four topics that are not only dear to me, but also chronicle the history of our research. Drs. Matthew Fisher and Glen Livesay organized the first session on Tissue Mechanics where my dear friend, Dr. Shu Chien gave a glowing introduction on the history of my career. He kindly bestowed high praises on how I have dedicated my life to education and to my family. I appreciate his words very much! Then, a video of Professor Y. C. "Bert"

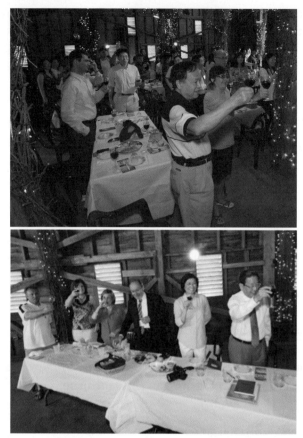

Fig. 1: Birthday celebration at a winery near Nemacolin Woodlands Resort

and Luna Fung was shown (thanks to Dr. Peter Chan), wishing me a happy birthday. Their appearance moved me to tears.

The second session was on the Application of Robotics, organized by Drs. Richard Debski and Hiromichi Fujie. Hiro gave a history of the development of robotic technology. Matt Fisher concluded the session by giving a polished talk on "Extracellular Matrix Bioscaffolds to Enhance ACL Healing". Even though the session extended well past 9 pm, the questions and answers continued like no one wanted it to end.

Early the next morning, we had our third session on Computational Modeling, which was put together by Drs. Zong-Ming Li and Thay Lee. It began with a tribute by Dr. Andy An on our contributions to the properties of biological materials, studies on joint function using robotics and the finite element analyses of the anterior cruciate ligament. His keynote lecture was followed by nice talks by Zong-Ming, Dr. Ken Fischer, and Dr. Guoan Li. Finally, the fourth session, entitled Functional Tissue Engineering, was organized by Drs. Al Banes and Cy Frank and was comprised of six talks given by international superstars on their cutting-edge research.

Needless to say, I was quite overwhelmed and little embarrassed by all the accolades and amplified praise bestowed upon me during these eight hours, since I can only take credit for a small fraction of what was said.

After the symposium, 80 of my students, research fellows and good friends from many countries gathered at the nearby Christian W. Klay Winery for a birthday party. The program was emceed by Zong-Ming and there were many wonderful toasts, kind congratulatory remarks, sweet reminiscences and moving commentaries given by Matt, Cy, Al, Andy and Drs. Harvey Borovetz, David Butler, Sanjeev Shroff, Tin-Kan Hung, Bob Nerem, and Rui Liang (Fig. 1).

Following all this, I found myself speechless and only able to say that Pattie and I were both deeply touched and sincerely thankful to everyone. I vowed to work harder to become the quality educator, caring mentor, exemplary role model and treasured friend that all have expected me to be.

2.2. *Birthday Parties from Assisi, Italy to San Francisco, U.S.A.*

On July 3, 2011, the celebration moved outside of the U.S. to historical Assisi – a small, old Italian town that is known for its stunning Papal Basilica of St. Francis of Assisi. My dear friend, Dr. Giuliano Cerulli hosted us in his summer villa surrounded by hundreds of olive trees and a stunning view of Assisi. Dr. Mario Lamontagne and his wife, Nicole, joined us along with Giuliano's faithful staff from his clinic and research institute. Throughout the years, we have become very close to him, his family (wife, Giuliana, and lovely daughter, Francesca) and his group. Eighteen of us swam and then dined on pasta *al dente* and barbequed meat while washing it all down with great wines from Tuscany. We then entertained each other with karaoke well into the summer night. After

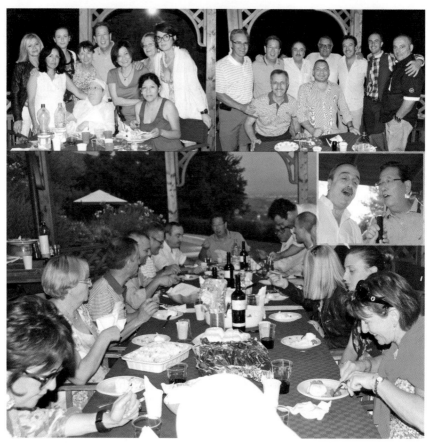

Fig. 2: Birthday celebration hosted by Dr. Giuliano Cerulli in Assisi, Italy

many songs, everyone gathered and sang Happy Birthday to me while presenting me with a well-decorated birthday cake with the greeting in Italian: "70 Buon Compleanno"! (Fig. 2)

From Italy, we traveled to San Francisco where my immediate family, my extended family and lifelong friends of forty-plus years gathered for a fabulous weekend of festivities. From July 22 - 24, 2011, the fifty of us had three days of nonstop celebration. Here, let me briefly describe this most memorable weekend.

We all stayed at the same hotel. After welcoming our guests upon their arrival, we had dinner at the nearby Embarcadero Ferry Building with a fantastic view of the San Francisco Bay. The food and wine mixed

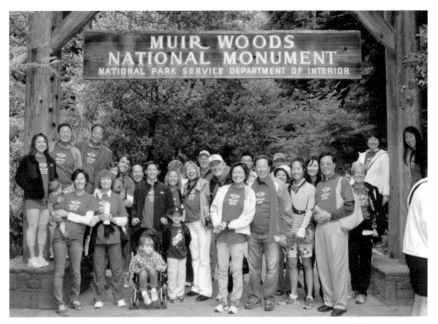

Fig. 3: At the entrance to Muir Woods

perfectly and it was a great opportunity for all to catch up on recent as well as not-so-recent happenings.

Day two was the main event! Our morning began with a breakfast buffet and then we went to Muir Woods – my favorite nature site in the Bay Area (Fig. 3). The cloudy sky with coastal fog made it a perfect day to walk amongst the sky-touching giant redwoods. After lunch by the scenic Golden Gate Bridge, we returned to the hotel for a short rest before the birthday cake. In the afternoon, we had a champagne toast followed by the presentation of an extremely beautiful cake, specially ordered by my daughter, Kirstin. It was decorated with grapes, vines and a bottle of wine at the top with a label that read, "SAVIO – 1941 - Aged to Perfection". (Fig. 4) Then, there was more humorous toasting by my two younger brothers, Stanley Lau-Po **(胡流波)** and Savio Lau-Ching **(胡流清)** and a number of precious gifts for me to treasure.

Dinner took place at my favorite Chinese restaurant in San Francisco, the R&G Lounge. Pattie planned an exquisite menu and Jonathan arranged the seating. The wine was flowing and everyone was talking and laughing aloud while eating and drinking. Kirstin made her "moving

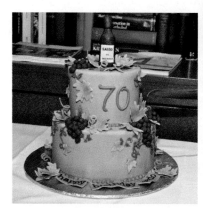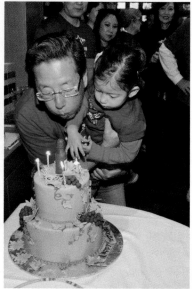

Fig. 4: My special birthday cake and Zadie helped to blow out the candles

me to tears" toast and presented me with a beautifully bound volume (that she made) containing memorable toasts from friends and family. Jonathan shared profound and humorous words from his heart.

On the third morning, we started the day with a pleasant walk along the Embarcadero and then had Sunday brunch together (Fig. 5). We went on to take a "Bridge to Bridge Bay Cruise" on a glorious, sunny, warm

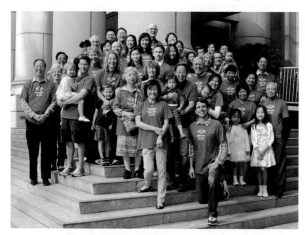

Fig. 5: Group photo in San Francisco

and calm day. The party wound down as a number of us departed for home. The ten remaining enjoyed a farewell dinner at a restaurant on the Bay. The view and the company were outstanding.

Never in my life have I imagined to be given a birthday celebration of this magnitude, for this duration of time and with so many who mean so much to me. Never have I been immersed in such an extraordinary amount of love and precious memories in a single setting. All the events were perfectly planned and executed by Kirstin with the help of Pattie, Jonathan and Adam. It is abundantly clear that I am a truly blessed husband and father!

2.3. *A Record Breaking Birthday Party in Taiwan*

The month of August came quickly. The Scientific Review Committees gathered in Taipei for a review of grant applications for the National Health Research Institutes (NHRI). On August 14, 2011, Dr. Cheng-Kung (Richard) Cheng, a dear friend and a member of the Medical Engineering Committee (fondly known as SRC-4) organized a dinner party in Hsinchu to celebrate my birthday. All ten members of my committee, plus friends and family were present. Chih-Hwa (Dr. Chen) also came from Taipei to join us. We enjoyed a beautiful buffet dinner, drank good wine and had a great time relaxing after a day of hard work (Fig. 6).

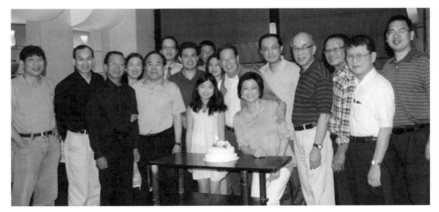

Fig. 6: Birthday party after the NHRI meeting

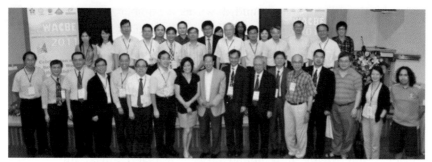

Fig. 7: The birthday symposium at the WACBE in Tainan, Taiwan

We then traveled south to Tainan for the 5th World Association of Chinese Biomedical Engineers (WACBE) Congress. Under the leadership of Dr. Fong-Chin Su and the hard work of his colleagues, staff and students, this congress was a huge success in terms of the record number of attendees, the high quality of papers and most importantly, an outstanding slate of plenary and keynote speakers.

On August 19, 2011, there was a special symposium organized by Cheng-Kung and Dr. Kai-Ming Chan to honor my birthday. Zong-Ming gave a glowing introduction and recapped all the celebratory events during the previous two months. Then, we enjoyed listening to six beautiful lectures given by Drs. Ching-Jen Wang, Hung-Mann Lee, Arthur Mak, James Goh as well as Chih Hwa and Fong-Chin. In addition, kind remarks were given by Cheng-Kung and Kai-Ming (Fig. 7). I was very pleased that such a beautiful symposium could take place during the 5th WACBE – a society that I founded with my colleagues.

The next day, Chih Hwa and my former fellows, Yin-Chih (Dr. Fu) and Shan-Lin (Dr. Hsu) had a private lunch with us (Fig. 8). A very special birthday cake was presented to serve as a prelude for the Congress banquet that evening. The banquet actually took place on the basketball court of the university's gymnasium, a space large enough to house about 1,000 delegates and students. We

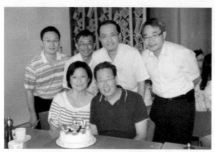

Fig. 8: Birthday luncheon with former fellows from Taiwan

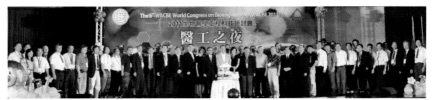

Fig. 9: On stage while being serenaded with the Happy Birthday song at the banquet

enjoyed delicious local cuisine and exciting cultural entertainment throughout the evening. In its midst, we were called onto the stage and presented with a three-tiered birthday cake. I was then serenaded with Happy Birthday in three different languages (Fig. 9). Having so many people singing to me was a record that will never be broken! We really enjoyed this special occasion and appreciate the kind efforts by all our hosts.

2.4. *Back to My Roots - Shanghai, China*

For the month of October, we returned to my birthplace – Shanghai, China for a family reunion and a tour of the historic Silk Road. All my siblings except my eldest sister were there, together with several of our first cousins. On October 8th, 2011, my sister Shu-Lee Woo (胡秀莲) planned a birthday party for me. There were eighteen of us including my nephew and two nieces. We were treated to a most elegant banquet that included many rare delicacies. My sister also ordered a beautiful and very tasty birthday cake and again, everyone sang happily and enthusiastically on my behalf (Fig. 10). It was a very moving evening for me as I reminisced that occasions like this are getting harder and harder to come by as years go on.

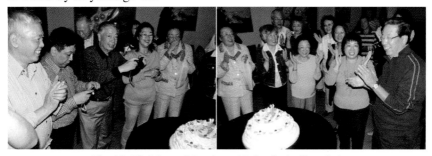

Fig. 10: Birthday celebration with family in Shanghai

3. The Woo Family: A Very Humble Beginning

The Woo family had a very modest beginning. My father, Mr. Kwok-Chong Woo (胡国章), was born in 1904 in a small town near Ningpo City in the Zhejiang Province of China to a family with little means. He was the second of four children. The family's financial situation became dire when his father died – my father was only eleven years old. Their only source of income was from his mother who did piecework as a seamstress. At fifteen, he sneaked onto ships as an unauthorized helper to the merchant marine sailors to earn a few coins. Eventually, he worked his way into a real job as a sailor, starting at the lowest rank. During this time, Dad's elder sister, whom he loved deeply and regarded highly, died prematurely. Throughout his life, he repeatedly told us how he cherished her while growing up. My father would respectfully light incense in her and his parents' memory each and every morning.

My mother, Mrs. Feng Xin Yu (虞鳳仙), was born in 1909 to a large family of fourteen children - she was the youngest of all the girls. Her father owned a single horse and carriage transportation business.

My parents' marriage was arranged by a matchmaker who did not earn any commission since my father's family was so poor. Interestingly, once my father learned whom he was going to marry, he - in his genius - found a way to take a sneak peek of my mother from a distance. Of course, he was quite content when he discovered that she was such a beautiful girl!

My parents' life together was very tough in the beginning as my father worked to support his family. Five family members were cramped in a tiny one-room loft and there was literally no space between them. Eventually, my father decided to immigrate to Shanghai in order for him and my uncle to find better opportunities. Lucky for us all, this was a wise and timely choice.

Even though times were neither easy nor simple, my parents made a great go at it in the great metropolis of Shanghai. Mom gave birth to twelve children, but only nine made it to adulthood. They were: three boys, three girls and three more boys in that order. With my father's brilliance, leadership qualities and hard work, he spearheaded many successful business ventures with his extended family and a group of close friends. A significant portion of his earnings was saved, while a smaller portion was used to support our large family plus a number of cousins and their families. With his example, we learned to live in modesty and appreciate everything we had.

My mother was busy raising her nine children, caring for her mother-in-law as well as being a very supportive wife to my father in his many business endeavors. She was extremely efficient, could multi-task naturally and had a great sense of humor! My father would regularly bring a group of business partners or guests home for dinner without giving my mother any advance warning (imagine any one of us doing that today!), and she would just go to the kitchen and put together a nine or ten course dinner effortlessly. She was also the best self-taught psychologist imaginable as she managed to make each of her nine children feel that he/she was the most loved. Even to this day, when my brothers and sisters gather together, we come up with stories to support our own argument that "*I* am Mom's most favorite child!!"

It may surprise you to know that neither of my parents had any formal education. Without ever setting foot in school, they only learned to print their initials and surnames in English in order to sign travelers' checks while visiting us in the U.S.! It is also amazing to note that in spite of never have taken a class on arithmetic, my father was always whispering numbers as he paced and calculated his earnings and savings in quantitative terms. My mother could tell me her monthly interest income accurately - not to the nearest week, but to the nearest day. Still, the fact that they had never had the means or the opportunity to go to school must have been difficult for them. As such, they made sure that we all got the best possible education and the primary priority for all of us was to bring home good report cards.

Growing up, I witnessed my parents observe Confucianism religiously, similar to most traditional Chinese families. They respected ancestry and revered my only living grandmother. In our home, we learned filial piety – respecting our parents and never questioning their authority. Siblings also had a strong order of governance; the older siblings had infinite authority over the younger ones. Surprisingly, this environment was conducive for us to share, learn and help each other while competing for limited resources and attention. We learned valuable lessons in preparation for our journeys in life and how to survive in the real world.

Our family underwent a huge change in 1949. In the late summer of that year, my father took my three elder brothers to Hong Kong for a business/pleasure trip. They were there when the new Chinese government came to power on October 1. Therefore, we - grandmother, mother, three girls and three younger boys - were summoned to leave Shanghai immediately. Led by one maternal uncle, we left almost everything behind and traveled by train to Hong Kong. We wore our oldest clothes to appear poor and avoid robbery during our journey. As a result, my family lost everything. The only valuables saved were a few pieces of my mother's jewelry hidden in my eldest sister's clothing.

My father worked extremely hard to restart new business ventures in Hong Kong. But without his team and his many connections, it was very difficult. Fortunately, my eldest brother, Mr. Liu-Ho Woo (胡流浩) stepped up for the family. He went to Kobe, Japan to start his import/export business. It was tough at first, but his ingenuity, hard work, and lessons learned from my father propelled him to great success. Through collaboration with my father in Hong Kong, his business flourished. My eldest brother's wife and business partner contributed generously to our family's well being during this time of transition. They actually provided complete financial support to our entire family for a while. Furthermore, my eldest brother, together with brother #2, Mr. Liu-Ching Woo (胡流澄), saved up enough funds to send me and my two younger brothers abroad for higher education at universities in the United States and Canada.

Brother #2 played an important role after we moved to Hong Kong as the trusted financial officer to my father and eldest brother. He was also a kind and generous man. More importantly, he and his wife took on the important duty of living with and caring for my parents for over twenty years! Two of their daughters, Nancy and Josephine were born when I was still home in Hong Kong and we have been close ever since.

Brother #3, Mr. Liu-Yun Woo (胡流泳) was the first to get a university education. He chose to return to Shanghai to pursue his Civil Engineering degree from Tongji University. I thank him for breaking the glass ceiling for us, as well as inspiring us to pursue higher education at universities even though they were thousands of miles away from home.

The remaining six of us grew up together in Hong Kong and were a very close-knit group. Sister #1, Shiu Cheng (胡秀珍) had the responsibility of watching over us. She was especially tough on me and we had many conflicts at that time. Nevertheless, I can thank her now for making me a better person. We all admire her tremendous devotion to her family. Sister #2, Bernadette Shiu-Ying (胡秀英) chose to devote her life in service to the Catholic Church. She is a great and caring educator and leader – something that I aspire to be. She is also the "glue" amongst us and has the best relationship with the younger generations. She has the ability to seek out what is inherently good and positive in everyone, even if it is (at times) disguised amid the negative. Sister #3, Shiu-Lee (胡秀蓮) is one beautiful and kind lady and she never forgets the hands that have fed her. The ultimate compliment I can pay to her is that she most resembles our mother!

My two younger brothers have led amazing lives. Brother #5, Dr. Stanley Lau-Po (胡流波) is the greatest planner and organizer. With his distinguished engineering skills, he led the effort to establish the rapid emergency response system for the city of Seattle. It is no wonder that the city loves him. He is also the most devoted father to his two sons. Brother #6, Dr. Savio Lau-Ching (胡流清) chose to travel along the same academic path as I – he even chose the same first name! He is brilliant, very accomplished, and a well-respected pioneer in the field of gene therapy.

Our two eldest brothers are now gone while the remaining seven of us are living all over Asia and North America. Each is still married to the same spouse (lucky for us!). Our spouses have been positive influences on us and have helped us to successfully raise our wonderful children. In recent years, we have managed to get together more frequently. I love all my siblings deeply – not only because we are family, but more importantly because they are outstanding human beings with unique, caring and admirable characters. I am sure that my parents are smiling "up there" when they see how well they have raised each and every one of us (Fig. 11).

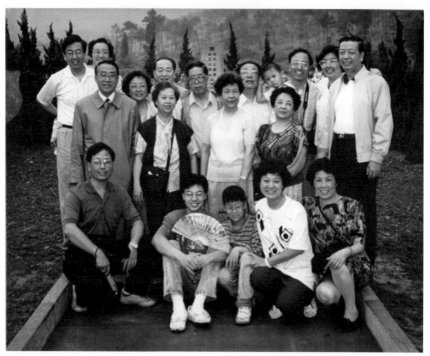

Fig. 11: All 9 Woo siblings and spouses (1991) Pattie & Emily not pictured

4. My Life – A Journey of Great Fortune

4.1. *In Hong Kong: 1950-1960*

There was a period of serious adjustment for me after we moved to Hong Kong. First and foremost was the language problem! I entered a small private primary school, but had no idea what the teachers and classmates were saying. My Shanghai dialect made my classmates glare and laugh at me like I was some strange person from another planet. A few months later, I learned to speak Cantonese and began to integrate with everyone better. But my grades were so poor that I was held back to repeat the third grade.

A few years later, I transferred to a larger middle school. At that time, I was more interested in playing football (soccer), basketball and table tennis than my studies. Being popular amongst the boys (and on rare occasions, with a few girls) was important to me. Academically, I managed to get by and was regularly ranked in the middle of the pack. During that period of time, I was also a bit rebellious and caught a lot of grief from my eldest sister. Messages on my uncooperative behavior frequently went up the chain to my parents. It was not a good thing!

A big turning point came when I transferred to Salesian School – an all-boys Catholic high school - to begin the second half of ninth grade. At the end of the year, we would be tested on every course taken during the three years of middle school. This made the transition especially challenging for me because there were big differences in the curricula between the two schools. For example, trigonometry had already been taught at Salesian but not yet at my old school. Fortunately, I befriended the physics teacher at Salesian and he, in three separate private lessons, tutored me on all the essentials of Trigonometry. To my own amazement, I was able to grasp all the "golden rules". I passed the examination without any problems. Being in a more demanding and competitive environment encouraged me to raise my game. In the process, I developed good study habits – including getting up early every morning while it was quiet in our very crowded flat to study. I grew up in a hurry and finally came to excel in my studies.

I also found that I enjoyed helping my classmates, especially those who were behind in their studies. One of my classmates with whom I played sports on a regular basis needed quite a bit of help. So, twice a week, I made him commit to study sessions where I would wake him up at 5:30 am to study. We reviewed lessons on algebra, geometry and calculus. It gave me great pleasure to see him doing better, making the grade on these classes and eventually graduating. I have always treasured this special memory. Certainly, this fulfilling experience helped to steer me toward a career in education and thankfully, that became my destiny!

4.2. *Coming to America*

I entered Hong Kong Technical College (now known as the Hong Kong Polytechnic University) in the fall of 1960 as a mechanical engineering student. After a couple of months, my father told me that he could afford to send me to America. So, I went to the library at the U.S. Embassy to search for universities that would accept foreign students. I found two that were attractive to me: Loyola University in Chicago (because it was Catholic and I had graduated from a Catholic high school) and Chico State College in Chico, California (because it was the cheapest). I applied to and was accepted at both but chose the latter for economical reasons, thinking that my two younger brothers would also need significant funding to follow me to study abroad. Of interest is that I had to comb through a number of maps of America before finding one that actually showed the city of Chico!

Meanwhile, I told the vice principal of the Technical College with regret that I was leaving. He was very very upset with me because my premature departure meant that my spot would be vacant for the next three years. I carried this guilt with me for many years. I have attempted to repay the College in a way via contributions to the Health Technology & Informatics and Rehabilitation Engineering Departments. For what little that I have done for them, their Academic Council rewarded me with a Doctor of Engineering Degree *honoris causa* in 2008 (Fig. 12).

I left Hong Kong for America on December 30, 1960 via the ocean liner *President Wilson*. After nineteen days at sea, I finally arrived underneath the Golden Gate Bridge in the early morning of January 17, 1961. A family friend and the only soul I knew in this new country met me by the dock and kindly accompanied me to the YMCA in Chinatown. After a brief stay, I took the Greyhound bus to Chico. When I arrived, I saw the city sign listing the population at 14,001. From then on, I frequently joked with friends visiting me that I represented that one!

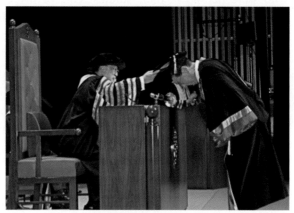

Fig. 12: Receiving Doctor of Engineering (honoris causa) from the Chief Executive of Hong Kong, the Honorable Donald Tseng

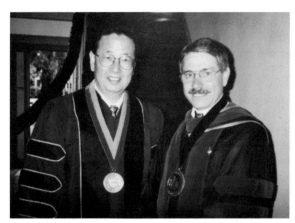

Fig 13: With President Manual Esteben after receiving honorary Doctor of Science from California State University system at commencement in Chico

Chico State turned out to be the best place for me to get an education. The student body was small and so was the class size. The professors were dedicated, reachable and supportive. To this day, the memory of their influence on me dwells deep in my heart. I called out their names in acknowledgement during my speech at Commencement in 1998 when the California State University System bestowed upon me an honorary Doctoral of Science degree (Fig. 13). These professors made such a deep impression that I yearned to be a caring professor – just like them.

The college campus was beautiful and the atmosphere was very conducive to learning. President Kendall was a fatherly figure who called me by my first name and the Dean of Students Carlson frequently sought my input on applicants from Asia, especially those from Hong Kong. My fellow students were warm and welcoming. It was easy for me to befriend a large number of them. I learned to sing many folk songs by joining in on hootenanny sessions. I also went to all the football and basketball games and enjoyed Monday morning quarterbacking with many varsity athletes and cheerleaders.

The tuition at Chico was $8.50 per semester credit for foreign students. The maximum charge per semester was 15 credits, but I could take as many as 21 credits for a total of $127.50. This would work out to be about 41 cents per 50 minute class. It was unbelievably affordable.

To support myself, I graded papers and tests (at $1/hr) for a number of professors, swept the aisles of the local National Dollar Store and washed dishes in a Chinese restaurant in San Francisco for two summers. During my junior and senior years, I was able to earn scholarships and worked as a consultant at engineering firms in the cities of Chico and nearby Redding. Financially, I became so well-to-do that I bought a very used 1953 Studebaker for $125!

During the summer of 1964, I was selected to attend the Space Technology Summer Institute at Cal Tech. It was an exciting program and I was delighted to be amongst the 50 students selected from the seven Western States. There, I also caught the first glimpse of the famous Professor Y.C. "Bert" Fung who, unbeknownst to us both, would later become my most respected mentor and friend! I also met a couple of students from the University of Washington, including my lifelong friend, Walt Federick and they encouraged me to consider it for my graduate studies. Knowing how much I loved sports, they put the exclamation point on the fact that the Huskies had gone to the Rose Bowl three of the last five years!

I have very fond memories of Chico State and the excellent education I received there. I have made an effort to give back by serving on the Advisory Board of the College of Engineering, Computer Sciences and Technology. Pattie and I also established a small endowment to provide an annual scholarship to the most deserving engineering students. We are thankful that Chico has continued to honor me by naming me as one of its distinguished alumni in 2000.

I graduated from Chico State in January 1965 and worked for the same consulting firm in Redding for eight months before going to University of Washington. It was my great fortune that I met Professor Albert S. Kobayashi who offered me a research assistantship. I learned to adopt the linear Fracture Mechanics theory to numerically calculate the zone of failure at the tip of a crack in metals (e.g., airplane cracks) and predict how it would progress under externally applied stresses. This project led to my M.S. thesis.

I must have done a decent job, as Albert asked me to go on to study the human eye with him. Together with the late Dr. Carteret Lawrence – a clinical scientist in ophthalmology, we determined the nonlinear mechanical properties of the human cornea and sclera and used the brand new finite element methods to model the corneo-scleral shell. We combined the nonlinear tissue properties that were measured to obtain a nonlinear intra-ocular pressure and volume relationship. We also used this validated model to evaluate the accuracy of clinical tonometric measurements in diagnosing diseases such as glaucoma and bulging of the cornea with keratoconus. These studies netted me my Ph.D. degree. It was indeed an exciting time as the field of Bioengineering was emerging and thanks to Albert, I was in its midst.

Since my departure in 1970, I have regularly returned to UW. On a number of occasions during the 1980s, I was being recruited to go back there as an endowed chair professor. In 2008, the School of Engineering recognized me with the inaugural Diamond Award for Distinguished Achievement in Academia. Last spring, I was honored again as I was selected to deliver the inaugural Kobayashi and Morrison endowed lecture. I did it proudly as Albert and Mrs. Morrison were in the audience.

Apart from receiving a great education at UW, I also enjoyed life as a graduate student. I made many lifelong friends and participated in countless hours of discussion/argument against those who were for the Vietnam war, and so on. Most importantly, I met, courted and married my lovely wife, Ms. Pattie Tak-Kit Cheong (张德潔)!

4.3. *K and J, How I Met Your Mother*

On a rare occasion in 1967, I visited the Far Eastern Library on campus after lunch to read about a special event happening in Hong Kong (internet was not yet available then). There, I was mesmerized by a most graceful and beautiful girl working as a clerk. Needless to say, I could not take my eyes off her, although I had to do so discretely. Then, I became a regular visitor to the library although I never got up enough nerve to start a conversation with her.

It was my great fortune that Pattie's housemate was the fiancé of a friend of mine. As soon as I discovered this, I rushed to his office and asked him to introduce us. After some trials and tribulations, we finally managed to "double date" to the Ice Capades on January 3, 1968. Unbeknownst to me, Pattie was under the impression that I was just the driver for the four of us! After a couple of weeks, I gathered up enough courage to call Pattie and got myself a real date with her. Since I knew that she was taking ice skating lessons, I asked whether she would like

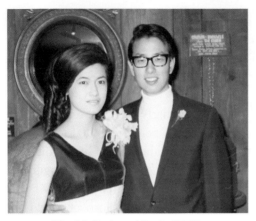

Fig. 14: Savio and Pattie (1968)

to practice what she was learning and she agreed. All the while, I was envisioning holding her hand (at least some of the time!) while we skated together.

For a little more than a year, we got together more and more frequently and our relationship flourished. Seattle is such a romantic city to pursue a lively and innocent young lady like Pattie (Fig. 14). However, the journey for me was not always easy, since she had many suitors! On March 2, 1969, I asked for her hand on a ferry boat ride and the rest is history! Actually, I really didn't take any chances as my parents had already met Pattie's parents, Mr. Antonio and Mrs. Tung Ho (何桐) Cheong in Hong Kong a month or so earlier and my mother had (successfully) proposed for me!

On September 6, 1969, we were married in Edmonds, Washington. Our marriage life began like a pair of new grinding stones. Even though we were made for each other, it does take years to grind out all the rough spots. Through the years, I have learned that Pattie got the best from both of her parents. She is one stunningly beautiful and graceful lady (both inside and outside) with a terrific personality. She is always positive, cheerful and encouraging and is a friend to everybody. She holds no grudges. Some of our friends have intimated to me the reason why I am successful is because they like Pattie! She listens to people's problems intensely and patiently (sometimes for hours) and always comforts them with genuine empathy. She also loves my students and opens our home to them. She has learned to be a creative and quality chef such that her family enjoys her fine cooking while students and friends happily come over to taste her creative cuisine as well.

For more than 42 years, she has been my most loving, caring, understanding and supportive wife and friend. I am also glad that she is so forgiving – the main reason why I have survived happily for so long! I also know that it was not easy for her to agree to move our family from the paradise of San Diego to Pittsburgh in 1990. But, she decided to pick up all our sticks, kids and all, and moved because she unconditionally supported what I hoped to accomplish.

To our daughter, Kirstin and our son, Jonathan, she is the mommy who has given her unconditional love. She guided them almost single-handedly while I devoted almost all my time to working and traveling. For all of us, she has always been there whether we needed consultation or consolation. She has been a pillar of strength for our family and "the wind beneath our wings". Although I didn't fully comprehend it in 1969, it has become abundantly clear that marrying Pattie was by far the very best decision I have ever made in my life!

4.4. *California Here We Come: 1970-1990*

In 1970, jobs for people with Ph.D. degrees were very scarce. Rumor had it that many were driving taxis in New York while waiting for any available post-doctoral positions. I was quite lucky that I had offers from Dr. Lawrence as well as from Chicago. But, the most attractive one was to be a junior research faculty member at the University of California, San Diego (UCSD). Here, I must thank Dr. Wayne Akeson, then a faculty member at UW, for giving me the opportunity to start my academic career with him and Professor David Amiel at UCSD. Indeed, it was a kind offer for which I remain grateful. Also, that I could be at the same institution with Professor Fung made my choice easy.

Meanwhile, Pattie was pregnant with our first baby and we were excited. Sadly, Angel was a stillborn at eight months. After we buried her in Seattle, I got permission to take my final examination for my Ph.D. degree so that I could start my position at UCSD right away. I would finish writing my doctoral dissertation in California.

The beginning of my academic career was interesting as well as challenging. I had to learn a lot about Orthopaedic Surgery and Medicine in a very short time as well as acquire some knowledge on biochemistry from my long-time collaborators: Wayne, David and a couple of years later, Dr. Richard Coutts. We worked well together and started a very strong multidisciplinary research group. In the early 1970s, this type of multidisciplinary research team was one of the first of its kind. Together, we performed exciting translational research that led to changes in the clinical management of musculoskeletal injuries – a paradigm shift from cast immobilization of joints to functional treatment.

The challenging part came as early as six months after we had started. We found out Wayne's active NIH grants were not favorably reviewed. We needed to borrow funds from the Department of Surgery to survive while we wrote amended applications and resubmitted them for review. Further, the then governor of California, Ronald Reagan, was not particularly kind to the state universities. He froze the faculty salaries for three years – putting special strains on young faculty and their young families.

Pattie and I could only afford to live in a modest two-bedroom apartment. It was sobering to discover that my income was lower than the average income of a white person living in Orange County – about 70 miles up Interstate 5! So, I sought additional consulting work with Gulf Atomic, a neighboring company to UCSD to supplement my income. One of our collaborators who was a senior staff member in that company, had introduced me to a group who was designing very thick concrete wall containers to house nuclear reactors. A young engineer interviewed me. I had suggested that my knowledge and experience with finite element analysis should be of help to the container design. To my chagrin, he quickly dismissed my idea and said that he didn't believe this numerical method would be useful. Needless to say, I was stung and thoroughly disappointed.

Following this rejection, I decided to focus on doing what I knew best. We wrote an additional NIH application on bone fracture healing with internal fixation plates. I also wrote an NSF grant on the Articular Cartilage of Human Femoral Head. Fortunately, all applications were funded! We gained a lot of confidence and had the means to go forward with our work. Meanwhile, the San Diego Veterans Hospital opened in 1972 and we were given a couple of new laboratories. We also got VA grants so that we could staff our laboratories with quality students and dedicated technicians and engineers. We also purchased new equipment for our experiments. We added a histology laboratory and fostered an environment that would enable us to forge ahead in collaborative research and education.

Pattie went to work as a technical staff member for the OB-GYN department at UCSD so that we could save her paychecks to buy our first condominium and then our first home in Encinitas. We grew very happy in San Diego – we made new friends and enjoying our work with the sunshine and ocean as our backdrop. We even got our first (and only) dog – an Irish setter we named Ferrous Oxide. We were living the American dream!

Then in 1975, Pattie became pregnant with Kirstin Wei-Chi (Wei-Wei) (胡玮琪) and on November 29, she delivered the loveliest bundle of joy of my life. Beginning on that day and for all of the next 36 years, I have loved, adored, admired and appreciated Wei-Wei. Whenever I reminisce about her - which is quite often - I am humbled (with a big grin on my face) by who she is and what she has accomplished! She has been a perfect child growing up, a loving and respectful daughter (well, most of the time!), a pretty singer and dancer, a beautiful writer, a polished public speaker, a born leader, a trusted friend to many, a creative artist and event organizer, a marathon runner, an award winning student (all through her K-12, at Brown University, University of Pittsburgh Medical School and UC San Francisco's OB-GYN residency program), a caring and well respected physician, a stunning beautiful bride (lucky you, Adam!), a loving and devoted "super-Mom" to our two darling granddaughters, Zadie Woo (慈欣) and Arden Pattie (慈慧) Frymoyer. There is literally an aura about her when she enters a room. One of the proudest moments of my life was when I was able to "hood" the new Dr. Woo at her medical school graduation ceremony (Fig. 15). I so appreciate how well Pattie has raised her and regularly brag to everyone

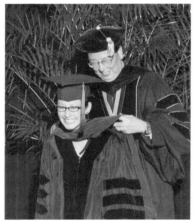

Fig. 15: Hooding Kirstin at graduation from Pitt medical school (2003)

"Kirstin, (my sweetie) is a perfect daughter that every (good) father deserves!"

For the next ten years, my colleagues at UCSD and I, with the help of our students, residents and fellows as well as my staff, especially my secretary of 18 years, Mrs. Lynette Fleck, were able to publish a series of fundamental studies on soft connective tissues, articular cartilage as well as long bone fractures. We found special ways to properly measure the properties of ligaments and tendons in addition to articular cartilage and how environment, maturation, ageing and exercise - or lack of it - changed these properties. We used the new knowledge gained on these tissues as the basis to evaluate the progress of their healing and repair following different treatment modalities. A number of our key findings were successfully translated into clinical use.

In the process, we also educated a number of students, residents and international fellows (see Appendix A). Many have become life-long friends and have gone on to be leaders in our field. Learning from mentors and colleagues, being advised by friends and being challenged by students – all of this enabled my academic career and my reputation to grow.

Apparently, my peers recognized our work in the field of bioengineering - orthopaedic biomechanics in particular. They also appreciated my passion to move this important field forward and chose me as their leader in three separate professional societies all around the same time (1985 to 1987). My friends also asked me to join the Scientific Advisory Committee for the Whitaker Foundation, where I served for ten years. When an opportunity arose, I was instrumental in keeping the Foundation's focus on Biomedical Engineering. I also helped to convince Dr. Peter Katona to join the Foundation, which culminated in his becoming its President. Also, together with Dr. Jody Buckwalter, we organized the first American Academy of Orthopaedic Surgeons symposium on soft tissues and edited the classic text on *Injury and Repair of Musculoskeletal Soft Tissues*. Thinking back, all these happenings must have helped me to solidify my philosophy as an educator and defined the academic that I have become.

On January 11, 1979, we were blessed with the arrival of our handsome son, Jonathan I-Huei (Jon-Jon) (胡裔晖). While he was growing up, I had to travel a lot and Jonathan would always miss me when I was not at the dinner table. Sometimes, he would even refuse to eat! He is sentimental and would, at a relatively young age, repeatedly ask me to tell him about my family and our history. He is a very sensitive person and I am proud that he has a great big heart.

When Jonathan was five or six years old, he surprised me with his comprehension of the concept of fractions. Years later, he worked with my formers students, Thay (Dr. Lee) and Pat (Dr. McMahon) at their VA Long Beach laboratory for a couple of years. He surprised me again when he came to the pre-ASB meeting in Pittsburgh in 1999 to give a talk on *in-vivo* measurements of shoulder motion in 6 DOF. I was the proud father sitting amongst the audience. He was poised and delivered his findings with clarity and answered the questions very well. His first lecture was certainly far better than the one I gave at the ORS in 1975 (see section 6)! In 2002, he became a co-author on a paper on gender differences on patellofemoral biomechanics that was published in Clinical Orthopaedics and Related research.

Jonathan has also been my companion to many sporting events – San Diego Chargers and Padres as well as Pittsburgh Steelers, Pirates and Penguins plus University of Pittsburgh Panthers football and basketball. We have also been regular supporters at the Panther's bowl games

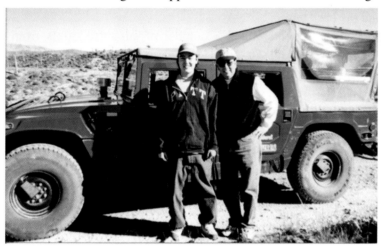

Fig. 16: With Jonathan on a desert tour in Arizona before going to watch Pitt play in the Fiesta Bowl (2004)

(Fig. 16). For a number of years, he comes home in July for my birthday and we would celebrate by going to a couple of Pirates' games together. It has become another great father-son thing!

Jonathan has chosen to forge his own path in becoming an upstanding young man. He is a talented manager/server/investor at a Steelers bar in San Francisco. All the patrons there love him and have the best things to say about him. Pattie and I enjoy going there as we love to see how positively all his customers relate to him. They even revere us like celebrities! Jonathan is such a people person as well as extremely generous to his friends. I only wish that I could have half of his admirable qualities. Jonathan's chosen path to life was so foreign to me and, although it took a while, I have finally learned to accept it and along the way, he has taught me to become a better parent.

My last five years at UCSD were the most gratifying – both at work and at home. Everything was falling into place for my family and me. On the other hand, I found myself becoming more and more restless. How could I teach more students, help more fellows, mentor more colleagues and make a higher impact in my fields of interest? Even leading the basic science faculty in the School of Medicine to challenge with the administration of the University of California system on unfairly changing our retirement benefits was not enough. I felt an urgent need to expand my horizons!

Indeed, I had entertained a number of attractive offers from fine universities. In the end, Dr. Jim Herndon and the late Dr. Thomas Detre of the University of Pittsburgh Medical Center, with the help of my dear friend T.K. (Dr. Hung), came calling. After a number of fascinating visits to Pittsburgh, I realized that they believed in my vision and wanted me to help to move their orthopaedic research and education program to the next level. I gladly accepted their kind and generous offer on July 3, 1990 to help lead the Department to newer heights. I could not wait to take on this new challenge!

4.5. *Pittsburgh or Bust: August 1990*

It was definitely not easy for any of us to leave the paradise of San Diego and our beautiful home. It was even harder to say good-bye to many close friends and colleagues. But, I was thankful that Pattie, Kirstin and Jonathan bravely flew to Pittsburgh with me without any signs of distress or verbal complaints. They were real troopers! Of course, we all knew that deep down, we would greatly miss the place where Wei-Wei and Jon-Jon were born and raised - where we had lived for 20 years! Indeed, we did miss San Diego even after we lived in Pittsburgh for a number of years. Whenever we would return to visit, we all became very sentimental. I would get a bit teary-eyed when I saw Pattie, Kirstin and Jonathan's wide smiles and how their faces lit up as soon as we landed and were met by our friends. Perhaps this is why both Kirstin and Jonathan chose to move back to live in California at the first opportunity.

My work at the University of Pittsburgh was filled with excitement. The new Musculoskeletal Research Center (MSRC) was born! Thanks to my staff, students and postdoctoral fellows who moved with me from UCSD, we got into full swing doing our research within a couple of months. We had all found renewed energy. Meanwhile, we were busy recruiting new faculty members and helping them set up their new laboratories.

By the end of our first year, the MSRC had grown to a total of 24 research faculty, graduate students, residents, fellows and staff working alongside five clinical faculty members. We started to develop novel bench and analytical skills for multidisciplinary and collaborative research while prioritizing high quality research. Our mantra was: "There is NO replacement for quality!" Our daily discussions were highly stimulating as they were elevated to higher intellectual. We also taught our younger investigators techniques on how to logically synthesize better study designs, how to perform experiments and collect as well as analyze the results, how to prepare grant proposals and how to write good manuscripts for publication. We also had a lot of fun together for a number of extracurricular activities. Colleagues, students, residents, fellows and staff were frequent visitors at our home (Fig. 17).

In 1995, the MSRC celebrated its 5th anniversary. By then, we had nine basic science faculty and 78 people divided into 12 research groups. Additionally, each clinical faculty member was paired with a basic science faulty member on bench to bedside research. One half of the eight orthopaedic residents also rotated through the MSRC for one to two

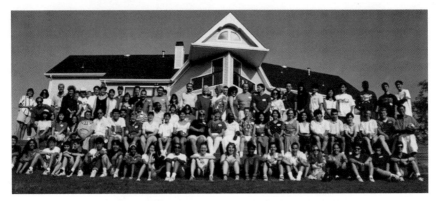

Fig. 17: MSRC summer parties at our home (1993)

years of research training. Each was assigned to a research group and worked with graduate students and research staff. We were also successful in securing a significant amount of extramural grant funds for our projects.

We invited a blue-ribbon panel of leaders to conduct an external review of the MSRC. After two and a half days, they wrote that they "were impressed by the professionalism and overall quality of the presentations...by the efficient organization...by the dedication of the students and staff, and by the magnificent laboratories, instruments and apparatuses available to pursue orthopaedic investigations. All this quality and competence is matched by the prodigious output of the MSRC over the last five years, and the overall quality of the research. It seems clear that the MSRC will continue to make major contributions... and to function with leadership capacity within the field." We were truly grateful for these encouraging remarks and used them to rededicate ourselves.

For the next five years, the MSRC was running almost a 7 days a week, 24 hours a day (well, at least 7-20) and I regularly had to ensure that everyone remembered to go home and do things unrelated to work. All participated actively in our Monday Morning Meeting (MMM) as well as seminars on Monday afternoons and Saturday mornings. Although, they also knew (and feared) that they would be subjected to many tough critiques and questions (which I casually named "training"), students and fellows all begged for an opportunity to show their work formally there. In this intense but supportive environment, members of all 12 groups worked together harmoniously and we were very productive.

Indeed, the most gratifying part was that the students and junior faculty from the MSRC were being recognized both nationally and internationally as they were winning many awards for their work. A complete list of awards can be found on the MSRC website under Two Decades of Excellence (http://www.pitt.edu/~msrc/awards). Many of our faculty members became better known for what they had accomplished and were regularly invited to give lectures as well as deliver instructional courses all over the world. It was such a pleasure to lead the MSRC as everyone there wanted to be there and everyone was happy - learning, doing and writing at a ferocious pace.

We were proud to be selected to host the 23rd Annual American Society of Biomechanics meeting in 1999. To further serve our profession, we organized the inaugural International Symposium of Ligaments and Tendons (ISL&T) at the dawn of the new millennium and throughout the years, this annual symposium has grown significantly both in quality and quantity. The ISL&T-XII in 2012 was the best yet! (Fig. 18) We also founded a second new society named the World Association of Chinese Biomedical Engineers (WACBE) and had our

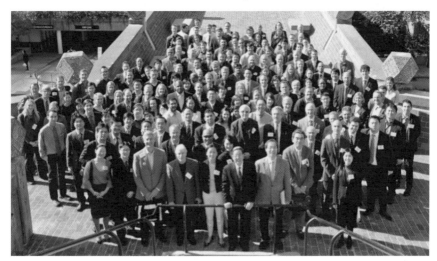

Fig. 18: Attendees of ISL&T-XII in San Francisco, California

first congress in Taipei, Taiwan in 2002. We returned to Taiwan in 2011 for a very successful 5th biannual congress in Tainan as I described earlier in Section 2.3.

On the lighter side, the MSRC functions like an extended family and we continually find occasions to have fun together. Our celebrations include monthly birthday parties, welcome and farewell parties, frequent lunches with Chinese food, and so on. Meanwhile, there have been several romantic connections between members of the MSRC that have ended up in matrimony. For some, this is fondly labeled as "the MSRC curse!"

4.6. *A Return to my Engineering Domain*

For the first thirteen years, a total of 393 students, residents and post-doctoral fellows became members of the MSRC family. We also had a number of notable accomplishments: $35 million of extramural funding including 33 NIH grants (19 were R01s) and 14 Whitaker Bioengineering Research Grants, 65 research awards, 974 referred journal papers, book chapters and review papers, abstracts and extended abstracts and conference proceedings plus 9 books. In addition, 2,268 visitors from all continents toured the MSRC.

There is a Chinese proverb: "Beneath the heavens, there is no banquet (or feast) that does not end." In 1998, Dr. Herndon left the University of Pittsburgh for Harvard and soon after, Dr. Detre retired. The Department of Orthopaedic Surgery as well as the School of Medicine underwent a leadership change and after a few years, I found that I was no longer a good fit. Since I had pretty much accomplished what I came to do in Pittsburgh, I thought seriously about moving back to California. We even put our beautiful home up for sale.

But, California was not meant to be! Chancellor Mark Nordenberg, Provost Jim Maher, School of Engineering (now the Swanson SOE) Dean Jerry Holder and Department of Bioengineering (BioE) Chair Harvey Borovetz refused to entertain the idea that I would leave Pitt. Together, they successfully moved me to the Swanson SOE as a member of the BioE faculty. Moreover, they generously provided me with the needed support so that the MSRC and a number of its members could

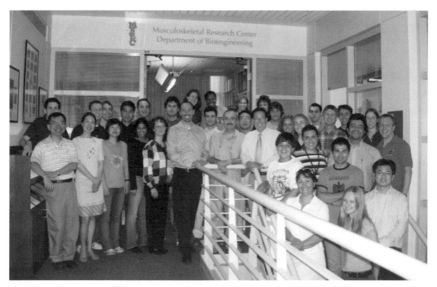

Fig. 19: The MSRC (2006)

move with me. Regrettably, I could not bring all my basic science faculty members and their staff and students along (although I wished that I could!), as there were only a limited number of tenure stream faculty slots available. Still, I was so grateful to receive such extraordinary collegiality and generosity from the University's leadership and vowed to do my very best in my new digs. I also made a conscious decision that I would no longer entertain other job offers in order to devote the rest of my academic career to Pitt (Fig. 19).

It was a perfect move! Everyone at the Swanson SOE and BioE was friendly and made us feel welcome. Our eyes opened wide in such a pleasant climate where faculty and staff actually like and aim to help each other. The spirit of cooperation was high, the politics were minimal and as a result, we have been able to focus our entire energy on our work! While I have benefited from and completely enjoyed my 34 years in the two Schools of Medicine at UCSD and Pitt, I am delighted to be in the Swanson SOE now. Its atmosphere is much more suitable for me at this stage of my academic life.

With the change in environment, we also determined that it would be in our best interest to narrow our scope to focus on ligament and tendon research and reorganized our laboratories accordingly. Several of the faculty members from the Department of Orthopaedic Surgery continued on our team and carried out their projects at the MSRC. International research fellows continued to arrive to study with me. We are now free to choose with whom we would like to help and with whom to collaborate. Many renowned and leading orthopaedic surgeons and basic scientists from around the world (all of whom also happen to be my best friends) are now collaborating closely with us.

With the advent of functional tissue engineering, we added a new and well-equipped mechanobiology laboratory to cover the spectrum of studies from cells to tissues to organs. Specifically, we applied extracellular matrix (ECM) as a bioscaffold to enhance the healing of the medial collateral ligament and patellar tendon and obtained improved quantity as well as quality of the newly formed tissues. We have moved onto a more challenging task: healing the injured anterior cruciate ligament (ACL). Much to our amazement, the ECM has successfully facilitated ACL healing with good neo-tissue. Still, much work remains to optimize ACL healing. We are excited about this possibility because of its significance for orthopaedic sports medicine. This could offer surgeons an alternate option in addition to ACL reconstruction for treating certain patients.

Recently, another good turn of events has transpired. We were invited to participate in a National Science Foundation application for an Engineering Research Center grant on Revolutionize Metallic Biomaterials (ERC-RMB). This exciting program involves a large number of investigators from a number of universities and industries working together to develop biodegradable and bioresorbable metallic materials. The principle is for them to provide the needed initial stiffness and strength to facilitate tissue healing. Once sufficient healing has taken place, these materials can be programmed to degrade such that the healing tissues would gradually take over and remodel to become better tissues. The ten years of funding from NSF allows us to work with and learn from many experts on the entire team. We are developing a magnesium alloy ring device to connect the two torn ends of the ACL in order to load its insertion sites immediately after surgery and to prevent disuse atrophy. The device will be used in combination with ECM and ECM hydrogels to accelerate ACL healing. The NSF site visiting team deemed the ERC-RMB very successful after the first three years and will fund the center for the remaining seven years. Therefore, our exciting ACL healing project will continue, which we hope will further impact the clinical arena. This project is sure to keep me busy for the remainder of my academic career.

5. Lessons I Have Learned

My parents, my parents-in-law, as well as my mentors have taught me a number of valuable lessons. Unfortunately, I have only been able to practice just a portion of them and am still working on the rest.

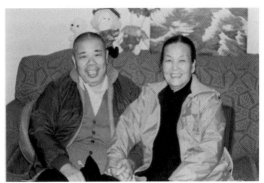

Fig. 20: My parents

Father and Mother (Fig. 20) were firm believers in Confucian values of selflessness, compassion, honor and rectitude. To honor my grandmother, they demonstrated filial piety to the extreme and we learned to think and behave the same way. To encourage us, my father would frequently quote a Chinese proverb (and I roughly translate): "When one is able to take suffering over suffering, then one becomes a person that is above another person". For someone who had never attended school, such a classic literary quote is quite amazing!

My parents were very generous in giving to others but not to themselves. They lived in modesty based on a model that when they earned $1, they would only spend 10 cents. Obviously, they did not find the need to "keep up with the Joneses". Although this model would definitely not go over well in today's "spend first" culture and "spend more" economy, our large family did thrive without suffering any severe financial hardship. For years, my parents were able to support and give generously to their extended family that included many who worked for my father.

Brother #3 (胡流泳) told me that my parents, once they became well to do, would set up stations at busy intersections around Shanghai to supply free "special barley tea" for rickshaw pullers and other hard laborers to quench their thirst as well as water for all passersby. This was one of their ways of giving back.

One of the most important lessons my parents taught us was to treat everyone equally with respect – no matter whether that person is rich or poor, a president or a janitor, and so on. I have taken this advice to heart and tried my best to follow that philosophy each and every day.

Finally, my being a perfectionist must have come from my mother! When I brought home a test score of 97, she would, in her sweet and humorous way say: "Well, this is great! I am so proud of you. But, what happened to the other 3 points?"

My father-in-law and mother-in-law (I fondly called them Gung Gung and Po Po since our children were born) were altruistic as well (Fig. 21). During the December 3, 1966 incident ("12-3 Riot") in Macao, a Portuguese province near Hong Kong, Gung Gung - the highest ranked Chinese officer in the government - was holed up with other leaders in the Governor's mansion. He helped to successfully negotiate a peaceful outcome and also authored the government's apology to its people in Chinese. The Governor gave him a medal to recognize his notable contribution and asked what he wanted as a reward. To that, Gung Gung's reply was that he did not want anything personally, but he wished for the small Department of Chinese Affairs to be elevated to a larger and more prominent division in the government. The Governor granted his wish!

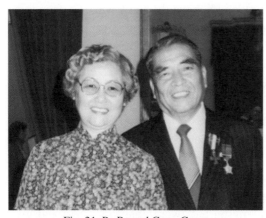

Fig. 21: Po Po and Gung Gung

Both were compassionate in helping people in need and they never asked nor accepted anything in return. Po Po was forever listening to the problems of friends and their children and then dispensed her sound advice generously – a character that Pattie has learned and also practiced. She was patient, concise and consistent in everything she did. She was a lady ahead of her time as she successfully combined what she learned from the east and the west. Together with her common sense, this selfless mother and grandmother was able to love, teach, guide and significantly influence her family.

Po Po took her time to examine people before passing any judgment. Perhaps that was why it took her a while to trust me, "the cradle robber"- Pattie is six years younger than me. But once she decided that I was worthy, she accepted me as her son and became my biggest fan for all her remaining years! Gung Gung, on the other hand, gave me a great big hug on our wedding day, and then proclaimed: "You are my son now!" He did so right after he had just given away his only beloved daughter. That was the magnanimous Gung Gung that everyone knew. I adored him ever since.

Gung Gung was very perceptive and frequently offered me much needed advice, followed by his beautiful poetry as encouragement. He participated with great pride in all the important events in my life and always had the best things to say about me. We had such a wonderful father-son relationship and in spite of my best efforts, I have yet to come close to adequately describing it. At his memorial service, I sobbed and said: "For 42 years, there was not one day that Gung Gung and I did not mutually admire each other!"

> "The beginning of education lies in imitation. Therefore, pick someone worth imitating"   Martin Fischer

I am lucky to have two ideal academic mentors: Professors Albert Kobayashi (see section 4.2) and Yuan-Cheng "Bert" Fung. Both have had profound influences on me. They are similar in many ways – both are outstanding human beings, caring teachers, true pioneers, visionaries and thrilled with new discoveries. Plus, they both have "bert" in their names! My closeness to them has allowed me to learn from them the importance of the process for proper research and how to teach it (Figs. 22, 23 and 24).

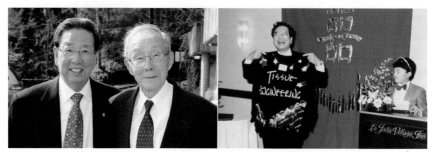

Fig. 22: With Prof. Kobayashi (2011)

Fig. 23: Celebrating Prof. Fung's 70th Birthday Party in La Jolla with Jonathan at the podium (1989)

Throughout my 20 years at UCSD, I followed Professor Fung like a dedicated disciple, and he became my respected mentor and cherished friend. By helping him establish new professional organizations and societies, I learned the importance of such endeavors as well as to how to be an effective leader. He and I had lunch together every Friday to talk about our lives both in and out of biomechanics. For years, I would look forward to our private luncheon every Monday morning!

Professor Fung always makes time for anyone who seeks his advice. He spent the whole of his workday seeing and advising people. Therefore, as I later learned, he ended up writing his textbooks at night. It is evident that young investigators truly have a special place in his heart. So, after I led the effort in a symposium to honor his 65th birthday in 1984, we were able to parlay the excessive funds (with the great help from Dr. Peter Chen, our treasurer) to establish the ASME Y.C. Fung Young Investigator Award in his honor.

By far the most important lesson that I have learned from my two mentors is the virtue of humility. They constantly resist the temptation of flaunting their successes at the first opportunity. It is

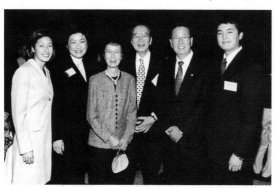

Fig. 24: My family with Prof. Fung and Luna at the ASB Conference in Pittsburgh (1999)

so natural for them to do so. They are secure with themselves; hence, they do not find the need to seek further admiration or praise from others, let alone go around advertising their achievements. At the risk of sounding old fashioned, I offer an idea that may be unlikely to be accepted by some, and might be unwelcome by many in today's "Madison Avenue/self promoting" society. Still, I maintain that one should remain humble and also share credits with others when one has success. Trust me, most people who are your true friends and those who have an interest in you would prefer it! Plus, it is a good thing to always keep one's feet firmly planted on the ground.

6. Lessons I Have Shared

The lessons I have shared with my students, residents, research fellow and junior colleagues stem from the lessons I have learned.

To all, I encourage, coerce, and - if that fails - demand *perfection*. By that, I mean paying attention to detail on everything that we do. I like to use professional sports competition as an example. The top-ranked teams have athletes that are of roughly the same skill level and ability. Winning really comes down to that one team whose coaches who have outlined and taught their system in detail and players who have bought into and executed the details effectively.

The other lesson involves *practice*. I still vividly recall my first presentation at a national meeting. I was quite nervous and unlike my son Jonathan (recall from Section 4.4.), I spent the entire 15 minutes covering all the fine points of our experiment and showing volumes of data. I had to speak much faster than my usual tempo to get through all the information. In the end, the audience did not grasp the main points. I decided right then and there that I must improve.

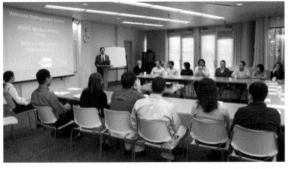

Fig. 25: A typical Monday Morning Meeting (MMM)

Now, with years of practice, I have gotten much better at giving talks - so everyone tells me. Today, I am still practicing and seeking perfection.

During our MMM, I frequently speak about the "three mores" with my students; i.e., think more, ask more and then do more (Fig. 25). Nowadays, information technology has given us help on numerous fronts. On the contrary, it has also made some of us less proactive in our thinking since almost everything is available with just a click on our computer or a tap on our Smartphone. Further, many of us spend so much time on computers and Smartphones (even during meetings) and use them exclusively for communication that it leaves precious little time for talking face to face with colleagues and collaborators. It seems that it is much easier and quicker to send an email or a text message.

In the laboratory, there is also a tendency to jump right into doing our experiments and analyses without the benefit of thinking through the study at hand. We do not always perform thorough searches, or carefully review (not just scan) the literature, or ask the appropriate research questions, or go through the experimental design. The theme of the "three mores" is designed to limit and prevent us from going down the wrong path from the get-go.

Years ago, my students gave me a book written by Dr. Carl Sagan. He wrote in <u>The Demon Haunted World</u> quite a bit on UFOs. The question people usually ask is "Do you believe in UFOs?" Rather, he advocated that the question that should be asked is "How good is the evidence that UFOs are alien spaceships?" So, we need to learn to ask the right research questions rather than just be whirlwinded into doing what is trendy and popular. That is why we continue to teach and learn biomechanics, as it is "a candle in the dark". It may not be flashy, but the quantitative data obtained on the behavior and function of molecules, cells, tissues, organs and the whole body are concrete and do have applicability and clinical relevance.

It is through discussion with colleagues and occasional heated debates with those who have the opposite opinion that we gain better perspective on what we are doing. This can be a great learning experience as well as fun! Professor Allan Bloom wrote in his 1987 book (way back then!) entitled <u>The Closing of the American Mind</u> about how rock music "ruins the imagination of young people" and with "the Walkman" (a very popular portable audio cassette player coupled with ear phones made by Sony) on, they cannot hear what the great tradition (liberal arts education) has to say. Today, there are so many people who have two thin, white cables coming from their ears while they are riding on buses and trains, walking across the street, cruising on their bicycles and while zipping in and out of traffic driving their cars. Certainly, they can hear precious little outside of the blasting sound from their earphones, nor are they completely aware of potential hazards around them. Many even wear the cables during their studies! All this makes me wonder how they are developing critical thinking, let alone developing the capacity to ask the right questions. At the very least, using the white cables to separate from one's surroundings is not conducive to discussion nor debate. Thus, the "three mores" might be a helpful way to reopen our minds!

My aspiration for the next generations, and especially for my own students, is to help them believe that they can become better and more accomplished than the generation before (Fig. 26). This is encapsulated in the saying: "The rear wave needs to be higher to push the one in the front." So, aiming high and dreaming big are what I encourage my students to aspire to. On a regular basis, my students are challenged to do better than their best even if it means asking them unreasonably tough

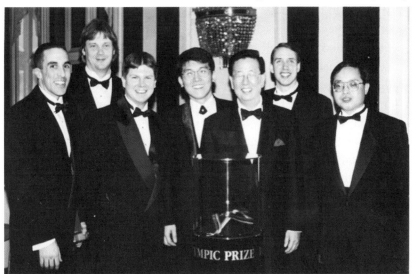

Fig. 26: At the ceremony for the IOC Olympic Prize in NYC (1998)

questions or challenging to their limit - pushing them to think harder and deeper. These days, I am very proud and happy that many of them are successful and famous, serving as department chairs, directors of institutes and leaders of professional societies as well as owners/CEOs of companies and law firms.

Here are a few addition items of "my philosophy" that I try to live by and regularly share with my students.

- Be uncompromising when it comes to the quality of work and the accuracy of data. There is no substitute for earning a good reputation such that all readers and competitors would always trust and respect your work and publications.
- Be very generous in giving time and sharing knowledge, and take pride and joy in helping colleagues and friends. Realize how lucky you are to be on the giving end. In the long run, you will reap much larger rewards.
- Be thoughtful by giving credit where it is due - to collaborators when giving talks or writing papers and especially when receiving awards and honors. It is the team that helped you get there and therefore, it should not be all about you.
- Be kind and courteous to everybody and good things will happen! Writing a brief note of congratulations, smiling while greeting others, opening doors for people, letting people out of the elevator first, and so on are all very small and easy things to do. But, when done habitually, the sum is huge! As a result, many will say and even do nice things for you in return – especially while you are not present or least expect it. They will genuinely appreciate your kindness and courtesy.
- Be sure to have only the best interest in mind for the person who seeks advice from you before dispensing any. Whatever you say should be beneficial to that person, even if your advice might be contradictory to helping you or your friends.
- Be respectful to people when talking with them. It starts with you giving them your full attention. Don't let your eyes wander around the room – like you are searching for someone more important.

A final point - whenever possible, chart a course for your life with a number of milestones for success that will result in going upward on a positive slope – similar to the nonlinear, concave upward, stress-strain curves for ligaments, tendons and articular cartilage. This is much more desirable than large fluctuations that could be joyous on the way up but miserable on the way down. The current housing crisis is a good reminder.

I hope for my students to practice the philosophy they have heard daily. I most wish that when they reach a fork on the road during their life's journey, they will have the wisdom to choose the right path.

7. Special Acknowledgement and Appreciation

Academia has showered me with many blessings! What a privilege it has been to teach and be inspired and challenged by such a large number of students, residents and post-doctoral fellows (see Appendix A). What an honor it has been to interact with so many inspiring colleagues and friends from all over the world. What a thrill it has been to meet royalties, dignitaries and professional sports superstars and Olympic gold medalists. What a surprise it has been to receive so many accolades, honors and awards for doing something that I love. For all this to happen, credit must be given to all of you who have kindly nominated, voted and facilitated for me. My simple words cannot come close to express my deep appreciation and affection. You all have shaped me to become who I am and I need to thank each and every one of you from the bottom of my heart. I trust that you will forgive me for not naming names – for sure, I will inadvertently forget a few. But, I know that you know who you are.

Still, there are three of my longstanding associates who need to be specially recognized for their immeasurable contributions to our success and my academic career. More importantly, they have helped me to make my academic life so much easier. The

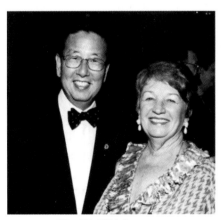

Fig. 27: With Lynnette

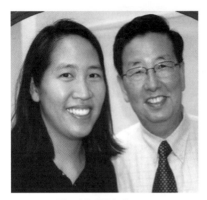

Fig. 28: With Serena

first person is Ms. Lynnette Fleck, who was my secretary for 18 out of my 20 years at UCSD (Fig. 27). She is a mother of five and also was the adopted mother of the laboratory. She is always calm and efficient, and metaphorically speaking, she is like a professional basketball player, - she could make the tough shots look smooth and easy. Lynnette played a crucial role in my early career and I am eternally thankful to her. She could not follow me to Pittsburgh on account of her family and it was extremely hard to leave her behind when we moved.

The second person is Mrs. Serena Saw (Fig. 28). Serena began as a graduate student of mine in 1993. After receiving her Masters degree, she stayed on as a staff member, helping me to run the MSRC. She is highly intelligent, efficient as well as extremely organized. Even with three children, I can always count on Serena to help me with a number of my duties. With her professional help, I know that all my assignments will be done promptly and professionally. If you liked my slides back then and appreciate my PowerPoint presentations now, it is to Serena's credit. She continues to work with us on a number of important projects even after she moved to New Jersey, and then on to North Carolina more than seven years ago.

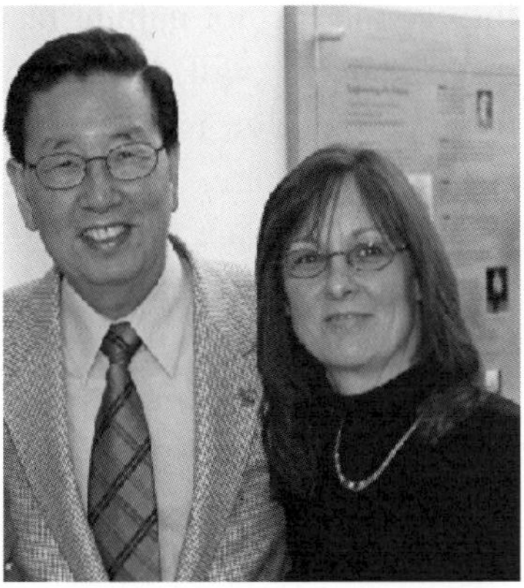

The third person is Mrs. Diann DeCenzo (Figs. 29 & 30). Diann has been working with me for nearly 21 years – first as the financial analyst for the MSRC and then as my executive assistant. She is my longest associate and as she now has broken Lynnette's longevity record, no one will ever break hers. Diann has the perfect temperament to do a great job to carry the MSRC forward through thick and

Fig. 29: With Diann (2008)

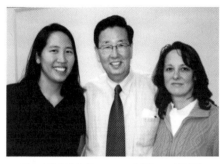

Fig. 30: With Serena and Diann (2005)

thin. No one in my professional life is more devoted to my well being, in addition to taking care of my administrative responsibilities. She is one sweet lady and is kind to everyone – especially to my students and foreign research fellows. To this day, Diann continues to work very hard in helping me to complete many tasks that I cannot (but should) say "no" to. She is so special that Pattie and I truly consider her a member of our family!

8. Back to the Future

During all the marvelous gatherings for my 70th birthday, many people asked me what I plan to be doing in the upcoming years. Such questions have led me to pause and reflect. So, here they are – although at 70, I am allowed to change my mind at any time.

For the immediate future, I want to continue what I have been doing at the University of Pittsburgh with the exception that I need to narrow my objectives somewhat - in order to free up time for new initiatives. One such initiative would be to help advance the skills of young surgeons and bioengineers from China. I have been asked by the Chinese Orthopaedic Association to chair a "blue ribbon" panel to evaluate worthy candidates for additional training by matching them with upstanding laboratories and clinics from all around the world. Another initiative would be to recruit a number of my good friends and former fellows to travel to China and teach surgical skills on a volunteer basis. There are a number of my colleagues who have similar interests and desires and we have already begun to work on setting the plan in motion.

Meanwhile, I want to spend as much time as possible to be with my own ever-growing family (Fig. 31). Pattie and I would love the opportunity to partner with Jonathan on his career advancement in business. We continue to find every possible opportunity to visit Kirstin and Jonathan – and most importantly, to hover over our two darling little

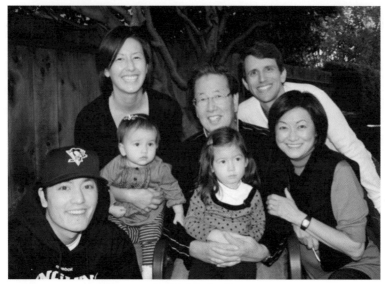

Fig. 31: My family

granddaughters. In 2006, Kirstin married Adam (Dr. Frymoyer). She met this bright young man during her first year of medical school and they have loved each other ever since. Adam comes from a family with great values and thanks to Holly and Bob, we now have a fine son-in-law. He has been working on his career as a clinical scientist – which is admirable. His expertise on conducting trials in pediatric pharmacology will undoubtedly help many children in the future. With all these loved ones living in the San Francisco area, Pattie and I are left wondering why we are still living in Pittsburgh.

In recent years, we have begun to do things together with my siblings and their families more regularly (Fig. 32). And in a couple of years, we will all become septuagenarians and some as octogenarians. So, we all want to make up for lost time and plan more trips and visits together.

Also, I want to find ways to meet with as many of my former students as frequently as possible – both in Pittsburgh and elsewhere. The legacy of a professor is really represented by his/her students. So, the yardstick to measure the success of a professor should be based on how well they are doing. For me, I am of the opinion that the more important yardstick would be whether one's students wish to return and visit with him/her or are happy to get together wherever and whenever possible.

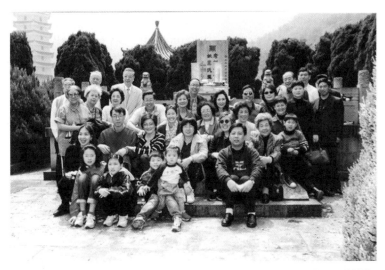

Fig. 32: Together with my siblings and their spouses, nieces, nephews (2003)

My granddaughters Zadie and Arden have brought me endless joy and have significantly changed my priorities! They are so cute and Pattie and I just love them (what an understatement)! We have found it necessary to travel to San Francisco to be with them almost every month. We truly appreciate the opportunity to witness how quickly both Z and A are able to learn new things (Fig. 33). We are privileged to be so involved in their lives as their Gung Gung and Po Po. Little Z, at age 3 not only tells me what to do and where to sit but also toys with my emotions as she flips between "I don't love you" to "I love you *this much*" (spreading her arms wide). I am especially touched that on our last visit, when I returned to Pittsburgh before Pattie, she asked Po Po whether her Gung Gung would be a little bit sad, knowing I would be alone! Arden Pattie, at 15 months knows what she wants and is persistent in getting it. This week, she has just learned to be coy with us.

With Z and A, I literally feel that my life has become so much more beautiful. It is no wonder that I possess the need to spend every possible moment with them - today, tomorrow and the next day, month, year and years after that! As much as I do savor what happens to them at present, I can envision how fun it will be to take them to kindergarten and (will surely) be so very emotional attending our first Grandparents' Day at their schools. I do look forward to be part of their lives and witness all the wonderful happenings with great anticipation – even though I know that before long, Z and A (like their mommy), will lovingly and subtly ask me to kiss them goodbye a couple of hundred meters before we are in the sights of their little friends and classmates!

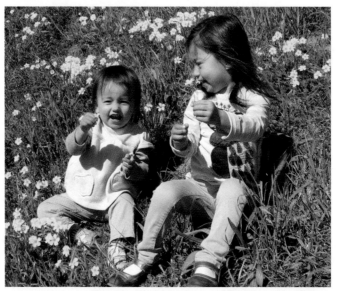

Fig. 33a: Arden and Zadie (2012)

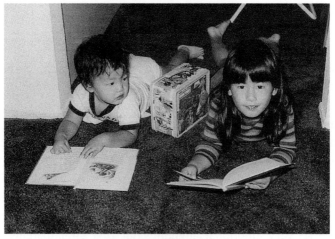

Fig. 33b: Jonathan and Kirstin (1980)

Chapter 7

Journey Down Memory Lane

Contributed by Pattie Woo

7.1. Childhood in Hong Kong

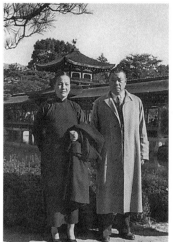

Woo parents in Kyoto (1952)

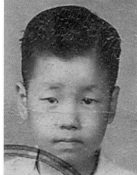

Moving to Hong Kong at age 9

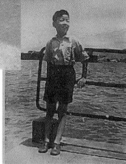

Little new immigrant

Teenage years

Graduating from high school

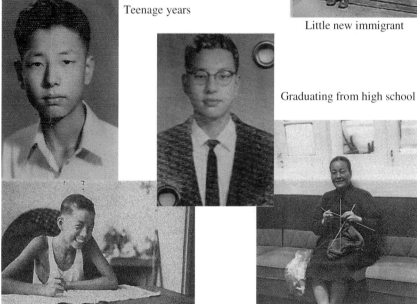

So HAPPY at homework time

Mama Woo's favorite pastime

7.2. Chico State and University of Washington

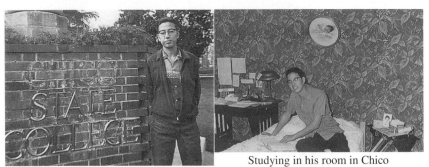

Arriving at Chico State College (1961)

Studying in his room in Chico

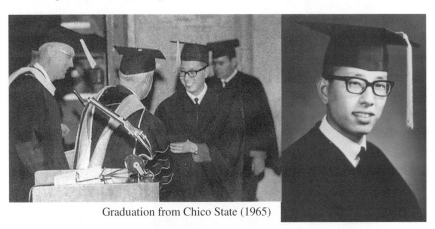

Graduation from Chico State (1965)

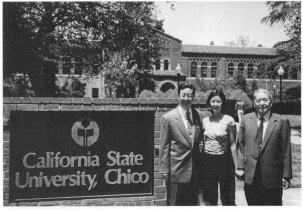

Back to Chico to receive an honorary degree 34 years later

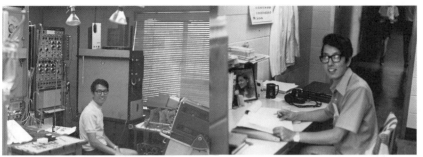

Doing experiments at the Bishop Eye Center

Promoted with Bruce Simon to a shared office for senior graduate students

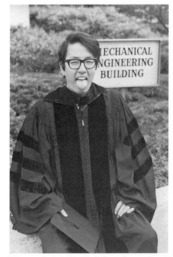

We made it! Graduation from the University of Washington with Bruce Simon

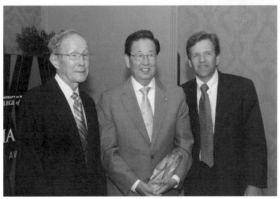

Receiving the Diamond Award from the University of Washington (2008)

7.3. Starting Our Own Family

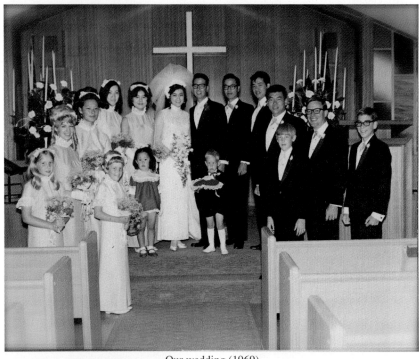

Our wedding (1969)

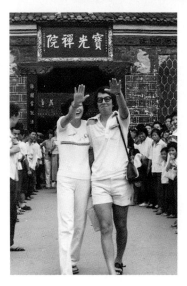

10th anniversary, first trip to China, reaching for blessings for the family

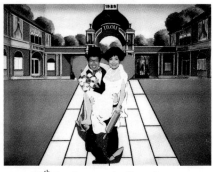

20th Anniversary in Copenhagen

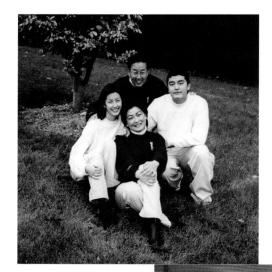

30th Anniversary

40th Anniversary

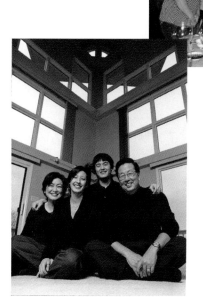

Family picture for Savio's 60th birthday

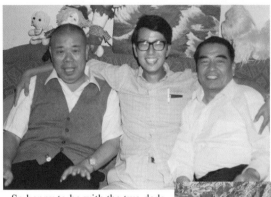

So happy to be with the two dads

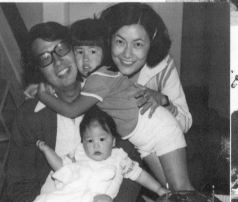

We were three

Then we were four

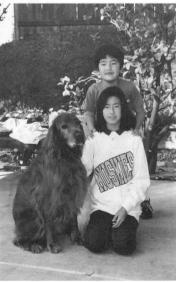

Our faithful companion for 13+ years, "Ferrous Oxide"

Father & son play

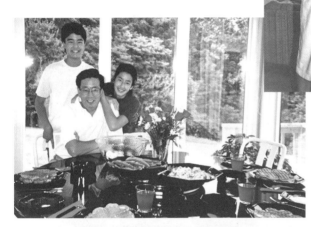

Special Breakfast
prepared by the kids
for our anniversary

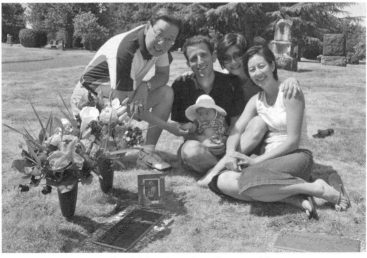

Zadie visiting Aunt Angel's graveside

7.4. Siblings

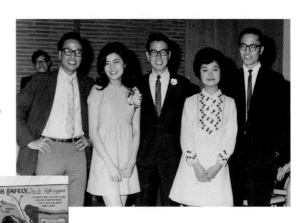

With brothers at our engagement party (1969)

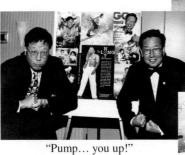

Crabbing on Oregon coast (1969)

NAE with family (1994)

"Pump… you up!"

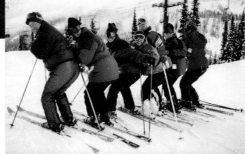

That certain special "Woo genes"

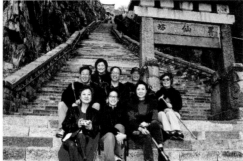

Climbing Mt. Tai together

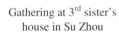

Gathering at 3rd sister's house in Su Zhou

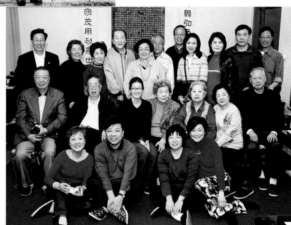

Family support at HKPU

On the road again - Silk Road fun

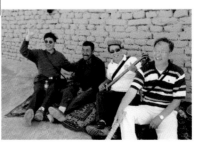

7.5. Fun and Travels

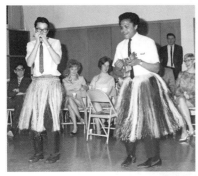

Duet with Caleb Otto in grass skirts

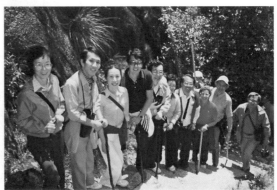

Climbing the Yellow Mountain

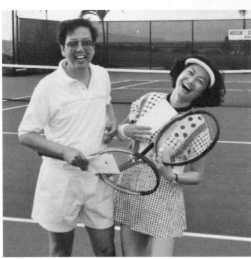

1st (and last) mixed doubles tennis championship

Journey Down Memory Lane

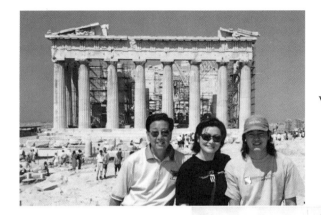

Visiting Acropolis with Jonathan

Yachting and sailing in Greece

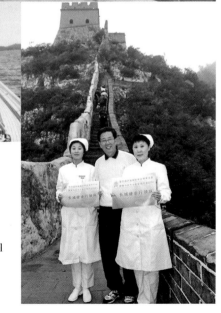

On the Great Wall

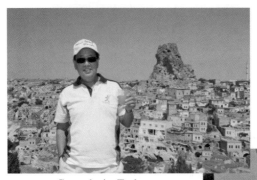

Cappadocia, Turkey

Giant mushroom, Florence

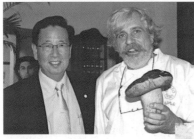

Breakfast fit for a king at a castle hotel in Cappadocia

Cruising Cinque Terre, Italy

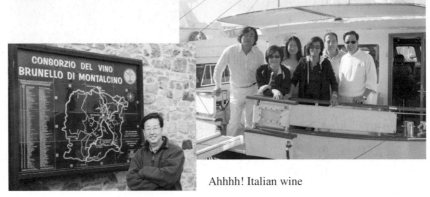

Ahhhh! Italian wine

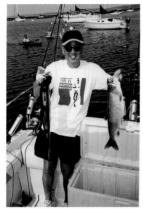
Quite a fisherman on
Lake Michigan

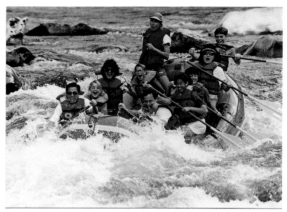
White water rafting with the Buckwalters

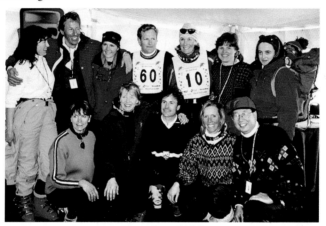
Olympians (1998)

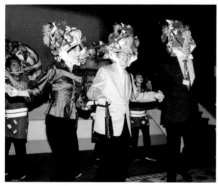
Hirosaki Dance, Japan

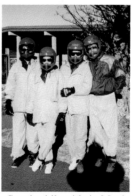
Sunrise bike ride in Maui

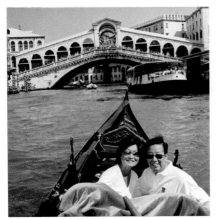

Anniversary in Venice

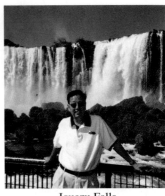

Iguazu Falls

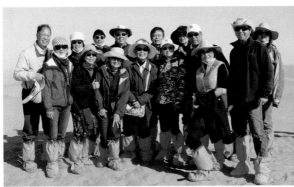

Silk Road tour

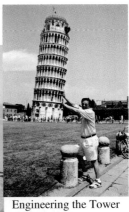

Engineering the Tower of Pisa

Temple of Heaven

Familiar early morning silhouette during travels

7.6. Sharing Good Times With Great Company

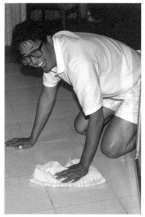

Clean up after parties

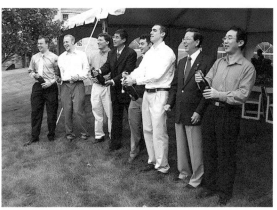

Popping the champagne for Kirstin & Adam

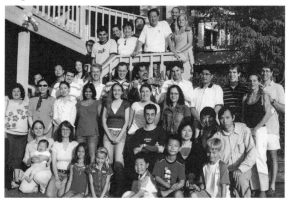

Summer parties

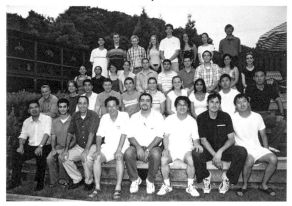

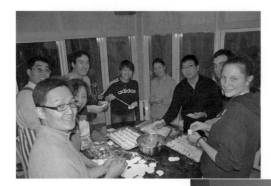

Dumpling party

Heritage dinner

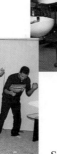

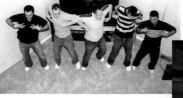

Students doing the chicken dance

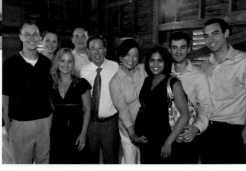

At the birthday party in Nemacolin

Journey Down Memory Lane

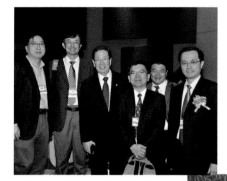

Taiwan fellows

European fellows in Oslo Nobel Prize hall

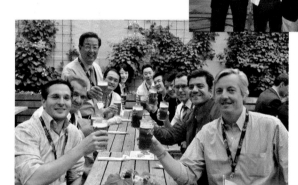

With fellows in Oslo

Hirosaki fellows and families

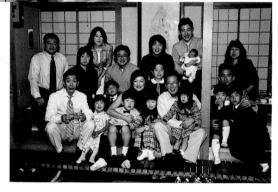

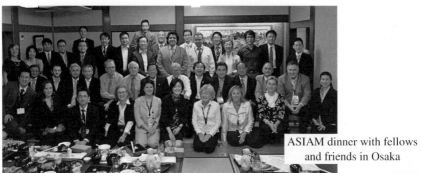

ASIAM dinner with fellows and friends in Osaka

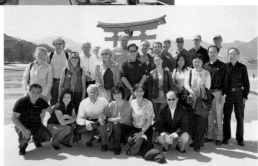

Day trip to Miyajima from Hiroshima

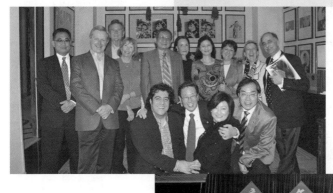

ASIAM board dinner in Las Vegas

ISL&T – XII banquet

Journey Down Memory Lane

With very special friends after receiving the Lissner medal (1991)

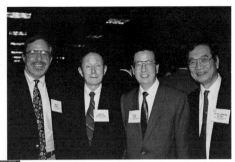

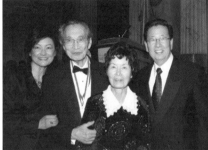

With the Fungs

At the Diamond Award with the Kobayashis

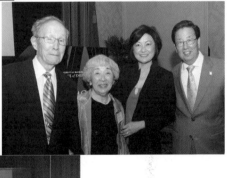

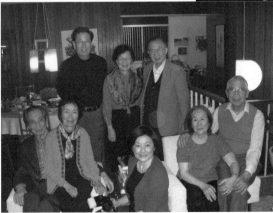

Our dear, dear friends in La Jolla: the Chiens, Fungs and Lins

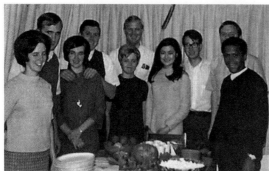

Gathering of our own fraternity (1968)

Friends from afar traveled to celebrate Kirstin's wedding with us (2006)

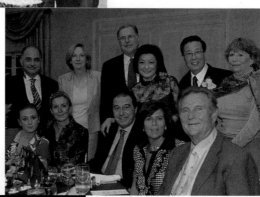

The Three Amigos

Touring Himeiji Castle near Kobe with friends (2009)

Annual meeting with our ski buddies in Vail

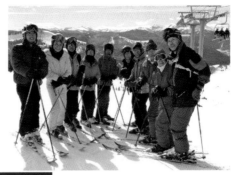

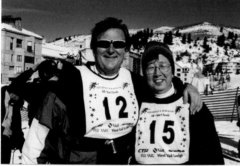

On Richard's team

Steadman Foundation ski classic, with Olympian Chad Fleischer

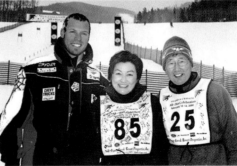

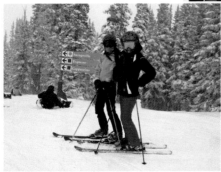

Skiing with sweet Audrey every year since 2008

7.7. Amazing Experience at the 1998 Nagano Winter Olympics

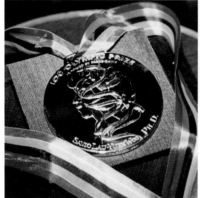

The Olympic Gold Medal for Sports Science (1998)

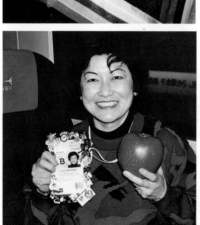

Receiving the medal from President Juan Antonio Samaranch and Prince Alexandre De Merode

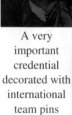

A very important credential decorated with international team pins

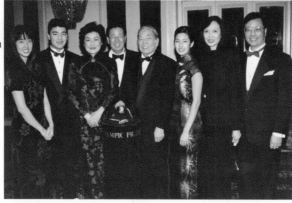

At the Olympic Prize celebration with family (Waldorf Astoria Hotel, NYC)

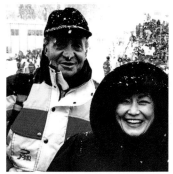
King Juan Carlos of Spain

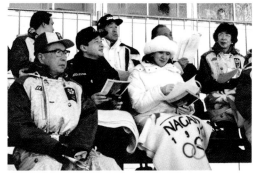
Crown Prince Naruhito & Princess Masako

Prince Albert of Monaco
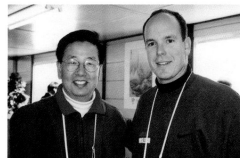

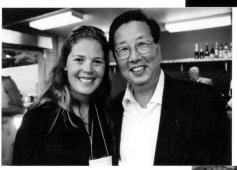
With Picabo Street - two gold medalists in Nagano Olympics

Guests of Juan Antonio Samaranch to visit the Olympic Museum
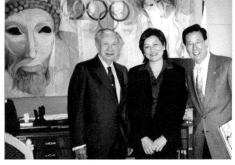

7.8. Encore Experience at the 2008 Beijing Summer Olympics – 10 Years Later

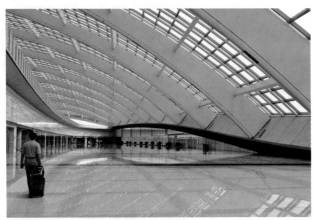

Beijing Airport

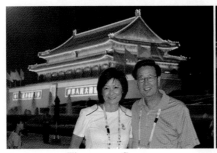

Tiananmen Square

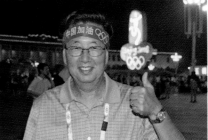

Let's go China!

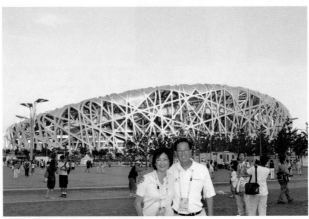

The Bird's Nest

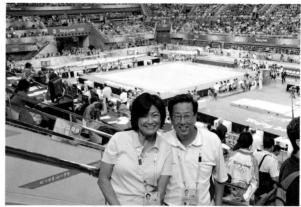
Gymnastics venue

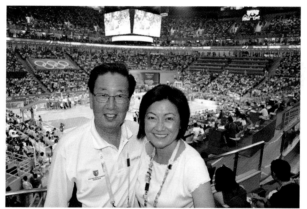
Basketball venue

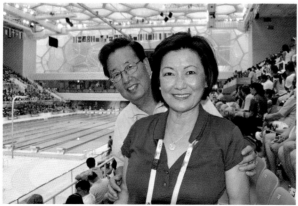
Swimming venue

7.9. Some Memorable Events

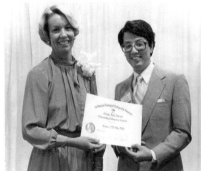

Elizabeth Lanier Kappa Delta Award at ORS/AAOS (1983)

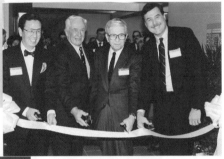

Opening of the MSRC (1990)

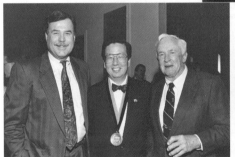

Endowed Chair Professorship with Drs. Herndon and Ferguson (1994)

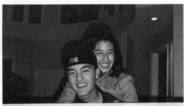

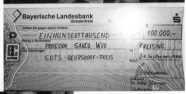

Inaugural GOTS award (1996)

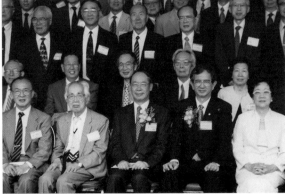

Academia Sinica (1998)

Distinguished Faculty with Drs. Mark Nordenberg and Jim Maher (1999)

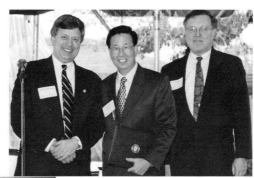

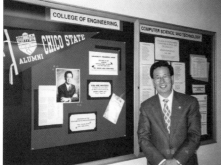

Distinguished Alumni at CSU, Chico, College of Engineering (2000)

Carnegie Centenary Professorship, Scotland (2002)

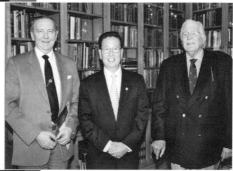

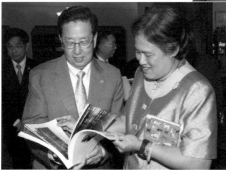

Guest of Princess Sirindhom of Thailand at her palace – The Princess presented her own photo book as a gift (2007)

7.10. Expanding Family – Pure Love and Joy

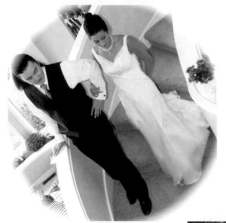

Jonathan presenting Kirstin to dad (2006)

It's time

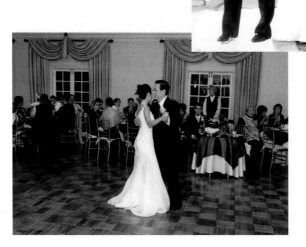

Father/Daughter dance

Journey Down Memory Lane

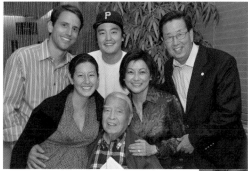

Zadie's on the way

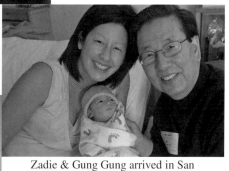

Zadie & Gung Gung arrived in San Francisco at the exact same time - NOON

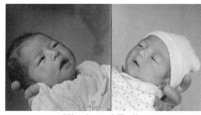

Kirstin and Zadie

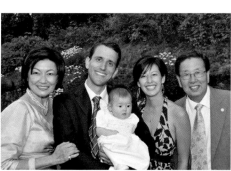

Presenting Zadie to family and friends in Seattle at 6 months

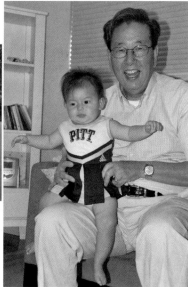

Future PITT cheerleader – Zadie at 10 months

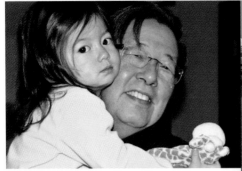
I love my Gung Gung

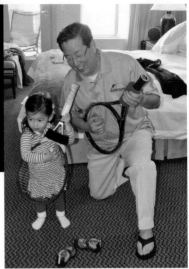
Let's do a duet

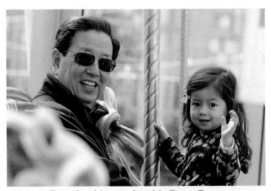
Favorite thing to do with Gung Gung

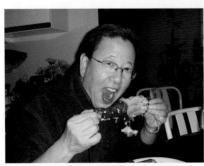
Gung Gung loves the drumstick

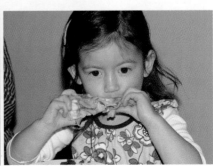
So does Zadie

Journey Down Memory Lane 467

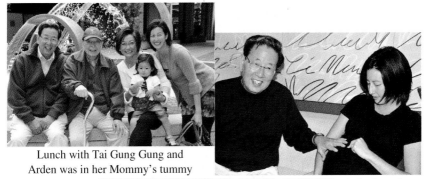

Lunch with Tai Gung Gung and
Arden was in her Mommy's tummy

Arden's saying
"HI" to
Gung Gung

Mother's Day

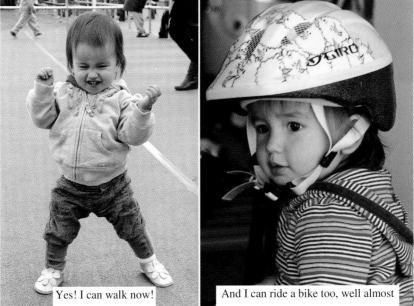

Yes! I can walk now!

And I can ride a bike too, well almost

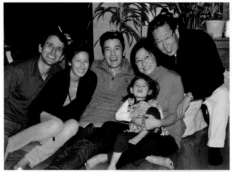

All together at Thanksgiving

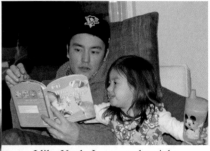

I like Uncle Jon to read tonight

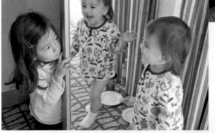

BOO! I got you Arden

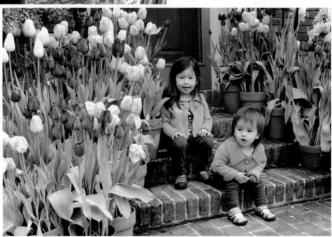

We are waiting for you Gung Gung

7.11. All Those Milestone Birthdays

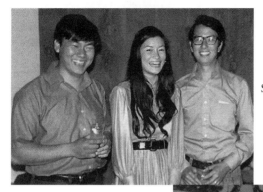

Surprise 30th birthday party, Vang's first visit to San Diego (1971)

40th birthday with Pattie's parents and the Seguchis in Kobe, Japan

Cure for midlife crisis? (1982)

50th birthday celebrated together with Ivan turning 3, in San Diego

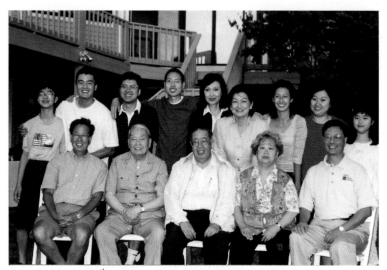

60th birthday celebration in Pittsburgh (2001)

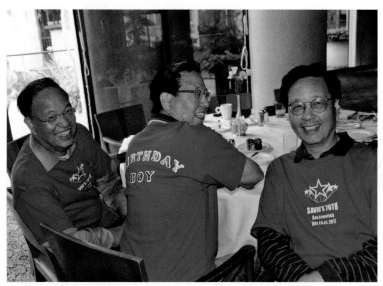

The birthday boy is turning 70, in San Francisco (2011)

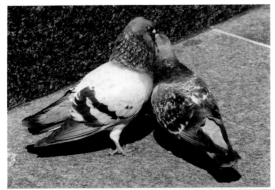

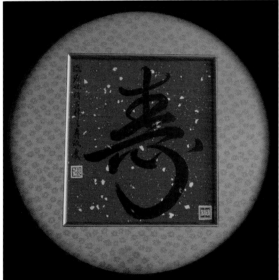

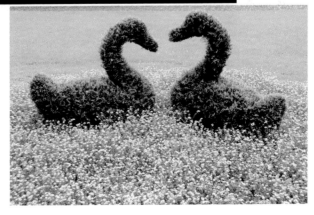

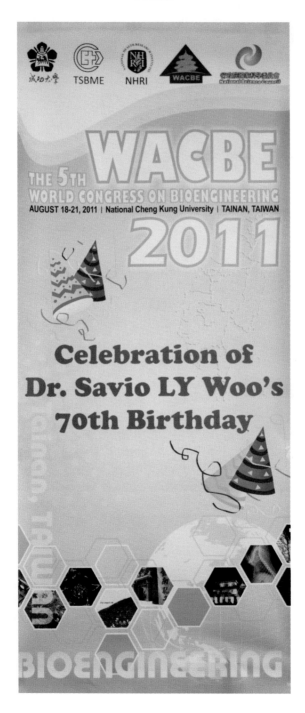

Appendix

Members of Dr. Woo's Team

at the

Orthopaedic Bioengineering Laboratory
University of California, San Diego
and
Musculoskeletal Research Center
University of Pittsburgh

University of California at San Diego (1970-1990)

Staff

Gil Jemmott	1972-1974
Lynnette Fleck	1973-1990
Chris Lawler	1975-1977
Mary Gonsalves	1975-1981
Mark Gomez	1977-1980
Wes Dillon	1978-1979
Norman Cobb	1978-1980
Kim Lothringer	1980-1983
Loren Van Hoy	1983-1984
Douglas Walker	1985-1986
Linda Kitabayashi	1985-1990
Karen Ohland	1986-1990
Doug Adams	1988-1990

Post-Doctoral Fellows

Young Kyun Woo, M.D.	1979-1981
Cyril Frank, M.D.	1981-1984
Steve Kuei, Ph.D.	1979-1981
Masahiro Inoue, M.D.	1985-1987
Hung Chang Lin, M.D.	1986-1987
Mark A. Gomez, Ph.D.	1986-1988
Shuji Horibe, M.D.	1987-1989
Shinro Takai, M.D.	1989-1990
Michael K. Kwan, Ph.D.	1987-1990
Nam-Yong Choi, M.D.	1990
Hiromichi Fujie, Ph.D.	1990
Masahiko Noguchi, M.D.	1990

Residents

John V. Matthews, M.D.	1972-1974
Ladd Rutherford, M.D.	1974-1975
David Doty, M.D.	1975-1976
Jess Boyer, M.D.	1976-1977
Donald A. Schmidt, M.D.	1977-1978
Steve R. Garfin, M.D.	1978-1979
Carol C. Frey, M.D.	1981-1982
Jon Fronek, M.D.	1982-1983
Jon F. Camp, M.D.	1983-1984
Dolois J. Bean, M.D.	1984-1986
Mark Abel, M.D.	1984-1985
Richard Roux, M.D.	1984-1985
Robert T. Ballock, M.D.	1985-1986
Terry J. Sites, M.D.	1985-1986
Roger M. Lyon, M.D.	1986-1988
Kevin J. Triggs, M.D.	1986-1987
Carlos J. Lavernia, M.D.	1986-1988
Peter O. Newton, M.D.	1988-1989
Edmond Young, M.D.	1988-1989
Eric J. Wall, M.D.	1988-1989
David R. Anderson, M.D.	1989-1990
Gregory D. Carlson, M.D.	1989-1990
Scott Kuiper, M.D.	1989-1990

Graduate Students

Larry L. Malcolm, Ph.D.	1971-1973
Neil G. Solomon, M.S.	1976-1978
Patrick Shoemaker, M.S.	1976-1978
Mark A. Gomez, Ph.D.	1980-1982
Grace Chuong Liao	1983-1985
Russell Mazelsky, M.S.	1983-1985
David Hawkins, M.S.	1983-1985
Erin McGurk-Burleson, M.S.	1983-1986

Joseph M. Hollis, Ph.D.	1983-1988
Robert Peterson, M.S.	1984-1986
Thay Q. Lee, M.S.	1984-1986
Jeff M. Spiegelman, M.S.	1984-1986
Edward Lee	1984-1986
Fred P. Field, M.S.	1985-1988
Jennifer S. Wayne, Ph.D.	1985-1990
Jeff Weiss, Ph.D.	1989-1990
Caroline Wei Hwa Wang, M.S.	1987-1988
Michael Danto, M.D.	1988-1990
Robert A. Hart, M.D.	1989-1990
Glen Livesay, Ph.D.	1989-1990

Undergraduate Students

Chris Farenbach, B.S.	1971-1973
Gil Jemmot, B.S.	1971-1973
Giullermina Velex, B.S.	1973-1974
Mark Van Veen, B.S.	1974-1975
Robert Mesdes Da Costa, B.S.	1975-1976
Debbie Yager, B.S.	1975-1976
Paul Lubock, M.S.	1975-1977
Joanna Schoon, M.S.	1976-1977
Mark Ritter, B.S.	1978-1980
Peter J. Pardee, B.S.	1978-1979
Jack M. Winters, Ph.D.	1978-1980
Christine Watt	1979-1980
Cheryl Endo, B.S.	1980-1981
Alan Vernac, M.D.	1980-1981
Eric Yum, B.S.	1980-1981
James St. Ville	1981-1983
Carlo Orlando, M.D.	1982-1984
Steve Y.C. To, B.S.	1984-1986
Frank W. Silva, B.S.	1984-1985
Kim Burton, B.S.	1984-1988
Richard Peindl, B.S.	1985-1986

Jim Marcin, M.D.	1986-1987
Alan Balfour, B.S.	1986-1987
Jeff Weiss, Ph.D.	1987-1989
Scott Harris, B.S.	1987-1989
David Tung, B.S.	1987-1990
Karen D. May, Ph.D.	1988-1989
Scott A. Hacker, M.D.	1988-1990
Deidre A. Mackenna, Ph.D.	1988-1990
Meena Joshi, M.S.	1989-1990
Mark Rasmussen	1989-1990
Hector Pacheo	1989-1990
Meredith Josephs	1989-1990

University of Pittsburgh (1990-Present)

Staff

Karen Ohland	1990-1993
Bonnie Zwarich	1990-1994
Cheri McCloskey	1990-1992
Diann DeCenzo	1991-Present
Dawn Tramaglini	1992-1995
Helene Marion	1992-1995
Polly Ionatti	1992
Nadine Reck	1992
Rich Sofranko	1992-1993
Ted Rudy	1992-2001
Barb Hepler	1992-1993
Colleen Weaver-Green	1993-1995
Jackie Barbour	1994
Greg Carlin	1994-1997
Vera Kornfeld	1994-2003
Sandra Antonucci	1994
Krista Lilly	1994-1995
Serena Chan Saw	1995-2005

Terri Moorcroft   1995-1996
Dave Smith   1995-1997
Nancy Mundy   1995-1997
Chari Clark   1996-1997
Chris Phillips   1997-2000
Debbie Peterson   1998
Becky Engel   1998
Tracy Vogrin   1998-1999
Colleen O'Hara   1998-2003
Mary Lou Clowes   1999
Andrea Cogley   1999-2000
Danyel Tarinelli   1999-2001
Brooke Spencer   2000-2001
Andy Van Scyoc   2000-2004
Mary Gabriel   2001-2004
Tony Montanaro   2001-2003
Jane Peart   2001-2004
Maribeth Thomas   2002-2004
Diane Budzik   2002-2003
Fengyan Jia   2002-2005
Ragan Brinkley   2004-2005
Joanne Barto   2005-2006
Guoguang Yang   2005-2010
Anna Goldman   2007-2008

Post-Doctoral Fellows

Hiromichi Fujie, Ph.D.   1990-1992
Masahiko Noguchi, M.D.   1990-1992
Nam-Yong Choi, M.D.   1991-1992
Greg Johnson, Ph.D.   1991-1994
Min Kocher, M.D.   1991-1992
Gail Blomstrom, Ph.D.   1991-1993
Donal McCarthy, M.D.   1991-1993
Shinji Kashiwaguchi, M.D.   1991-1993
Kuo-pin (Joseph) Kuo, M.D.   1992-1993

Kazunori Ohno, M.D.	1992-1994
Shuhei Morifusa, M.D.	1992-1994
Harutaka Aizawa, M.D.	1992-1994
Takeshi Kusayama, M.D.	1992-1993
Christian Jantea, M.D.	1993
Daniel Baker, Ph.D.	1993-1994
Yoshitsugu Takeda, M.D.	1993-1994
Emin Taskiran, M.D.	1993-1994
Tomoo Yamaji, M.D.	1993-1995
Kyoung Soo Kim, M.D.	1993-1994
Yasuyuki Ishibashi, M.D.	1993-1995
Stefano Zaffagnini, M.D.	1993-1994
Takeshi Marui, M.D.	1993-1996
Jiang-ming Xu, M.D.	1993-1997
Rupinder Grewal, M.D.	1994-1996
Andreas Imhoff, M.D.	1994-1995
Panayotis Giannakopoulos, M.D.	1994-1995
Ryoma Saito, M.D.	1994-1996
Mehmet Demirhan, M.D.	1994-1995
Riccardo Marinelli, M.D.	1994-1995
Kwong-Won Lee, M.D.	1994-1995
Masataka Sakane, M.D.	1995-1997
Goo-Hyun Baek, M.D.	1995-1996
Chih-Hwa Chen, M.D.	1995-1996
Gregoris Mitsionis, M.D.	1995-1996
Kevin Hildebrand, M.D.	1995-1997
Anton Plakseychuk, M.D.	1995-1997
Jaime Bastidas, M.D.	1995-1996
Masataka Deie, M.D.	1995-1997
Juergen Hoeher, M.D.	1996-1997
Asbjorn Aroen, M.D.	1996-1997
Kotaro Nishida, M.D.	1996-1999
Ko Adachi, M.D.	1997
Franklin Sechriest, M.D.	1997-1998
Jyh-Horng Wang, M.D.	1997-1998
Ioannis Gelalis, M.D.	1997-1998

Christos Papageorgiou, M.D.	1997-1999
Sven Scheffler, M.D.	1997-1998
Sokratis Varitimidis, M.D.	1997-1999
Nobuyoshi Watanabe, M.D.	1997-1999
Akihiro Kanamori, M.D.	1997-2000
Masayoshi Yagi, M.D.	1998-2000
Gustavo Azcona-Arteaga, M.D.	1999-2000
Yukihisa Fukuda, M.D.	1999-2001
Eiichi Tsuda, M.D.	1999-2001
Fengyan Jia, M.D.	1999-2002
Andreas Burkart, M.D.	2000
Stefano Brue, M.D.	2000
Akin Uzumcugil, M.D.	2000
Robert Giffin, M.D.	2000-2001
Volker Musahl, M.D.	2000-2002
Yasuhiko Watanabe, M.D.	2000-2001
Takatoshi Shimomura, M.D.	2000-2002
Rajesh Jari, M.D.	2001-2002
Yuhua Song, Ph.D.	2001-2002
Tomoyuki Sasaki, M.D.	2001-2002
Yoshiyuki Takakura, M.D., Ph.D.	2002-2004
Yuji Yamamoto, M.D., Ph.D.	2002-2004
Xinguo Ning, Ph.D.	2003-2004
Wei-Hsiu Hsu, M.D.	2003-2004
Robert Kilger, M.D.	2003-2004
Rui Liang, M.D.	2003-2010
Kazutomo Miura, M.D., Ph.D.	2004-2005
Tan Nguyen, M.D.	2004-2007
Yin-Chih Fu, M.D.	2004-2005
Ozgur Dede, M.D.	2005-2007
Fabio Vercillo, M.D.	2005-2006
Sinan Karaoglu, M.D.	2005-2006
Ping-Cheng Liu, M.D.	2005-2006
Alejandro Almarza, Ph.D.	2005-2008
Changfu Wu, Ph.D.	2006-2007
Chin-Yi Chou, M.D.	2006-2007

Giovanni Zamarra, M.D.	2007-2008
Xianna Guo, M.D.	2007
Muqing Liu, M.D.	2008
Ho-Joong Jung, M.D.	2008-2009
Shan-Ling Hsu, M.D.	2008-2009
Huinan Liu, Ph.D.	2009-2010
Matteo Tei, M.D.	2010-2011
Matthew Fisher, Ph.D.	2010
Andrea Speziali, M.D.	2011-Present
Norihiro Sasaki, M.D.	2012-Present

Residents

Gary Anderson, M.D.	1990-1991
Richard Berger, M.D.	1990-1991
Anthony DiGioia, M.D.	1990-1991
J. Scott Doyle, M.D.	1990-1991
Carolyn "Sis" Engle, M.D.	1991-1992
Jim Jamison, M.D.	1991-1992
Les Schwendeman, M.D.	1991-1992
Pat McMahon, M.D.	1991-1992
Chris Schmidt, M.D.	1992-1993
Bill Thompson, M.D.	1992-1993
Brian Smith, M.D.	1992-1993
Jim Dowd, M.D.	1992-1993
Mike Pappas, M.D.	1992-1993
Bill MacCauley, M.D.	1993-1994
John Xerogeanes, M.D.	1993-1994
Doug Boardman, M.D.	1993-1994
Steve Scherping, M.D.	1993-1994
Jeff Stone, M.D.	1994-1995
Prakash Patel, M.D.	1994-1995
Carl Hasselman, M.D.	1995-1996
Ross Fox, M.D.	1995-1996
Christy Allen, M.D.	1996-1997
Chuck Cha, M.D.	1996-1997

Benjamin Ma, M.D.	1997-1998
Moby Parsons, M.D.	1997-1998
Jim Fenwick, M.D.	1998-1999
Mark Knaub, M.D.	1998-1999
Ezequiel Cassinelli, M.D.	1999-2000
Ronald Hall, M.D.	1999-2000
Mi Lee, M.D.	1999-2000
John Loh, M.D.	2000-2001
Jamie Pfaeffle, M.D., Ph.D.	2001-2002
Peter Tang, M.D., MPH	2001-2002

Graduate Students

Glen Livesay, Ph.D.	1989-1996
Franz Shelley, M.S.	1990-1992
Rich Sofranko, M.S.	1990-1992
Rich Debski, Ph.D.	1991-1997
Todd Doehring, Ph.D.	1991-2000
Amy Pomaybo, M.S.	1992-1994
Becky Levine, Ph.D.	1992-1996
Meena Joshi, M.S.	1992-1994
Greg Carlin, M.S.	1992-1994
Serena Chan Saw, M.S.	1993-1995
Rafi Neiman, M.D.	1993
Jamie Pfaeffle, M.D., Ph.D.	1993-1996
Greg Przybylski, M.D.	1993-1994
Brian Taylor, M.S.	1994-1995
Dan Latt, M.D., Ph.D.	1994-1995
Tom Runco, M.S.	1994-1996
J.P. Romano, M.S.	1995
Terry Koo, B.S.	1995
Chuck Kovach, M.S.	1995-1998
Venkatesh Balasubramianian, Ph.D.	1995-1998
Maria Apreleva, Ph.D.	1995-1999
Ted Clineff, M.S.	1996-1998
Ted Manson, M.S.	1996-1998

Jason Lessard, B.S.	1997
Tracy Vogrin, M.D.	1997-1998
Ling Liu, M.S.	1997-1998
Marsie Janaushek, M.S.	1997-1999
Eric Wong, M.S.	1997-2000
Jennifer Zeminski, M.S.	1997-2001
John Withrow, M.S.	1998-1999
Jorge Gil, M.S.	1998-2001
Chris Celechovsky, M.D.	1998-2000
Steven Abramowitch, Ph.D.	1999-2004
Thomas Gilbert, Ph.D.	2000-2003
Jing Lei, Ph.D.	2000-2001
Shon Darcy, Ph.D.	2000-2003
Jesse Fisk, M.D.	2001-2004
Sarah Brown, B.S.	2002-2003
Scott Hanford, B.S.	2002-2003
Daniel Moon, M.D.	2002-2004
Li Zou, M.D., Ph.D.	2002-2004
Brooke Coley, Ph.D.	2003
Sarita Maheedhara, M.S.	2004-2006
Sabrina Noorani, M.S.	2004-2007
Richard Stoner, B.S.	2004-2005
Noah Papas, M.S.	2005-2007
Matthew Fisher, B.S.	2005-2010
Xiaoyan Zhang, Ph.D.	2005-2008
Lauren Hellmann, B.S.	2006
Serena Augustine, B.S.	2006-2008
David Torick, B.S.	2006
Oneximo Gonzalez, B.S.	2007-2008
Christopher Richardson, B.S.	2007-2008
Kwang Kim, B.S.	2008-Present
Ben Rothrauff, B.S.	2010
Kathryn Farraro, B.S.	2010-Present

Undergraduate Students

Wayne Bayer	1990-1991
Mark Schatz	1991
Steven Biancuilli	1991
Vince Spotts	1991
Victor Rozynblyum, B.S.	1991-1993
Mary Ann (Mimi) Battista, B.S.	1992
Mark Brositz, B.S.	1992
Serena Chan Saw, M.S.	1992
Eric Yun	1992
Ben Maher	1992-1993
Scott Hudson	1992-1993
Duane Morrow, M.S.	1992-1995
Greg Bijak, M.D.	1993
Jennifer Burgess	1993
Brian Holzer, B.S.	1993
Brian Anderson, B.S.	1993
Keith Lobel, B.S.	1993
Dan Beatty, B.S.	1994
Chee-Hahn Hung, B.S.	1994
Anat Galor	1994
John Pacella, B.S.	1995
John Herndon	1995
Sharon Bansal	1995
Eric Wong	1995-1996
Jorge Gil	1995-1998
Jonathon Bishop, B.S.	1996
Steve Yang	1996
Walter Chang	1996
Amy Kastner, B.S.	1996
Brian Kilpela, B.S.	1996-1997
Amber Patterson	1997
Alexander Feng	1997
Lindsay Johnson	1997
Despina Hages	1997

Christine Fitzgerald	1997
Jon Woo	1997
Tim Nolan	1997
Marc Brozovich	1997-1998
Lance Brunton	1997-1998
Marshall Kuremsky	1997-1998
Rob Svitek	1997-1999
Damion Shelton	1997-2000
Umang Patel	1998
Tiffany Sellaro	1998
Kimberly Griger	1998
Jennifer Olewnik	1998-1999
Susan Ney	1998-1999
Jonathan Fischer	1999
Beth Kirkpatrick	1999-2000
Amaury Rolin	1999
Michael Williams	1999
Maura George	2000
Kristina Goodoff	2000
James Chung	2001
Katie Yoder	2001
Bradley Stokan	2001
Charles Vukotich	2001
Greg Frank	2001
Allison Westcott	2001
Christina Casella	2002
Casey Castner	2002
Kristen Moffat	2002
Mara Schenker	2002-2003
Kelly Baron	2003
Lily Jeng	2003
Kevin Suzuki	2003
Hillarie Stern	2003
Stephanie Bechtold	2003-2004
Mary Zettl	2003
Selina Brownridge	2004

Molly Curran	2004
Erik Frazier	2004-2005
Sylvia Kang	2004
Emily Sieg	2004
David Shin	2005
Shawn Burton	2005-2006
Dana Irrer	2005-2006
Amanda Roof	2005
Christopher Carruthers	2006
Noah Lorang	2006-2008
Emily Engel	2006
Tobias Long	2006
Caressa Watson	2006-2007
Sarah Henderson	2006
Mitchell Kosowski	2007
Danielle Dukes	2007
David Gladowski	2007
Ryan Prantil	2007
Kristin Frawley	2007
Rayna Nola	2007-2008
Collin Edington	2008
Alexandra Cirillo	2008
Kristen Klingler	2008
Megan Ferderber	2008
Thomas Chase	2008
Wendy Shung	2009
Austin Borisy	2009
Philip Manor	2009
Christine Hall	2009
Gautam Vangipuram	2009-2010
Fei Yan Lin	2009-2010
Daniel Perchy	2009-2010
Nicole Scarbrough	2010
Elizabeth Chen	2010
Nachshon Rothman	2010
Eran Goldberg	2010

Nadav Bramson	2011
Joseph Kromke	2011
Aimee Pickering	2011-Present
Hunter Eason	2011-Present
Jonquil Flowers	2011-Present
Jillian Cheng	2012
Wai-Ching Yu	2012
Bonnie Leung	2012

Author Index

Abramowitch, Steven 110
Akeson, Wayne 224
Alaseirlis, Dimosthenis 149
Almarza, Alejandro 114
Amiel, David 226
An, Kai-Nan 243
Andriacchi, Thomas 244
Apreleva-Scheffler, Maria 108
Arnoczky, Steven 247
Au, Sister Agnes 23
Azcona Arteaga, Gustavo Miguel ... 178

Banes, Albert 233
Banes, Elizabeth 233
Bartlett, John 258
Borovetz, Harvey 292
Brubaker, Cliff 203
Buckwalter, Jody 246
Buckwalter, Kitty 246
Budinger, Thomas 216
Burkhart, Steve 383
Butler, David 248

Canata, Gian Luigi 360
Caplan, Arnold 264
Carlin, Greg 143
Carruthers, Christopher 155
Cerulli, Giuliano 252
Chan, Helen 30
Chan, Irene 30
Chan, Kevin 30
Chan, K.M. 275
Chan, Nancy 30
Chang, H.K. 197
Chao, Ed 209
Chen, Chih-Hwa 79
Chen, Peter 228
Chen, Shiyi 333
Cheng, Richard Cheng-Kung 326
Cheong, Anna 24
Cheong, Antonio 15

Cheong, Eileen 26
Cheong, Paulo 24
Cheong, Vang 26
Chien, Shu 191
Chow, James 266
Cohen, Moises 378
Cugat, Ramon 287

Dai, Kerong 219
Debski, Richard 145
DeCenzo, Diann 83
DeFrate, Louis 136
Dieck, Ron 54
Doehring, Todd 100
Doral, Mahmut 260
Dye, Scott 286

Espregueira-Mendes, João 358

Farraro, Katie 157
Feagin, John 279
Feola, Andrew 161
Fischer, Ken 150
Fisher, Matthew 98
Flatow, Evan 384
Fleck, Lynnette 46
Fleming, Braden 350
Frank, Cy 37
Frymoyer, Bob 33
Frymoyer, Holly 33
Fu, Yin-Chih 96
Fujie, Hiromichi 67
Fukubayashi, Toru 379
Fukuda, Yukihisa 128
Fung, Luna 189
Fung, Y.C. 189

Gil, Jorge 85
Gilbert, Thomas 122
Goh, James 329
Goldstein, Steven 217

Gomez, Mark ... 39
Green, Jr., William ... 305
Guilak, Farshid ... 337
Guo, X. Edward ... 373
Guo, Xia ... 141

Handl, Milan ... 369
Hart, Robert ... 55
Hawkins, David ... 59
Herndon, James ... 300
Hildebrand, Kevin ... 147
Ho, Chien ... 314
Ho, Monto ... 312
Holder, Gerald ... 201
Hollis, J. Marcus ... 41
Horibe, Shuji ... 48
Hsu, Robert ... 348
Hsu, Wei-Hsiu ... 93
Hu, Wei-Shou ... 328
Hung, Chee-Hahn ... 183
Hung, Shunan Cho ... 242
Hung, Tin-Kan ... 242
Huylebroek, Jose ... 262

Ishibashi, Yasuyuki ... 163

Jari, Rajesh ... 181
Jia, Fengyan ... 170
Johnson, Robert ... 284
Jokl, Linda ... 289
Jokl, Peter ... 289
Jones, Barbara ... 223
Jones, Jeremy ... 223
Joshi, Meena ... 73

Kanamori, Akihiro ... 112
Kanamori, Jennifer (Zeminski) ... 112
Kang, James ... 309
Karaoglu, Sinan ... 132
Katona, Peter ... 268
Kibler, Ben ... 283
Kibler, Betty ... 283
Kim, Kwang ... 106
King, Albert ... 212
Kitabayashi, Linda ... 57

Kobayashi, Albert ... 193
Kobayashi, Betty ... 193
Kocher, Mininder ... 118
Kuo, Catherine ... 343
Kuo, Ken ... 380

Lai, James ... 31
Lai, Joshua ... 32
Lai, Michael ... 381
Lamontagne, Mario ... 273
Langrana, Noshir ... 377
Lee, Abraham "Abe" ... 322
Lee, Eva ... 236
Lee, Thay ... 44
Lee, Wen-Hwa ... 236
Leibowitz, Becky (Levine) ... 167
Leong, Kam ... 320
Leung, PC ... 382
Li, Guoan ... 120
Li, Tingye ... 220
Li, Zong-Ming ... 290
Liang, Rui ... 94
Liang, Zhi-Pei ... 318
Livesay, Glen ... 69
Loughlin, Patrick ... 302
Lovell, Michael ... 195
Lu, Helen ... 341
Lyon, Roger ... 62

Ma, C. Benjamin ... 153
Maffulli, Nicola ... 364
Maheedhara, Sarita ... 173
Maher, James ... 199
Mak, Arthur ... 331
Mann, Gideon ... 383
Mao, Jeremy ... 327
Maquirriain, Javier ... 339
McGurk, Erin ... 54
McMahon, Patrick ... 77
Miura, Kazutomo ... 130
Moffat, Kristen ... 104
Moon, Daniel ... 121
Morrow, Duane ... 87
Mueller, Werner ... 256

Author Index

Nakamura, Norimasa 362
Nerem, Robert 210
Nguyen, Duy Tan 89
Nigg, Benno 282
Noorani, Sabrina 114
Nordenberg, Mark vii

Ochi, Mitsuo 346
Ohland, Karen 65

Papageorgiou, Christos 81
Papas, Noah 139
Philippon, Marc 306
Pluim, Babette 367
Pope, Malcolm 249
Prantil, Ryan 91
Provenzano, David 184
Puddu, Giancarlo 288

Rainis, Carrie (Voycheck) 116
Redfern, Mark 301
Reider, Bruce 277
Renström, Per 253
Rodeo, Scott 366
Root, David 281
Rothrauff, Ben 175
Rubash, Harry 308
Russell, Alan 303

Sakane, Masataka 126
Sankar, Jag 304
Saw, Serena Chan 102
Saxon, Linda 27
Saxon, Mark 27
Scheffler, Sven 108
Schenker, Mara 137
Schmid-Schönbein, Geert 214
Schmidt, Christopher 152
Schultz, Jerome 298
Seguchi, Ikuko 241
Setton, Lori 337
Shimomura, Takatoshi 159
Shroff, Sanjeev 294
Shuman, Larry 307
Shung, K. Kirk 324

Simon, Bruce 28
Song, Yuhua 168
Soslowsky, Lou 352
Sowers, Brad 239
Sowers, Loretta 239
Steadman, Richard 250
Stehle, Jens 182
Su, Fong-Chin 335

Takai, Shinro 50
Takeda, Yoshitsugu 124
Tei, Matteo Maria 177
Teixeira da Silva, Rogerio 376
Thomassen, Tim 221
Tibone, James 375
Torry, Michael 356
Tsai, Daisy 316
Tsang, Priscilla 238
Tsang, Winston 238
Tsuda, Eiichi 180
Turner, Michael 367

Vercillo, Fabio 134
Verdonk, Rene 280
Vorp, David 296

Wang, Caroline 56
Wang, Ching-Jen 382
Warner, Jon JP 308
Watson, John 218
Wayne, Jennifer 42
Weinbaum, Sheldon 207
Weiss, Jeff 60
Winters, Jack 52
Wong, Eric 185
Woo, Bernadette 21
Woo, Jonathan 7
Woo, Kirstin 3
Woo, Liu-Yun 19
Woo, Pattie 11, 435
Woo, Savio L-Y 385
Wu, Changfu 171
Wu, Cheng-Wen (Ken) 310
Wu, Theodore 205

Xerogeanes, John 71

Yagi, Masayoshi 166
Yamamoto, Yuji............................... 174
Yang, Guoguang 144
Yang, King....................................... 371

Yen, Michael.................................... 230
Young, Edmond (Ned)...................... 61

Zaffagnini, Stefano.......................... 164
Zernicke, Ron.................................. 270
Zheng, Nigel 354

Excerpts from the Woo Family Genealogy Book

胡氏宗譜 卷二房

種德堂編輯

民國甲申年重修

胡氏宗譜

誠心堂石鐫

胡氏世裔源流

胡氏生於媯墟故以媯為姓舜時有虞氏陳時有陳氏周武王封公滿於陳建安定胡公之諡也子孫蔟祭葬紫黃黎之墓惑之亂者同為十一皆故老所傳以來我胡氏之由南渡者也

余始祖舜帝位傳於周代凡幾易姓而得姓於唐末節度使奉川望族又定海金塘山殷陸木胡駛之派同家也

余又諱直我公有子二人長者居歙邑之橫河京兆公徒小山殷陸金塘藏及冊千百長白總源十槁

余胡氏始祖諸侯君子徒居多不可考允武略再傳至臣公徒今昌國之蔦嘉溪海梅墪千百族木胡駛之派

余胡徵為胡子孫繁衍星羅地異有居橫河京兆公徒今海木胡駛之派

余居安定公之支派於後世武力超群戰破川之一支定海金塘藏及冊千百長白總源十槁

故譜牒數十而世遠年湮不可悉載者

余胡氏始遷為胡其後得姓而後數世使有奉川嵌鴒公遷居奉川之梅溪嵌鴒公再徒居於奉化之凇北嵌鴒公徒居於奉化之凇小山殷陸金塘藏及冊千百族

余公之後散居奉川者有遷居歧川者有居歧川者徙居金塘藏者小山殷陸金塘藏及冊千百族木胡駛之派同家也

余倣歐蘇二公之例謹列世裔於前而詳譜系於後源流清楚昭穆不素族無不亂宗族曆千載

如一日云

第四十五世孫雲楣撰

算山胡氏宗譜卷首　種德堂

宗規六條

一、崇祀以敦孝思
一、睦鄰以同宗風
一、讀書以蕭家業
一、擇術以務本業
一、勤儉以厚民生
一、作不孝論

後世子孫遵此者

第四十五世黎雲樹軍錄

算山胡氏宗譜 卷之 宗規 四十貳頁 華壹百三十叁 種德堂

明忠榮
信法永子
生於同治十三年癸酉十
月初六日亥時
卒於民國五年丙辰五月

懷良祖
長子明忠
字國章
生於光緒三十年甲辰十
一月初四日寅時

浩流
長子懷良
字鑑定
生於民國十四年己巳
八月初四日申時

流澄

良懷次子字禮銓生於民國十九年庚午二月廿二日丑時

民國己卯宣統元年七月初九日巳時流澤流源

生於光緒三十年甲辰十二月廿二日辰時卒於光緒三十年十二月

聞氏生於光緒十二年丁亥十二月廿一日亥時卒於民國十四年乙丑二月十有四日戌時墓在有野祥鯉洞

流泳

良懷三子字禮齡生於民國二十二年癸酉十二月初六日戌時

嚴女一適王書鎮海良墾子懷二良

流源

良懷四子字禮萼生於民國三十年辛巳閏六月初三日辰時

流波

We gratefully acknowledge the financial support of the
Asian ♦ American Institute for Research & Education (ASIAM)

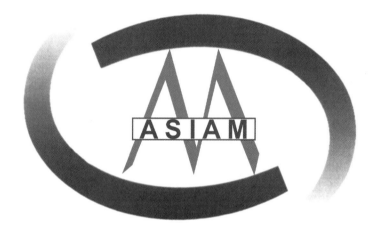